Counseling & Diversity

Devika Dibya Choudhuri
Eastern Michigan University

Azara Santiago-Rivera
University of Wisconsin-Milwaukee

Michael Tlanusta Garrett
Eastern Band of the Cherokee Nation, Counselor and Private Consultant

D1568438

BROOKS/COLE
CENGAGE Learning™

Australia • Brazil • Japan • Korea • Mexico • Singapore • Spain • United Kingdom • United States

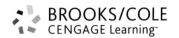

BROOKS/COLE
CENGAGE Learning™

Counseling & Diversity
Devika Dibya Choudhuri, Azara Santiago-Rivera
and Michael Tlanusta Garrett

Acquisitions Editor: Seth Dobrin

Developmental Editor: Shelley Murphy

Assistant Editor: Naomi Dreyer

Editorial Assistant: Suzanna Kincaid

Program Manager: Tami Strang

Marketing Assistant: Gurpreet Saran

Marketing Communications Manager:
Tami Strang

Content Project Management:
PreMediaGlobal

Design Director: Rob Hugel

Art Director: Caryl Gorska

Print Buyer: Paula Vang

Rights Acquisitions Specialist:
Roberta Broyer

Production Service: PreMediaGlobal

Cover Designer: Caryl Gorska

Compositor: PreMediaGlobal

© 2012 Brooks/Cole, Cengage Learning

For product information and technology assistance, contact us at
Cengage Learning Customer & Sales Support, 1-800-354-9706.

For permission to use material from this text or product,
submit all requests online at **www.cengage.com/permissions.**
Further permissions questions can be e-mailed to
permissionrequest@cengage.com.

Library of Congress Control Number: 2010943399

ISBN-13: 978-0-618-47036-5

ISBN-10: 0-618-47036-0

Brooks/Cole
20 Davis Drive
Belmont, CA 94002-3098
USA

Cengage Learning is a leading provider of customized learning solutions
with office locations around the globe, including Singapore, the United
Kingdom, Australia, Mexico, Brazil, and Japan. Locate your local office at
www.cengage.com/global.

Cengage Learning products are represented in Canada by
Nelson Education, Ltd.

To learn more about Brooks/Cole, visit **www.cengage.com/brookscole**

Purchase any of our products at your local college store or at our preferred
online store **www.cengagebrain.com**.

Printed in the United States of America
1 2 3 4 5 6 7 15 14 13 12 11

CONTENTS

6 Age   153

PREFACE

OVERVIEW AND PURPOSE

Multicultural counseling has become a critical course in many counseling programs. Teaching for multicultural competency becomes more significant as counselor education programs increasingly incorporate requirements for specific courses in multicultural counseling (Ridley, Espelage, & Rubinstein, 1997).

There are a number of texts that deal with the issue of multicultural counseling, in terms of theories, approaches, interventions, and research. Sue, Arredondo, and McDavis (1992) identify three dimensions of multicultural counseling competency: awareness, knowledge, and skills. Pedersen (1993) identified a common flaw in multicultural training: an overemphasis on any one dimension of the three areas to the detriment of the others. For example, an exclusive emphasis on multicultural awareness may well guide students to become aware of their own shortcomings as well as environmental inadequacies. However, it leaves them with little direction on how to effectively advocate and counsel. On the other hand, emphasizing knowledge with huge doses of information fails to convince the student of the legitimacy or importance of applying the information in counseling.

In addition to the three dimensions of competency, Swigonski (1996) argues that no course on multicultural issues is meaningful without an exploration of the system of oppression and an understanding of the ways in which privilege serves to reinforce existing social structures. Without such a basis, learning cultural attributes of various ethnic groups becomes an act of exotic tourism with students unable to know the importance of such information. Identifying sociocultural and ethno-psychological differences between groups, without any grounding in their sociopolitical history and environment, becomes a trivial pursuit of data collection.

Multicultural counseling emerged in response to recognition that the needs of members of certain social groups were unmet as well as actively discriminated against by traditional forms of counseling (Sue, Ivey, & Pedersen, 1996). The efforts of multicultural counseling theorists and researchers are aimed at improving counseling forms so as to empower people who have been discriminated against and stigmatized by society (Pedersen, 1994). It is essential to develop constructive conversations about power differentials and the resulting social structures to educate counselors-in-training about the needs of the diverse clients they encounter (Locke & Faubert, 2003).

As counseling students, we learn that human beings exist in relationship. In multicultural counseling courses, we learn that identities of race, ethnicity, gender, age, sexual orientation, physical and mental ability, socioeconomic class, and religion create a complex of social identity that defines relationships between human beings. But we also need to understand that for each of these identities, societies tend to value one manifestation and devalue or "other" the complementary identity. For example, in American society, European American identity is normalized as American, whereas other ethnic identities are marginalized as "hyphenated-Americans." Similarly, in terms of sexual orientation, heterosexual identity is privileged as normative and preferred, to the extent that the process of developing a heterosexual identity is never questioned, whereas that of developing a gay, lesbian, or bisexual identity is constantly interrogated.

The systemic classification of groups of people and its effects on institutional frameworks, social structures, as well as community and family and interpersonal interactions, goes beyond discrimination to become oppression. To work effectively with people from oppressed groups, counselors need to understand these concepts in both their personal and professional dimensions (Ridley et al., 1997). Furthermore, because most counselors are themselves members of both privileged and oppressed groups, it becomes all the more important that they understand the impact of such membership on their own worldviews as well as on the relationships they form with clients.

The goal of this text is to address the three dimensions of multicultural counseling competency with a focus on understanding the constructs of oppression and the structures of power. We provide an overarching framework for developing multicultural competency across the dimensions of social identity. The usefulness of the central text as a teaching tool is enriched by two important sets of ancillaries: (a) a "satellite" series of monographs, titled *Counseling & Diversity Primers*, which provide students with an introduction to issues in counseling with specific populations and (b) an active *Online Instructor's Resource Center*, which enables instructors who use the textbook to access and share teaching ideas and materials.

The chapters of this text provide you with a historical, sociopolitical, and psychological overview of each aspect of identity that will have resonance in counseling and psychotherapy. You will be encouraged to apply some of the information and analyses to the ways in which you understand and experience those aspects of identity in yourself as well as in the range of people you will be helping.

What we will not offer you in this text is a set of recipes on how to work with diverse clients. However, the application of skills and specific strategies and means of understanding diverse groups is critical. For that purpose, this text is accompanied by a series of monographs that address those practitioner issues. With those, you will get greater exposure to specific issues in counseling different ethnic groups such as African Americans, Asian Americans, Native Americans, Latino/a Americans, and Arab Americans. Additionally, you will get further information on specific issues in counseling gay, lesbian, bisexual, and transgender populations; and in forthcoming monographs examine counseling issues with people with disabilities; as well as elders.

ORGANIZING AND PEDAGOGICAL FEATURES

Each chapter contains the following elements:

- An opening quotation or excerpt from original literature that brings up the issues to be covered
- An introduction to the chapter and the concepts to be covered
- Definitions of the key concepts as needed
- Exploration of the concepts with an interwoven review of the literature
- A section on opening the dialogue designed to provide impetus for exploration of the chapter content in session with clients
- Glossary of key terms
- Conclusion and implications for practice
- References with additional resources

Woven throughout each chapter are the following:

- Boxed excerpts from relevant original sources
- Boxed reflection and personal growth questions that help you apply concepts to your own experience
- Boxed case study examples with case discussion questions and summary

ANCILLARIES

Supplementary Monograph Series: *Multicultural Counseling Primers*

A series of monographs accompany the central text. Whereas the textbook describes themes, critical concepts, and central constructs in multicultural counseling, the "satellite" series of monographs provide students with an introduction to issues in counseling with specific populations. The monographs cover the subject areas in greater depth than can be accomplished in a single textbook chapter while offering choices in which specific populations the instructor may wish to emphasize in the course. Although the monographs may be purchased separately, they will be discounted when purchased along with the central text. Included in the series are the following:

Counseling & Diversity: African Americans

Counseling & Diversity: Arab Americans

Counseling & Diversity: Asian Americans

Counseling & Diversity: Latino Americans

Counseling & Diversity: LGBTQ Americans
Counseling & Diversity: Native Americans

I. Demographics

Introduces the population to the reader in terms of numbers, diversity of origin, migration patterns and geographic settlement areas (where applicable), educational attainment, income levels, poverty levels, age cohorts, occupations and professions, and so forth with use from the latest census data.

II. Sociopolitical History

Provides a brief coverage of the population's history in the United States, with some attention to origin; includes social movements, legal issues, and critical incidents that have impacted the group; demonstrates how oppression has structured the group's participation and access in society through a description of the institutional barriers to advancement.

III. Current Status

Describes the group's current status and issues facing this group as well as social advocacy and empowerment movements; discusses resiliency and strengths as well as areas of pain and poverty; discusses common presenting problems and issues that clients holding membership in this group bring.

IV. Cultural Systems

Provides an overview of the major cultural values that hold true for the group, with caveats of specific subgroup differences; addresses critical issues with this group, identifying the dynamics of gender socialization, attitudes toward sexuality, beliefs about family and marriage, parenting and childrearing styles, socioeconomic class consciousness, and religious beliefs; includes ways in which beliefs about health and illness influence help-seeking attitudes and behaviors; discusses ways in which oppression has manifested and impacted values, beliefs, identity, and cultural responses.

V. Counseling Dynamics and Interventions

Addresses the critical counseling dynamics, with the use of case illustrations that describe entry into counseling, factors and issues leading to premature termination, appropriate counselor stance and approaches, and development and maintenance of the counselor–client relationship; addresses same group as well as different group pairings of client and counselor; describes particular interventions and approaches that are effective as well as some discussion of ways in which internalized oppression issues may manifest.

VI. Resource List for Further Reading

Offers a list of resources for further study for practitioners.

Online Instructor's Resource Center

Given the myriad issues with which multicultural counseling is concerned, instructors are often faced with the impossible directive of inculcating multicultural counseling competency in the course of fifteen weeks or so. In addition, resistant institutions, general counseling theory courses that are not infused with multicultural awareness, and relatively homogeneous populations of counselor education students are some of the realities with which multicultural counseling instructors struggle.

For these reasons, this unique resource for instructors, accessible through the text website, is available, and we will be updating it frequently to reflect the most current information. Ultimately, the Resource Center will include not only standard "instructor's manual" materials but also contributions of teaching ideas and activities from a wide variety of instructors experienced in teaching the course. This active support center will enhance the structure and direction that an instructor can take, while providing a rich assortment of helpful activities, additional readings, films, Internet sites, and other curricular material that would enhance the learning process for multicultural competency.

ACKNOWLEDGMENTS

Jelane A. Kennedy, College of St. Rose; Aneneosa A. G. Okocha, University of Wisconsin, Whitewater; Lakota L. Brown, Northern Arizona University; Sandra I. Lopez-Baez, University of Virginia; Carmen F. Salazar, Texas A&M University; Carlos P. Zalaquett, University of South Florida; Dana Griffin, University of North Carolina, Chapel Hill; Simone Alter-Muri, Springfield College; Sarita Sankey, Bowie State University; Shawn Patrick, Texas State University, San Marcos; Mary Fukuyama, University of Florida; John Queener, University of Akron; Chuck Reid, University of Texas, Pan American; Margaret Miller, Boise State University, Arpita Ghosh, University of Wisconsin-Milwaukee, as well as those who participated in reviews but did not wish to be acknowledged.

REFERENCES

Locke, D. C., & Faubert, M. (2003). Cultural considerations in counselor training and practice. In F. D. Harper and J. McFadden (Eds.). *Culture and counseling: New approaches* (pp. 324–338). Needham Heights, MA: Allyn & Bacon.

Pedersen, P. B. (1993). *Culture-centered counseling and interviewing skills: A practical guide.* Westport, CT, US: Praeger Publishers/Greenwood.

Ridley, C. R., Espelage, D. L., & Rubinstein, K. J. (1997). Course development in multicultural counseling. In D. B. Pope-Davis and H. L. K. Coleman (Eds.). Multicultural counseling competencies: Assessment, education and training, and supervision. Multicultural aspects of counseling series, Vol. 7. (pp. 131–158). Thousand Oaks, CA, US: Sage.

Swigonski, M. E. (1996). Challenging privilege through Africentric social work practice. *Social Work, 41*(2), 153–161.

Sue, D. W., Arredondo, P., & McDavis, R. J. (1992). Multicultural counseling competencies and standards: A call to the profession. *Journal of Multicultural Counseling and Development.* 20(2), 64–88.

Sue, D. W., Ivey, A. E., & Pedersen, P. B. (Eds.). (1996). *A theory of multicultural counseling and therapy.* Belmont, CA: Thompson Brooks/Cole.

CHAPTER 1

Orientation to Counseling and Diversity

The whole object of travel is not to set foot on foreign land; it is at last to set foot on one's own country as a foreign land.

—G. K. Chesterton

A good traveler has no fixed plans, and is not intent on arriving.

—Lao Tzu

I soon realized that no journey carries one far unless, as it extends into the world around us, it goes an equal distance into the world within.

—Lillian Smith

THE JOURNEY

All Aboard!

In the early 1900s, one of the most celebrated trains was the *Orient Express*, traveling across the length of the Eurasian continent. Travelers boarded the train for the experience of the journey rather than the destination. We use this metaphor of a journey to imagine you, the reader, getting on board this "multicultural express" while we, the authors, and perhaps your instructors play the role of conductors. As on all such journeys, you bring baggage with you: some that you will need along the way, and some that may prove to be obstacles rather than assets. You may also be boarding with a mixture of emotions. You may experience excitement as you look forward to new experiences while also having apprehension as you imagine the difficulties that arise when one is a stranger someplace new. Perhaps you will not be able to communicate effectively, or you may not understand. Conceivably you will be homesick. Let us explore this, speaking directly now of the journey that lies before us.

Because we have conducted this multicultural tour so many times, we can predict that along the way you will probably experience some rather strong feelings. We ask that you neither suppress your feelings nor label them as right or wrong. Instead, we encourage you to recognize and work with them as you consider the material presented in this book.

Feelings

Let us examine some of the feelings you may experience in this journey:

Excitement

Like many travelers, you may be looking forward to this journey as an opportunity to learn about diversity. You may have the perception that you live a very ordinary life and that you are finally going to be seeing the more exotic ways of living. The positive part of this reaction is that you are pretty open to taking the tour. The negative part is that you may not be open to learning anything from the tour. This multicultural journey has been incorporated into your professional training for good reason. You cannot simply be a sightseer. It is important to accept that your learning will be about not just others but also yourself. Unlike the *Orient Express*, this train has an important destination: your effectiveness as counselor in a diverse world.

Anxiety

Like some other travelers, you may be coming aboard with a host of apprehensions. You fear you will not be able to cope with encountering differences. These fears are common among students who have lived in the majority. You look around at your classmates, the professor, and the course topics, and you feel fearful. You fear that you don't know enough and that you are going to offend others. You fear having your ignorance publicly displayed. You might even feel that the best way to cope is to keep your head down and hope to avoid attention. Although such caution protects you, your fear prevents you from taking the risks that oftentimes lead to growth. As you peer downward looking for the pitfalls, you forget to look ahead to the horizon.

Cynicism

Cynical travelers believe that the journey is important, but don't believe that it will change anything. Do you consider yourself a cynical person? Do you believe that society is the way it is, people are the way they are, and no course is going to make a difference in your life or in the lives of others? We believe that people become cynical after being disappointed. Perhaps you have seen in your life that in spite of the Herculean efforts of many good people, poverty, violence, and hate are as present in the world today as they were when you were young and had high hopes for the future. Perhaps you have tried to make change happen in some arena of your own life, but it didn't work. You got hurt, and you hide your scars behind a façade of despair. There are two problems with this. The first is that it may act as a self-fulfilling prophecy, where you give up on yourself, your peers, or the material. We invite you to consider that there are different battles we wage on a daily basis, and that although you have every right to not want to get hurt again, you will not heal by retreating from the battlefield.

Vulnerability

Some travelers approach this journey from a different vantage point. Unlike the anxiety of facing new experiences, this is the approach of "Been there and done that." Those of you who have experienced being discriminated against may feel that this journey will be more of the same except in a concentrated form. In many ways, you see yourself as being here not for your own learning but to provide learning for others at your expense. We would like to say to you that although few of the places we go on this journey may be completely new, as you revisit them on this train, with your instructor and this book as your guides, this time around you may well find new perspectives and understandings of that familiar terrain.

Hostility

Some travelers feel forced to get on the train and don't want to be here. Do you believe this is neither important nor valid, and, in fact, think it might well be a conspiracy to blame you or hold you responsible? Do you feel that a lot of this stuff is whining from a bunch of losers who can't make it? As much as possible, we would like you to consider that this journey is in the interests of being effective with people. You have been learning in your other coursework that the key to effectiveness in the helping professions is the ability to listen. If you are unable to bring yourself to hear different perspectives, can you really be helpful? The other aspect to consider is that anger can be a defense to prevent you own pain. If, in this course, you came to acknowledge that there are ways in which other people are hurt over and over again by the same system that helps you, what would it mean for you? We are all, by and large, good people who are well intentioned, and no one likes to think of themselves as causing hurt. You may find by the end of this journey that you want to make changes in your life, even if they cause you discomfort. Or you may not. We ask only that you put aside your hostility and stay open to the possibilities.

As you consider what you bring on this journey, we urge you to look around at your fellow passengers thoughtfully. A critical component that will shape this experience for you is the diversity of experience, opinion, values, and attitudes that your peers bring in their baggage. An environment of honesty, authenticity, and congruence is very important in facilitating successful multicultural learning experiences (Torres-Rivera, Phan, Maddux, Wilbur, & Garrett, 2001).

In addition, we invite you to notice your responses to your course instructor, who is a significant person in facilitating your journey (Estrada, Frame, & Williams, 2004). Often, instructors of such courses are themselves persons of color. Many are women. Regardless, your course instructor is charged with being the messenger of course content that is powerful, provocative, and challenging. Sometimes, the discomfort of the message is transferred to the instructor, and students end up being extremely critical of the

REFLECTION EXERCISE **1.1**

Your Emotional Travel Pack

From time to time, we will invite you to do some self-reflection. It will be helpful if you keep a journal to document and put all your reflections in one place.

For now, start the journal by making some notes about your responses
to these questions:

Think about the idea of learning about multicultural issues as a train
journey:

- What emotions and thoughts might you pack into your baggage? You
  may examine this from past history when you have been confronted by
  change or risk. How do you tend to react or respond?
- What emotions or thoughts would you want to pack that might be
  useful? How might they be useful as you enter this process?
- What emotions or thoughts do you now think would be best left
  behind? How may they get in the way?

instructor. We are not necessarily accustomed to being in positions where a
person of color, particularly a woman of color, has authority and evaluative
power over us. Sometimes, our hidden negative reactions to women or people
of color also get added to the mix, increasing our criticism and hostility. On
the other hand, if the instructor is a European American man, we may deny
the uncomfortable messages by delegitimizing his authority to teach on such
a subject. Attend to and notice if this begins to happen to you, reflecting on
whether your discomfort or unease with the content of the course is shaping
your attitude toward the instructor. One way to think through your responses
is by identifying your triggers.

Triggers and Responses

According to Griffin (1987), situations in which we feel diminished, offended, stereotyped, discounted, blamed, or attacked trigger an emotional response. Such
responses can include hurt, confusion, anger, fear, surprise, or embarrassment.
The way we respond is based on our inner resources and our previous experiences as well as the dynamics of the situation. The following guide is intended to
assist you in recognizing your habitual responses to triggers as well as offer a
fuller repertoire of possible responses so you will be able to intentionally respond
most effectively. It is not supposed to be complete or in order of preference.

- *Retreat from the trigger*: We physically remove ourselves from triggering
  situations.
- *Avoid potential triggers*: We avoid potential encounters with triggers and
  withdraw emotionally from those people or situations that might trigger us.
- *Respond to triggers with silence*: We do not openly respond to triggers,
  even though we feel upset, but endure them without saying or doing
  anything.

- *Deflect the blow*: We notice the trigger but choose to let it go by without admitting to ourselves any need to respond.
- *Attack the triggering person*: We respond with the intention of hurting whoever triggered us.
- *Internalize the trigger*: We absorb the content of the trigger. We believe it to be true.
- *Rationalize the trigger*: We avoid confronting the trigger by convincing ourselves that we misinterpreted or overreacted to the trigger and that the triggering person's intention was not to harm us.
- *Misinterpret as a trigger*: We are so ready to be triggered that we misinterpret what is said or done and are triggered by our misinterpretation rather than what actually happened.
- *Respond to a trigger with confusion*: We feel upset but are not clear about why we feel that way. We are not sure whether we feel angry, hurt, offended, or all of the above. We just don't know what to say or do about it.
- *Respond to a trigger with shock*: We are caught off-guard, unprepared to be triggered by this person or situation, and have a difficult time responding.
- *Name the triggering person*: We attribute what is upsetting us to the triggering person or situation.
- *Engage the triggering person in a discussion*: We declare the trigger and invite discussion about it.
- *Confront the trigger*: We name the triggering person or situation, and demand that the offending behavior or policy be changed.
- *Surprise the triggering person*: We respond in an unexpected way, for instance with a joke that makes the triggering person laugh.
- *Strategize*: We work with others to develop a programmatic or political intervention to address the trigger in a larger context.
- *Choose discretion*: Because of the dynamics of the situation such as power differences or risk of physical violence or retribution, we decide that it is not in our best interest to respond to the trigger at that time, but choose to address it differently at another time.

 REFLECTION QUESTIONS 1.1

- In what types of social situations are you most likely to be triggered?
- Which responses are most typical of you when triggered?
- Which responses would you like to use now or would like to either stop using or use more effectively?
- Which responses would you like to add to your repertoire? (Griffin & Bell, 1987)

ABOUT THE AUTHORS

As we begin this journey, we would also like to introduce ourselves as your conductors. As we ask you to take risks in learning and challenging yourselves, it seems only fair that we begin by taking some risks of self-disclosure. In the following section, each of us will share an aspect of who we are and how we have come to this journey.

Devika Dibya Choudhuri

I will start with a story about myself that may tell you many things about me. I grew up going to 16 different schools. With my father in the Indian Army, we moved every year or so across India. I learned to throw myself into every new school situation and quickly join in. In kindergarten, I was 5 and proud to be given a role in the school play, a tale of a king unable to sleep because he was harassed by bedbugs every night. Finally, under the advice of his wise prime minister, his loyal soldiers set up guard and caught the bedbugs creeping out at night, and victoriously drove them away and saved the king. I had been awarded the role of chief bedbug, an undersized skinny child in tights and tunic dyed brown by my mother, and a wire antenna cap on my head.

The evening of the play, all went well until the climactic moment when the soldiers attacked. Before the hilarious amazement of assembled parents and teachers, I decided to fight back at the injustice. Leading a charge of the bedbugs, we created a shambles of the play, with cowering soldiers having their cardboard swords wrestled away, and the child king wailing in the middle of his bed. Triumphant, the bedbugs gathered on stage, and, brandishing my captured sword, I shouted out that bedbugs deserved a home, too. The audience was wiping tears of laughter from their faces, and my father, in a rare moment home from the battlefront, was beaming with pride. My family never let me forget it.

I am a middle child, one of three daughters whose untraditional Indian mother announced with pride that she was glad to have only daughters, and as you can see, I am fiercely passionate about injustice. At the age of 17, I came to the United States, leaving everyone I knew 10,000 miles away, to go to college. My first brushes with ethnocentrism started the day I entered the elite Ivy League college, when a young White woman wanting to make conversation with the poor foreigner standing bewildered in the cafeteria, brightly commented, "It must be so nice for you to have all this food available." The hallowed institution was no stranger to racism, and there were incidents of hate and discrimination that ended up with the FBI and the U.S. Civil Rights Commission being called in. I was a student activist and, working with other people of color, soon became a facilitator, leading workshops on racism. I continued this work after graduation and entered a master's counseling program, where yet again we were targeted.

As a counselor-in-training, every counseling encounter for me was inescapably a cross-cultural one. I found little preparation for it in the curriculum and invented ways to make sense of it. I focused on multicultural counseling during my PhD training, wanting to prepare myself and also wanting to learn how to teach the topic to others. My ultimate commitment has always been to the clients. When I teach counselors-in-training, what I imagine as I challenge and educate them is the impact of the clients with whom they are going to come in contact. I believe that counselors come into the profession to do good and prevent harm. I believe that when we know that what we do is hurtful because we are delegitimizing parts of a person's identity, we want to learn to behave differently—even when the cost of that learning is to be changed ourselves. I once wrote a poem, an angry one, which had the lines "And home is a nowhere place, halfway between wishful longing and the other side of despair" to express that sense of exile from the comfortable. I understand that what we ask of you has a high price: to notice, to confront, and to unlearn the walls that we live within, sometimes making such walls unfit for habitation again. I want to share with you that I myself continue to make that journey of discomfort, of being somewhat of a stranger to myself in the quest to be a comfort to others.

Azara Santiago-Rivera

I am Latina of Puerto Rican heritage, born to parents who immigrated to the United States during the mid-1940s. I was born in the United States and raised in this country a good part of my childhood and early adolescence. There are many experiences in my life that have shaped who I am today. Because my father was in the U.S. Army for many years, I had the good fortune of traveling and living in different places both in the United States and abroad while growing up. From an early age, my friends were from many diverse ethnic and cultural backgrounds. In retrospect, I learned about differences in language, traditions, and foods, and differences in physical features very early in my life—so much so that diversity was a part of my everyday world. Although these early experiences were positive, I have also experienced overt racism and discrimination and know firsthand how it feels. I have vivid memories of being called a "spick" by many Anglo Americans. Another unpleasant memory is being told by an Anglo American high school counselor that I was not "college material," and as a result I did not get the proper guidance about options to further my education. I remember feeling angry, hurt, and hopeless.

I am the oldest of three siblings. I was taught at an early age to care for my younger sisters and set a good example. My parents were loving but very strict with us. My mother took her duties as a wife and mother very seriously and in many ways was the carrier and transmitter of Puerto Rican traditions in our lives. She taught us the value of education and instilled in us the importance of hard work in order to achieve, despite the obstacles that she knew we would face in this society as women of color. It is because of her that I was the first in my family to attend college.

I chose the counseling profession as my career for the same reason that most people do—to help make a difference in people's lives. Unlike many of the current counselor education programs, my academic training did not include multicultural perspectives. As one of very few students of color in most of my classes, instructors often targeted me to "serve as the voice of minorities." I struggled with understanding how traditional counseling theories applied to the unique life experiences of oppressed people. A commitment to multiculturalism is not easy. We must be willing to take risks, change our beliefs, and be open to new experiences. It is much safer to stay in a familiar place rather than explore new territory. The irony is that as counselors, we encourage our clients to try new ways of thinking and behaving, and yet we may not be willing to change our own ways. I hope you are ready to join us in this journey.

Michael Tlanusta Garrett

People have often asked me questions like, "What is your culture?" "What is your religion?" or "What is Native spirituality and Indian medicine?" and I have struggled at times to pick just the right words in just the right way to best describe something that is so meaningful in my life and has been so critical to the survival of my family and nation across generations. As you read my words here, it is important for you to know who I am as a member of the Eastern Band of Cherokee and the son of an Eastern Band of the Cherokee enrolled tribal member from western North Carolina and his wife, who, German by heritage, is the daughter of a Methodist minister and his wife from Ohio, a family of farmers for many generations back. When I think about who I am, where I have come from, and where I am in life now, I know that I come from people on both sides of my family who care about people, care about the land, and value life for the gift that it is. I became a counselor for several reasons, not the least of which was a very practical need filled by tribal scholarship and family support that allowed me to choose something that I really loved and was passionate about. I have lived in many different places, connected with people from many different backgrounds over the years, and worked professionally in school, community, and university settings in a variety of capacities that always somehow come back to the simple truths of what it means to connect, heal, and learn from the inside out. In some ways, I feel as though I have not only crossed worlds but also lived many lives in one so far.

There is a Cherokee story about the old medicine man who was walking in the forest when he came upon a young man sitting on the ground. He asked the young man, "Why is it that you are sitting here like this?" sensing that the young man was troubled by something. "I am sitting here because I don't know which way to go, so I'm listening and waiting to be moved by having my direction come to me," answered the young man. "Oh, OK," said the old man, and he kept going on his way. A year went by, and the old man found himself walking through the same woods where he, once again, came upon the young man still sitting in the same spot he had been a year before. So, he asked the young man, "Have you been sitting here in the same spot all of this time?" The young man replied, "Yes, I am still listening and waiting to be moved by having my direction come to me." The old man sat with the young man and reminded him of the lessons offered by each of the Four Directions. He suggested that the young man spend 4 days and 4 nights fasting in order to seek the lessons in each of the different directions, one for each night. On the morning of the fifth day, the young man was to nourish his body and resume his journey in the direction that seemed best as revealed in his vision. "How will I know if I am moving in the right direction?' asked the young man. "Home is wherever you are," said the old man, smiling. "Seek harmony and balance in your life's journey, and allow the many helpers that come to you to guide you as you walk the path of Good Medicine, being a helper to others as you go."

Now, when asked, "What is Native culture and spirituality?" I simply say that it is a feeling. I tell them that it is a breath of life that just moves through you somehow, and just is a way of knowing that things are what they need to be at any given point in time, and a way of connecting with the essence of life.

THE IMPORTANCE OF MULTICULTURALISM IN COUNSELING

By the year 2050, over half the population of the United States will be people of color (U.S. Census, 2004). The term **people of color,** as used in the Census, means people who belong to ethnic groups identified as African American, Hispanic, Asian, and Native American peoples (another term sometimes used in describing all of these peoples is the acronym AHANA). We (the authors) don't use the term *non-White* to describe this collection of people—though, in many ways, it includes all peoples other than Europeans and their descendants—because we do not wish to name a constellation of peoples based on who they are not.

The United States has had a long history of conflict based on adversarial relationships, hostility, and conflict between groups of people. Although we glorify and mythologize our country as being one of immigrants and opportunity, we often downplay and mystify the negative aspects. When we speak about this country as being a nation of immigrants, we forget to acknowledge Native Americans, who are descendants of the dispossessed first Americans. We also forget to acknowledge that most African Americans are descendants of persons who did not come here of their own accord. The legal enslavement of Africans and their descendants started in 1619, with the arrival of a Dutch slave trader in Jamestown, Virginia, and continued until the end of the Civil War. In the 1800s, much of the land mass of Mexico was taken and made a part of the United States, but the original inhabitants were not welcomed along with the natural resources. Finally, we forget to acknowledge so many other groups of people, such as the Chinese Americans, who chose to come here and were exploited for their cheap labor but were not welcomed into the fabric of American communities.

The point is that the idealized American melting pot where successive groups have joined to live in harmony can be viewed at best as a work in progress. On the other hand, given the changing demographics as well as the global context, it becomes increasingly important that we continue to find ways to bridge our differences and work together. We need to make a paradigm shift to interact effectively and find common ground and mutual enrichment across our differences (J. L. White, personal communication, 2003).

In addition to aspects of race and culture, a focus on diversity also acknowledges other significant aspects of a person's identity by which they define themselves, or are grouped by society, and share a collective experience based on their group membership. These other aspects include social class, gender, religion, disability status, sexual orientation, and age.

MULTICULTURALISM AND THE HISTORY OF COUNSELING APPROACHES

In the last several decades, there has been extensive criticism of traditional counseling theory and practice for its lack of attention to issues of multiculturalism (Robinson & Morris, 2000; Weinrach & Thomas, 1998). The criticism of traditional counseling can be categorized into three interrelated concerns: the intrapsychic counseling model, the development of verbal counseling approaches, and the counseling process variables that ignore sociopolitical forces (Atkinson, Morten, & Sue, 1993). First, traditional models of counseling have invariably focused on individuals, assigning both the locus of pathology and the ability to change to the individual. Second, counseling approaches have been developed along verbal lines, which necessitate a shared language and, more subtly, an understanding of commonly shared beliefs between the counselor and the client. Third, sociopolitical forces are as prevalent within the process of counseling as anywhere else, and counselors are not immune to bias and prejudice against clients who are members of socially discriminated groups (Atkinson et al., 1993). By refusing to examine the possibility of bias in any systematic way, the biased process has been allowed to flourish.

The above criticisms of counseling, as traditionally practiced, have primarily arisen because it is embedded in European American cultural systems, and excludes members of other cultures. For instance, the pioneers in psychology who influenced the field of counseling such as Sigmund Freud, Carl Jung, Alfred Adler, John Watson, B. F. Skinner, and Carl Rogers are all men of European heritage. The field, shaped and transformed by their contributions, reflects that heritage. Any area of study that grows out of a particular heritage will reflect the cultural constructs of that heritage. Counseling in its present form has developed primarily in the West, and reflects the cultural values and belief systems of Western culture. Western culture embodies the confluence of European traditions and belief systems that were brought to America by European colonizers and immigrants, and that hold a dominant place in the United States' mosaic of cultural systems (Atkinson, 2004). These cultural value systems have implications not only for clients from different cultural systems but also for clients from the same cultural system who occupy a negative status in that system in terms of their access to services and of the efficacy of such services. Therefore, clients from African, Asian, Latino, and Indigenous cultural traditions were expected to conform to Western cultural values and beliefs. Additionally, clients who are poor or working class; gay, lesbian, or bisexual; disabled; or otherwise either invisible or negatively perceived within Western cultural traditions are also ill served (Liu et al., 2004; Smart & Smart, 2006; Phillips, Ingram, Smith, & Mindes, 2003).

Traditional developmental theory assumed that psychosocial development occurred in a linear fashion and that cultural identity was subsumed in importance to these universal human processes. Kohlberg's stages of moral development (Berk, 2007) and Piaget's stages of cognitive development (Huit & Hummel, 2003) exemplify these linear stage theories. These stages were perceived as universal for every child regardless of specific cultural contexts. Universalist assumptions such as these were then incorporated into theoretical models and put into practice. However, the structures of this relationship, framed in the particular contexts of Western normative expectations of mental health and sickness, have not been traditionally helpful to clients from underrepresented groups (Atkinson, 2004). Clients who did not fit the theoretical models, and who were "uncooperative" in practice, were usually from different cultural systems. Such systems sometimes designated as collectivist, non-Western, or (more specifically, for example) Afrocentric in their worldview were deemed to be incompatible with the individualistic, linear perspective of Western forms of counseling. Clients from such cultural systems also had a record of not seeking counseling as exemplified in the Western cultural tradition (Sue & Sue, 2008).

As a matter of course, counseling historically gave minimal attention to clients who did not flow smoothly through the established theoretical systems. According to Casas (1984), although there are many reasons for this seeming disinterest, the existence of subtle yet complex forms of bias and prejudice against these groups was a major factor. Counselors preferred to work with clients with characteristics similar to themselves because these factors were often correlated with more successful outcomes (Casas, 1984). Because members of culturally different groups have been historically underrepresented in the counseling field (Russo, Olmedo, Stapp, & Fulcher, 1981), there was little challenge to the dominant Western cultural perspective of the profession.

Following the psychodynamic, behavioral, and humanistic traditions in the field of counseling, the "fourth force" (Pedersen, 1990) of multicultural counseling has engendered an extensive literature detailing both the biases of traditional counseling theories and remedies for those biases. This large body of work has taken the form of comprehensive research on people of different races, ethnicities, cultures, genders, ages, abilities, and sexual orientations. As well, attention has been given to developing theoretical stances that counselors can take in working with clients from different groups, and critiques and reframing of counseling techniques for use with such clients (Helms & Cook, 1999; Atkinson, Morten, & Sue, 1993; Casas, 1984). Extensive recommendations have been made in the preparation and training of counselors, and counselor education programs have initiated changes in both content and structure to reflect these concerns (Atkinson, 2004).

The experience of gay, lesbian, bisexual, and transgender clients serves as an example of the ineffectiveness of traditional counseling with members of its own culture. As with culturally different clients, same-culture clients who deviate from the norm are often ill-served by counseling professionals. There has been a long history of condemnation of minority sexual orientation in Western society. Psychiatry viewed homosexuality as a mental illness, and both psychoanalytic and behavioral treatment usually focused on changing the client's sexual orientation to one of heterosexuality. In 1973, the American Psychiatric Association declassified homosexuality as a mental illness except for individual clients who were subjectively distressed with their orientation. In the revised third edition of the *Diagnostic and Statistical Manual of*

Mental Disorders (American Psychiatric Association, 1987), used to diagnose psychological disorders, *ego-dystonic homosexuality* was subsumed under the category of sexual disorders as a "persistent and marked distress about one's sexual orientation" (p. 296). The categorization was finally removed in the next edition of the DSM (American Psychiatric Association, 1994). The attitude of professionals was merely a reflection of the profound lack of acceptance of society and continues to vary (Boysen, Vogel, Madon, & Wester, 2006). This negative societal attitude is related to a variety of problems for gays and lesbians (Barret & Logan, 2002), including poor self-esteem, depression, violent assault, as well as discrimination and inadequate legal protection. Lesbians and gays seek counseling proportionately 2 to 4 times more often than do heterosexuals, and a significantly greater percentage report dissatisfaction with their treatment compared with heterosexuals (Chernin & Johnson, 2002).

Much of counseling literature has dealt with issues in *coming out*, a term referring to the process by which an individual acknowledges, initially to self and gradually to others, a sexual orientation of being gay, lesbian, or bisexual (Chernin & Johnson, 2002). Clinical experience and research have shown that this process is a complex, one of intrapersonal and interpersonal transformations, often beginning in adolescence and leading well into adulthood (Perez, DeBord, & Bieschke, 2000).

Similarly, the volume of literature focusing on the concerns of women is tremendous. Responding to the ways in which women have been ignored in psychological research, stereotyped in theory, and discriminated against in practice, the field of the psychology of women has grown rapidly. Sociopolitical forces linked many movements in the United States: The civil rights movement recharged the struggle for women's liberation, sparking, in turn, the gay rights struggle. The development of alternate modes of theory and practice has consequently piggybacked on each other's efforts. Issues in working with clients with disabilities, engaging in effective therapy with elders, and dealing with diverse spiritual and religious belief systems are all fields that have sprung up as the consciousness of clients and practitioners from these populations is raised (Lee, 2008).

APPROACHES TO MULTICULTURAL COUNSELING

A way to conceptualize two major avenues of multicultural counseling theory and research has been to describe the *etic* and *emic* approaches. Derived from the linguistic terms *phonetic* (referring to the underlying structure of language) and *phonemic* (referring to the meaning of a unit of language), the etic perspective looks at culture in universalistic terms, whereas the emic perspective examines the specifics of a particular cultural system (Draguns, 2008). One way to think about this is to distinguish between appreciating culture as an aspect held universally by all humans (etic) versus appreciating the specific ways in which an individual constructs his or her humanity within his or her cultural system (emic). In the first instance, culture becomes a commonality across humans, whereas in the second, culture distinguishes between humans. Both approaches diverge and converge on one another as this field grapples with the issues and problems of meeting the needs of clients effectively.

Etic Approach

To have a coherent, universally applicable theory of multicultural counseling, counselors have to identify principles that are common to helping relationships and that can also be applied to clients from different cultures. *Etic* refers to a common factor perspective that the therapeutic properties of counseling pertain not to theoretically unique components, but to elements common to all counseling approaches. Vontress (1988) adapted a framework emphasizing the shared human experience of existence. He described it by three concepts that divide experience into the physical (*umwelt*), interpersonal (*mitwelt*), and inner (*eigenwelt*) environments. These interacting elements provide counselors a basis from which to judge their clients' modes of existence. Sue and Zane (1987) identified other universal elements of the counseling relationship as the credibility of the helper and the effectiveness of the counseling encounter to the client.

One way to operationalize client constructs of culture and identity is through cultural worldviews as mediating variables (Ibrahim, Roysicar-Sodowsky, & Ohnishi, 2001). Worldviews suggest the possibility of cultural shaping of concepts such as mental health or mental illness. Sue (Sue, 1978) first proposed the idea of worldviews as a counseling construct and stressed their importance. His model for understanding clients who are culturally different from the counselor consisted of two dimensions—*locus of control* and *locus of responsibility*—that can be used to make attributions about clients. The interaction of these dimensions creates four possible worldviews. Once the client's worldview is understood, the counselor can develop an appropriate therapeutic system of treatment.

A broader conceptualization of worldview, based on earlier work in value orientations and emphasis, was developed by Ibrahim (in Ibrahim, Roysicar-Sodowsky, & Ohnishi, 2001). Using a values perspective that views worldview and cultural identity as mediational forces in individual lives, Ibrahim's model placed both the counselor's and the client's identities under scrutiny. These identities are a complex interacting combination of identities of ethnicity, culture, gender, age, life stage, socioeconomic status, education, and philosophy. Another etic model of examining cultural differences and creating universal applications is to look at identity development among members of different groups and work from a specific counseling approach that is based on advocacy and social justice (Ellis & Carlson, 2009).

An offshoot of the etic approach has been to examine the main feature of transcultural counseling: effective communication. Various theories have been developed to conceptualize cross-cultural communication within a universal framework (Pedersen, Crethar, & Carlson, 2008). The most basic component of transcultural features of counseling is language. Embedded in, arising from, and a seamless part of a cultural system, language is important in defining and labeling reality according to the cultural worldview. Fukuyama (1990) cautions that it is necessary to remember that mere ability to speak a language is not enough. There are subtle dimensions to language use that may lead to miscommunication and assumptions on the parts of both the counselor and the client.

Emic Approach

This approach in multicultural counseling involves studying specific cultures and adapting previous techniques or creating new ones to work with these groups. The emic perspective suggests that in counseling ethnic minority clients, to be effective in meeting their needs, counseling strategies must be congruent with the cultural characteristics of a particular client group. Although cross-cultural research studies have been plentiful, Ivey (1977) was one of the first to focus on cultural expertise as a salient feature in multicultural counseling. By this theory, the counselor would be effective in two cultures; his or her own as well as another. Because no counselor would be able to be expert in all cultures, the emic approach suggests counselor specialization.

The rationale for a culture-specific model is that whereas a general philosophy of multiculturalism is necessary for awareness, the next steps of knowledge and skills inevitably need to be specific. If the etic approach has shown all counseling to be culture-based and value laden, the emic approach goes further. The emic approach recognizes values within multicultural counseling dependent on three interrelating factors: the culture within which the counseling occurs, the identity and belief systems of the client as well as the counselor, and the interaction of the first two factors (Locke, 1990). Traditionally, counseling has been perceived as seeking to answer questions about human behavior from a universalist position (Leong & Blustein, 2000). Although focusing on specific cultures might seem more appropriate to counseling than focusing on patterns of cultural impact, Fischer, Jome, and Atkinson (1998) felt that there was significant evidence for the common factors approach in multicultural counseling and that it might well be possible to bring both perspectives together. Viewing individuals as unique within the context of their primary cultural group affirmed both the client's ethnicity and the client's individual humanity.

A major objection to the etic approach was that it began with a European American cultural frame (Nwachuku & Ivey, 1991). Multicultural and cross-cultural approaches seek to adapt existing methods and theories to different cultures. Beginning from a culture-specific approach, however, would enrich counseling by taking on the position of the client culture. For instance, Native American cultures view solving an individual problem within the context of family and community (Witko, 2006). Therefore, instead of attempting to fit traditional models to Native American clients, it might be more effective to derive theory and practice from Native American value structures. Instead of trying to adapt the traditional individualistic one-on-one approach to a community-based client, one could create a community-based theory that incorporates the individual. Culture-specific study could inspire new ways of conceptualizing the helping relationship simply by expanding the boundaries of what is possible through studying other cultures.

The emic approach is also relevant to the issue of diagnosis. Diagnosis is typically done by an "expert" observing and interpreting a client's behavior. The interpretation of behavior is based on the expert's cultural frame of reference rather than the client's. Behavior diagnosed as "pathological" in one culture may be deemed "adaptive" in another. Ridley (1995) discussed African American "cultural paranoia" as a healthy development that has its roots in life experiences in a hostile society. The determination of normality and abnormality is therefore intimately associated with the cultural standards used, and is therefore relative across cultures.

Locke (1990) paraphrases Carl Rogers's sixth condition of the client perceiving the counselor's empathic understanding and unconditional positive regard in relation to multicultural counseling. The counselor needs to be perceived by the culturally different client as "positive, serious, and capable of helping the devalued person or group in this situation, not as protecting the dominant group" (p. 21).

Comparison and Critique of Multicultural Counseling Approaches

There has been criticism of both etic and emic approaches. One criticism of the emic approach is that a counselor could fail to see the individual client as a whole person. The culture-specific information could very well be interpreted as a package that describes every member of that group, reducing the individuality of a client to a set of stereotyped cultural definitions. The other identities held by the client, such as gender, age, life experience, sexual orientation, and so on, would then be overlooked. Instead of increasing understanding, this approach holds the dangers of narrowly defining human beings in rigid cultural systems. Another criticism is that focusing so narrowly means that a counselor can only be of service to a limited population of clients.

The etic approach, on the other hand, has been criticized as being so broad in its focus so as to lose sight of specific cultural dynamics. Counselors dealing with clients who are culturally different from them would be ineffective in understanding these specific dynamics and the ways in which they affected the therapy. The social systems perspective of the etic approach, although acknowledging the complexity of individuals and the cultural components of all people, focuses on ways to universalize culture and ends up focusing on only the surface of culture. The emic approach focuses on behavior and custom, observable features that are only reflections of the deeper system. In developing theoretical models that seek to categorize any cultural constructs of the client into units amenable to the European American counselor's analysis (Christensen, 1989; Vontress, 1988), the emic approach also deals only with the surface aspects of culture. The surface manifestations of culture are subject to change and are affected by time and space (Jackson & Meadows, 1991).

Specific multicultural models have also emerged in response to the concerns raised (Ponterotto, Fuertes, & Chen, 2000). Table 1.1 summarizes the major aspects of each model for you. In later chapters, you will receive a more thorough exploration of these models and perspectives.

TABLE **1.1**
Models of Multicultural Counseling

Period	Model	Main Proponent	Major Tenets
Foundational models of the early 1980s: These have undergone extensive conceptual elaboration and have been empirically researched.	Multicultural competencies model	D. W. Sue et al. (1982)	Organized into three broad areas of counselor awareness of own values, biases, and attitudes; knowledge of the culturally different client; and skills in appropriate interventions and strategies.
	Racial identity model	J. Helms (1990)	Focusing on a developmental approach to racial identity, specific to various groups, that examines the movement of an individual from lack of awareness to a complex and flexible awareness and knowledge of their own racial identity.
1990s: Emerging models of multicultural counseling, which focus in on clinical intervention and treatment that are theoretically sophisticated but also less empirically validated.	Three-dimensional model counseling racial and ethnic minorities	Atkinson, Morten, & Sue (1993)	The counselor's role shifts based on the client's position along three dimensions of low to high acculturation, internal or external locus of problem etiology, and prevention versus remediation goals of counseling.
	Change in counseling through using worldview	J. G. Trevino (1996)	Using worldview as an internally coherent system derived from shared cultural and unique personal experiences, the model looks at counselor–client congruency in general perceptions and values, together with encouraging differences across specific cognitive levels to generate alternative client conceptualizations and solutions.
	Cultural sensitivity model using perpetual schemata	C. R. Ridley et al. (1994)	A cognitive process model that examines the counselor's cultural sensitivity to five subprocesses of self-processing, gains a meaningful understanding of the client's experience, maintains flexibility to avoid stereotyping, attends actively to cultural stimuli, and demonstrates a willingness to engage in the process.
	Integrative model of cross-cultural counseling	F. R. Leong (1996)	Based on a tripartite model of personality on the three levels of universal, group, and individual that interact in a dynamic manner, this model attends to cultural schemata in the context of the

(continued)

TABLE **1.1** (*continued*)

Period	Model	Main Proponent	Major Tenets
			counselor–client interpersonal relationship, unfolding on all three levels to enhance the counselor's cultural complementarity and mindfulness.
	Model of universal healing factors and cultural specificity	A. R. Fischer et al. (1998)	Examining culture within the context of universal healing factors that include the therapeutic relationship, a shared worldview between counselor and client, meeting client expectations, and using appropriate ritual and intervention, this model attempts to bridge universalist and culture-specific approaches to multicultural counseling.

Source: Adapted with permission from Ponterotto, J. G., Fuertes, J. N., & Chen, E. C. "Models of Multicultural Counseling," in S. D. Brown & R. W. Lent (Eds.), *Handbook of Counseling Psychology (3rd edition)*. Copyright © 2000 by John Wiley & Sons.

MULTICULTURAL COUNSELING COMPETENCIES

All of the helping fields have developed standards and ethical guidelines that affirm a commitment to addressing and respecting diversity (American Counseling Association [ACA], 2005; American Psychological Association, 2003; National Association of Social Workers [NASW], 1999). Social workers are asked directly to be sensitive to cultural and ethnic diversity and to work with the clear goals of bringing an end to injustice and oppression (NASW, 1999). Professional counselors are asked to appreciate diversity and adopt a cross-cultural approach that is sensitive to the cultural context in which clients are located (ACA, 2005). The field of counseling psychology is committed to promoting multicultural competence and working for social justice (Toporek, Gerstein, Fouad, Roysircar, & Israel, 2006). Multicultural counseling competence is essentially the ability of a counselor to recognize, acknowledge, and respond sensitively and appropriately to clients in their cultural contexts.

In an influential paper, Sue and others (Sue et al., 1982) developed a construct of multicultural competency. Under the aegis of the Association for Multicultural Counseling and Development, Arredondo and others (1996) clarified and operationalized these fundamental competencies. Essentially, competency lies in three domains of multiculturalism (awareness, knowledge, and skills) across three areas of the self of the counselor, the client, and the therapeutic relationship [See Table 1.2]. We are asked to develop awareness of ourselves, in the context of our own aspects of social identities, and pay attention to our own cultural and sociopolitical foundations. From such surer ground, we are better able to meet a client who will inevitably be different from us on some aspect of race, culture, gender, age, sexual orientation, disability, or religion, or perhaps in just their unique experience of that social identity. So, an African American woman counselor would need as much competency in making sure she understands her African American female client and not simply assume similarity, as would a European American male counselor working with an Asian American woman. Although these multicultural counseling competencies focus primarily on race and cultural identity, other aspects have also been attended to in various guidelines. For instance, the American Psychological Association (2009) issued a task force report with recommendations on gender identity and gender variance and the need for professionals to be sensitive to various aspects of the experience of transgender persons.

 REFLECTION QUESTIONS 1.2

- What does it mean to you to be multiculturally competent?
- What is the difference, if any, in your mind between being competent and being effective in multicultural counseling?
- What are areas of strength and limitation for you regarding multicultural awareness, knowledge, and skills?
- How can you work to build on areas of strength and improve areas of limitation?

TABLE **1.2**
Multicultural Counseling Competencies

	Awareness	Knowledge	Skills
Counselor	1. Culturally competent counselors have moved from being culturally unaware to being aware and sensitive to their own cultural heritage and to valuing and respecting differences. 2. Culturally competent counselors are aware of how their own cultural background and experiences, attitudes, and values and biases influence psychological processes. 3. Culturally competent counselors are able to recognize the limits of their competencies and expertise. 4. Culturally competent counselors are comfortable with differences that exist between themselves and	5. Culturally competent counselors have specific knowledge about their own racial and cultural heritage and how it personally and professionally affects their definitions and biases of normality–abnormality and the process of counseling. 6. Culturally competent counselors possess knowledge and understanding about how oppression, racism, discrimination, and stereotyping affect them personally and in their work. 7. Culturally competent counselors possess knowledge about their social impact on others. They are knowledgeable	8. Culturally competent counselors seek out educational, consultative, and training experiences to enrich their understanding and effectiveness in working with culturally different populations. 9. Culturally competent counselors are constantly seeking to understand themselves as racial cultural beings and are actively seeking a nonracist identity.

(continued)

TABLE **1.2** (*continued*)

	Awareness	Knowledge	Skills
	clients in terms of race, ethnicity, culture, and beliefs.	about communication style differences, how their style may clash or facilitate the counseling process with minority clients, and how to anticipate the impact it may have on others.	
Client	10. Culturally competent counselors are aware of their negative emotional re-actions toward other racial and ethnic groups that may prove detrimental to their clients in counseling. 11. Culturally competent counselors are aware of their stereotypes and preconceived notions that they may hold toward other racial and ethnic groups.	12. Culturally competent counselors possess specific knowledge and information about the particular group that they are working with. They are aware of the life experiences, cultural heri-tage, and historical back-ground of their culturally different clients. This partic-ular competency is strongly linked to the racial-ethnic minority development mod-els available in the literature. 13. Culturally competent counselors understand how race, culture, and ethnicity may affect personality formation, vocational choices, manifestation of psychological disorders, help-seeking behavior, and the appropriateness or inappropriateness of counseling approaches. 14. Culturally competent counselors understand and have knowledge about sociopolitical influences that impinge upon the life of racial and ethnic minorities.	15. Culturally competent counselors should familiarize themselves with relevant re-search and the latest findings regarding the mental health and mental health disorders of various ethnic and racial groups. 16. Culturally competent counselors become actively involved with minority individuals outside the counseling setting (via community events, social and political functions, celebrations, friendships, neighborhood groups, and so forth) so that their perspective of minorities is more than an academic or helping exercise.
Counseling Relationship	17. Culturally competent counselors respect clients' religious and/or spiritual beliefs and values about physical and mental functioning.	20. Culturally competent counselors have a clear and explicit knowledge and un-derstanding of the generic characteristics of counseling and therapy (i.e., that it is culture bound, class bound,	25. Culturally competent counselors are able to engage in a variety of verbal and nonver-bal helping responses. They are able to send and receive both verbal and nonverbal messages accurately and appropriately.

(*continued*)

TABLE **1.2** (*continued*)

Awareness	Knowledge	Skills
18. Culturally competent counselors respect indigenous helping practices and respect minority communities' intrinsic help-giving networks. 19. Culturally competent counselors value bilingualism and do not view another language as an impediment to counseling (monolingualism may be the culprit).	and monolingual) and how they clash with the cultural values of various minority groups. 21. Culturally competent counselors are aware of institutional barriers that prevent minorities from using mental health services. 22. Culturally competent counselors have knowledge of the potential biases in assessment instruments, and use procedures and interpret findings keeping in mind the cultural and linguistic characteristics of the clients. 23. Culturally competent counselors have knowledge of minority family structures, hierarchies, values, and beliefs. They are knowledgeable about the community characteristics and the resources in the community as well as the family. 24. Culturally competent counselors are aware of relevant discriminatory practices at the social and community levels that may be affecting the psychological welfare of the population being served.	They are not tied down to only one method or approach to helping but recognize that helping styles and approaches may be culture bound. 26. Culturally competent counselors are able to exercise institutional intervention skills on behalf of their clients. 27. Culturally competent counselors are not adverse to seeking consultation with traditional healers or religious and spiritual leaders and practitioners in the treatment of culturally different clients when appropriate. 28. Culturally competent counselors take responsibility for interacting in the language requested by the client; this may mean appropriate referral to outside resources. 29. Culturally competent counselors have training and expertise in the use of traditional assessment and testing instruments. They not only understand the technical aspects of the instruments but also are aware of the cultural limitations. This allows them to use test instruments for the welfare of clients from diverse cultural, racial, and ethnic groups. 30. Culturally competent counselors should attend to as well as work to eliminate biases, prejudices, and discriminatory practices. They should be cognizant of sociopolitical contexts in conducting evaluations and providing interventions, and should develop sensitivity to

(*continued*)

TABLE **1.2** (*continued*)

Awareness	Knowledge	Skills
		issues of oppression, sexism, and racism. 31. Culturally competent counselors take responsibility in educating their clients to the processes of psychological intervention such as goals, expectations, legal rights, and the counselor's orientation.

Adapted from Arredondo et al. (1996).

It is important to notice how complex this endeavor to build competency is. In many ways, we are aspirational in this process because we cannot ever say we have arrived at competency. The landscape of cultures and diversity is at once complicated, vast, and dynamic—it changes as we speak, as history progresses, and as experience and understanding and ascribed meaning change. What multicultural competency is not, however, is much simpler to understand, though it may be uncomfortable for us to accept. It is not a memorized list of behaviors, values, and facts assigned to persons by virtue of their membership in groups. It is not an idealized understanding of people's heritage as expressed through music, dance, folklore, or myth, though many of these are useful and powerful directions. It is not a belief that one has sufficient knowledge about groups that is arrived at through depictions of groups in television, film, and other media. Although it might be comforting to imagine one knows about a group of people, when one works with a member or members of a group (whether that group is defined by race, culture, gender, sexual orientation, age, disability, or religion), one has to negotiate the delicate balance between using awareness, knowledge, and sensitivity, knowing that they are necessarily limited, to strive toward developing understanding of the unique set of contexts and issues present in the life of that person. In cross-cultural work, competency is essentially an endeavor to engage in relationship building, based on an understanding of both the contexts and the dynamic individual response to those contexts.

Another inescapable aspect of acquiring competency is that although it is necessary to go through acquiring information through resources such as this and other courses, it can only actually be tested in practice. Vereen, Hill, and McNeal (2008) found that counselor trainees rated themselves significantly higher on multicultural competency when they had actually worked with diverse clients and received clinical supervision during the process that assisted them in developing greater awareness and skills.

Much research has examined the issue of multicultural counseling competency, and it has increased over the last 20 years (Worthington, Soth-McNett,

& Moreno, 2007). One of the problems in this area has been that much of it has focused on trainees and depended on self-perception or self-report. However, other aspects have examined the intrapersonal aspects of the counselor in terms of demographics, attitudes, training, and personality; client outcomes such as reported satisfaction, attrition, or level of self-disclosure; as well as client perceptions of their counselors' competency, credibility, or trustworthiness. Acquiring multicultural competency is helpful in having clients rate counselors as more satisfactory, having them return for more sessions, enabling them to communicate concerns relating to culture or race, and, in general, improving counseling process and outcomes across clients of diverse backgrounds (Worthington, Soth-McNett, & Moreno, 2007).

A multiculturally competent practitioner takes on many roles in responding to the client's needs. The traditional notion of counseling has often depicted a counselor as a neutral helper who helps the client focus on an internally understood issue, this helping being conducted in a neutral space removed from the messy dimensions of both the helper's and client's lives. However, multicultural counseling assigns the counselor many more roles and avenues of intervention depending on the client's needs. These include the following:

Advisor: For low-acculturated clients who have limited experience in dealing with the U.S. mainstream society, and whose problems stem largely from external sources.

Advocate: Appropriate with low-acculturation clients who need remediation of a problem that results from oppression and discrimination.

Facilitator of Indigenous systems: Working with low-acculturated clients whose intrapersonal and interpersonal problems appear to have an internal locus. Requires awareness of and a relationship with community networks.

Facilitator of Indigenous healing: Referring clients to an indigenous system that better serves their needs, either by referring clients to a healer within the culture or by the use of indigenous healing techniques directly.

Consultant: Working with acculturated clients who seek to prevent externally caused problems. Most appropriate for organizational counseling.

Change agent: Working with acculturated clients to help them change the discriminatory environment.

Counselor: A preventive and developmental role focusing on the needs of highly acculturated clients.

Psychotherapist: Working primarily with psychologically minded, highly acculturated clients who are looking for relief from problems with internal etiology.

In working with different clients, the practitioner may have diverse goals. Some of these include the following:

1. Support with multiple stressors
2. Coping with posttraumatic stress

3. Assisting acculturation and adaptation
4. Avoiding further marginalization
5. Addressing discrimination and developing coping strategies
6. Assisting clients to manage cross-cultural relationships
7. Assisting clients to manage intergenerational conflict
8. Assisting long-stay transients and expatriates
9. Assisting with gender role and equality issues
10. Assisting with sexual orientation and coming-out issues
11. Assisting with adjustment to disability issues
12. Facilitating spiritual questioning
13. Assisting with self-actualization and personal growth (adapted from Nelson-Jones, 2002)

IMPLICATIONS FOR LEARNING

There are a plethora of texts available on multicultural counseling. This is a welcome change from the days when it received little attention and publishers were reluctant to accept manuscripts on multiculturalism (Atkinson, 2004). One of the primary ways in which this text is different from the others is the focus on theoretical constructs of multiple social identities. Rather than examining diverse groups, we start with the premise that striving to be multi-culturally competent is to address and respond to the ways in which marginalization and alienation occur across society. As helpers, we wish to be sensitive and responsive and not simply revictimize people who have already had such experiences.

All counseling is cross-cultural when it takes place between a counselor and client who may both share social identities while experiencing them differently, or differ from each in other aspects of identity (Pedersen, 1990). Therefore, an Asian American male counselor must attend to the cultural differences between himself and his Latino client. Such considerations are as critical when both the counselor and client are European American men who may appear similar, but come from different socioeconomic status and ethnic backgrounds, sexual orientations, or ages that lead to experiential differences that will shape the course of the relationship. However, the focus of developing alternate models and practices of counseling has concentrated on those peoples who are somehow different—in essence, those groups who are different from the dominant group. Whether they are labeled *culturally different*, *hyphenated-Americans*, *multicultural populations*, *minorities*, *special education folks*, *homosexuals*, or *the poor*, the purpose of the label is to distinguish them from the normative mass of supposedly generic people.

Through this text, we offer you a framework for thinking about the aspects of identity that are important to consider in working with any client. We explicitly articulate each aspect of identity in terms of oppression, acknowledging that our identities become important as points of difference primarily because difference has been perceived negatively and experienced in terms of access or denial to opportunity and social power. For instance, we think of race as an important aspect of identity. However, if you were the only human being on the planet Jupiter, your race would be singularly unimportant. Race is important because the race we are assigned has implications of power and privilege or, conversely, discrimination and denial in society and in the context of our relationships. The same is generally true of culture, gender, sexual orientation, socioeconomic class, age, religion, and disability. For purposes of study, we will take each characteristic of identity, but only to highlight and focus on it rather than to isolate it.

We will start with the foundational construct of culture in Chapter 2. We then move on to the notion of individuals experiencing a complex of identities and developing a worldview that is shaped by those identities in Chapter 3. Following this, in Chapter 4, we will describe and articulate the concept of oppression to offer you a beginning analysis of the structures of society that have implications for you as a helper as well as those whom you help. Chapter 5 will address the historical impact of race and ethnicity and their influence on various groups in U.S. society. We then examine specific constructs of identity, examining age in Chapter 6, gender in Chapter 7, sexual orientation in Chapter 8, social class in Chapter 9, spirituality and religion in Chapter 10, and disability in Chapter 11. In Chapter 12 we return to the issue of multicultural counseling competency, exploring it in greater depth and using the work we have done in previous chapters to examine how it may work in practice.

The chapters in this text will provide you with a historical, sociopolitical, and psychological overview of each aspect of identity that will have resonance in counseling and psychotherapy. You will be encouraged to apply some of the information and analyses to the ways in which you understand and experience those aspects of identity in yourself as well as in the range of people you will be helping.

What we will not offer you in this text is a set of recipes on how to work with diverse clients. However, the application of skills and specific strategies and the means of understanding diverse groups are critical. For that purpose, this text is accompanied by a series of monographs that address those practitioner issues. With those, you will get greater exposure to specific issues in counseling different ethnic groups such as African Americans, Asian Americans, Native Americans, Hispanic Americans, and Arab Americans. Additionally, you may get further information on specific issues in counseling gay, lesbian, bisexual, and transgender populations; people with disabilities; and elders through continuing monographs.

Counseling Implication

We offer you, as a counselor, a way to conceptualize client issues in a way that neither generalizes identity nor ignores its many dimensions.

At this point, we invite you to notice the complexity of striving to make sense of the issues presented. Through the course of this textbook, we will be offering you points of information to use as analysis in thinking through the race, culture, gender, sexual orientation, socioeconomic class, or religious issues. The above case study is to demonstrate to you that in the process,

CASE STUDY **1.1**

The Case of Susie Dinh

Susie Dinh: A Vietnamese American Teenager

Sixteen-year-old Susie is a Vietnamese American girl in a predominantly European American high school. She lives at home with her parents. Her parents came to the United States in the late 1970s, but Susie was born here much later. She knows she had an older brother who died before she was born. The family owns and operates a Laundromat, and Susie spends most of her after-school hours working there. She is doing well in school, and also takes piano lessons twice a week. Susie has come in to see you, the school counselor, reluctantly on the urging of some of her friends.

Susie says she is sad. She spends time with her few close friends in school, because of having no time out of school. All of her friends are Asian, but only girls. She cannot date like her peers do, because her father will not allow it. However, she reports that she wouldn't want to date boys anyway, though she feels embarrassed to say that. She enjoys the piano lessons, but her piano teacher, a young Russian American woman, is the real reason she keeps going. According to Susie, she is the one person who seems to really understand her. She reports feeling like crying most of the time, but is unable to really think of a reason. "After all," she says, "it's not like some tragedy has happened. Actually, nothing has changed except me." She reports that her parents are concerned and urge her to work harder, but they would never understand about counseling. She considers them very traditional, and though she does not want to fight them, she often feels that they do not understand what life is like for her as an American.

Case Discussion
Thinking About This Case
1. How do you make sense of Susie?
2. What do you think her presenting problem is?
3. What aspects of her presentation do you consider significant?

As you read the above description, notice that Susie's ethnic and racial identity play a role in her sense of self and depression. That she is a girl of 16 is no doubt significant, bringing in issues of gender and development, within the context of conflicting cultural clashes between school and family. Sexual identity is an issue, of which sexual orientation may well play a role as Susie begins to figure out her reluctance to engage with boys, her father's prohibition to do so, and her intimacy with her teacher. Her family came as immigrants, and they may well have come with refugee status. The struggle to build a life in a new country and culture, and to develop the family-owned business, is significant to Susie's sense of belonging and security, and invokes socioeconomic issues that need to be taken into account. If her family follows any traditional spiritual beliefs, she may well inherit the mantle left by her deceased older brother. The circumstances of his death and his age at the time of death, as well as the family's reaction and response to the death of the oldest son, might offer clues to Susie's malaise.

you must not let any aspect of identity become the only salient one that takes your attention. Although different clients may well focus on or be aware of certain aspects, your task as counselor is to notice the details on a wider landscape so that, in turn, your responses and interventions can be rich and engaged with the full range of who the client is.

Please read the following poem, which describes the breathtaking and sometimes terrifying demands that a journey of developing multicultural competence makes on us. Please know that it is seldom about getting it right and most often about continuing to risk, to care, and to grow.

Good luck on your journey.

REFLECTION EXERCISE **1.2**

The Invitation

The Invitation

By Oriah Mountain Dreamer

It doesn't interest me what you do for a living.
I want to know what you ache for
and if you dare to dream of meeting your heart's longing.
It doesn't interest me how old you are.
I want to know if you will risk looking like a fool for love
for your dream for the adventure of being alive.
It doesn't interest me what planets are squaring your moon...
I want to know if you have touched
the centre of your own sorrow
if you have been opened by life's betrayals
or have become shriveled and closed from fear of further pain.
I want to know if you can sit with pain mine or your own
without moving to hide it or fade it or fix it.
I want to know if you can be with joy mine or your own
if you can dance with wildness and let the ecstasy fill you
to the tips of your fingers and toes without cautioning us to be careful
to be realistic
to remember the limitations of being human.
It doesn't interest me if the story you are telling me is true.
I want to know if you can disappoint another to be true to yourself.
If you can bear the accusation of betrayal and not betray your own soul.
If you can be faithless and therefore trustworthy.
I want to know if you can see Beauty even when it is not pretty every day.
And if you can source your own life from its presence.
I want to know if you can live with failure yours and mine
and still stand at the edge of the lake and shout to the silver of the full moon,
"Yes."
It doesn't interest me to know where you live or how much money you
have.
I want to know if you can get up after the night of grief and despair
weary and bruised to the bone and do what needs to be done to feed
the children.
It doesn't interest me who you know or how you came to be here.
I want to know if you will stand in the centre of the fire
with me and not shrink back.
It doesn't interest me where or what or with whom you have studied.
I want to know what sustains you from the inside when all else falls away.
I want to know if you can be alone with yourself and if you truly like
the company you keep in the empty moments.

CONCLUSION AND IMPLICATIONS

This chapter began with a metaphor of the journey that challenged you, the reader, to visualize this process of learning about multicultural counseling as a journey of learning and healing that is ever present and always happening, requiring active, intentional participation along the way to make it meaningful. We then introduced not only ourselves as professionals who offer to you our experience and expertise in the area of multicultural counseling, but also our lives as people of color, who see ourselves traveling the path of the journey moving alongside you. We discussed the importance of multicultural counseling based on the long history of conflict in the United States based on adversarial relationships, hostility, and conflict between groups of people, and the resulting effects of this on clients' lives and needs in counseling. We offered a view of the history of multiculturalism in the profession of counseling and various models of multicultural counseling that grew out of that long, rich tradition, intended to help you, the constantly growing practitioner, along your journey.

GLOSSARY

Culture: Culture is the personification of a worldview through learned and transmitted beliefs, values, and practices, including religious and spiritual traditions and psychological processes. It is a way of living shaped by historical, economic, ecological, and political forces on a group. All individuals are cultural beings and have a cultural, ethnic, and racial heritage.

Emic: A view of culture as specific and distinguishing between humans.

Ethnicity: Similar to the concepts of race and culture, the term *ethnicity* does not have a commonly agreed upon definition, but includes sociocultural heritage based on commonalities represented in such dimensions as collective history, common ancestral origin, religion, nationality, and language.

Etic: A view of culture as a commonality shared by all humans.

Multicultural and diversity: The terms *multiculturalism* and *diversity* have been used interchangeably to recognize the broad scope of dimensions of race, ethnicity, culture, language, sexual orientation, gender, age, disability, class status, and religious and spiritual orientation as critical aspects of an individual's personal identity.

Multicultural counseling competence: The ability of a counselor to recognize, acknowledge, and respond sensitively and appropriately to clients in their cultural contexts.

People of color: A term used, primarily in the United States, to describe persons who are not of European heritage. In other words, people who belong to ethnic groups identified as African American, Hispanic and Latino/a, Asian, and Native American peoples. The term is meant to be inclusive, emphasizing a commonality of experience, particularly with racism.

Race: The categories to which individuals are assigned based on physical characteristics, such as skin color or hair type, and the generalizations and stereotypes made as a result. Although race may have some basis in shared genetic history and heritage, there is much empirical evidence that there are as many within-group variations as there are across so-called racial groups, leaving it a powerful social construct rather than a biological one.

REFERENCES

American Counseling Association (ACA). (2005). *ACA code of ethics*. Alexandria, VA: Author.

American Psychiatric Association (APA). (1987). *Diagnostic and statistical manual of mental disorders* (3rd ed.). Washington, DC: Author.

American Psychiatric Association (APA). (1994). *Diagnostic and statistical manual of mental disorders* (4th ed.). Washington, DC: Author.

American Psychological Association. (2003). Guidelines on multicultural education, training, research, practice, and organizational change for psychologists. *American Psychologist, 58,* 377–402.

American Psychological Association, Task Force on Gender Identity and Gender Variance. (2009). *Report of the Task Force on Gender Identity and Gender Variance*. Washington, DC: Author.

Arredondo, P., Toporek, M. S., Brown, S., Jones, J., Locke, D. C., Sanchez, J., et al. (1996). *Operationalization of the multicultural counseling competencies.* Alexandria, VA: AMCD.

Atkinson, D. R. (2004). *Counseling American minorities* (6th ed.). New York: McGraw-Hill.

Atkinson, D. R., Morten, G., & Sue, D. W. (1993). Counseling American minorities: A cross cultural perspective (4th ed.). Madison, Wisconsin: Brown and Benchmark.

Atkinson, D. R., Thompson, C. E., & Grant, S. K. (1993). A three-dimensional model for counseling racial/ethnic minorities. *Counseling Psychologist,* 21, 257–277.

Barret, B. & Logan, C. (2002). *Counseling gay men and lesbians: A practice primer.* Pacific Grove, CA: Brooks/Cole.

Berk, L. (2007). *Development through the Life span* (4th ed.). Allyn & Bacon.

Boysen, G. A., Vogel, D. L., Madon, S., & Wester, S. R. (2006). Mental health stereotypes about gay men. *Sex Roles,* 54, 69–82.

Casas, J. M. (1984). Policy, training, and research in counseling psychology: The racial/ethnic minority perspective. In S. D. Brown & R. W. Lent (Eds.), *Handbook of counseling psychology* (pp. 785–831). New York: John Wiley.

Chernin, J. N., & Johnson, M. R. (2002). *Affirmative psychotherapy and counseling for lesbians and gay men.* Thousand Oaks, CA: Sage.

Christensen, C. (1989). Cross-cultural awareness: A conceptual model. *Counselor Education and Supervision,* 28, 270–287.

Draguns, J. (2008). Universal and cultural threads in counseling individuals. In P. Pedersen, J. Draguns, W. Lonner, & J. Trimble (Eds.), *Counseling across cultures* (6th ed., pp. 3–21). Thousand Oaks, CA: Sage.

Ellis, C. M., & Carlson, J. (Eds.). (2009). *Cross cultural awareness and social justice in counseling.* New York: Routledge.

Estrada, E., Frame, M. W., & Williams, C. B. (2004). Cross-cultural supervision: Guiding the conversation toward race and ethnicity. *Journal of Multicultural Counseling and Development,* 32, 307–319.

Fischer, A. R., Jome, L. M., & Atkinson, D. R. (1998). Reconceptualizing multicultural counseling: Universal healing conditions in a culturally specific context. *Counseling Psychologist,* 26, 525–588.

Griffin, P. (1987). Introductory module for the single issue courses. In M. Griffin, L. A. Bell, & P. Griffin (Eds.). *Teaching for diversity and social justice* (pp. 61–81). New York: Routledge.

Helms, J. (Ed.). (1990). *Black and White racial identity: Theory, research, and practice.* Westport, CT: Greenwood.

Fischer, A. R., Jome, L. M., & Atkinson, D. R. (1998). Reconceptualizing multicultural counseling: Universal healing conditions in a culturally specific context. *The Counseling Psychologist,* 26, 525–588.

Fukuyama, M. A. (1990). Taking a universal approach to multicultural counseling. *Counselor Education and Supervision,* 30, 6–17.

Helms, J. E. & Cook, D. A. (1999). *Using race and culture in counseling and psychotherapy: Theory and process.* Needham Heights, MA, US: Allyn & Bacon.

Huitt, W., & Hummel, J. (2003). Piaget's theory of cognitive development. *Educational Psychology Interactive.* Valdosta, GA: Valdosta State University. Retrieved October 28, 2010 from http://www.edpsycinteractive.org/topics/cogsys/piaget.html

Ibrahim, F. A., Roysicar-Sodowsky, G., & Ohnishi, H. (2001). Worldview: Recent developments and needed directions. In J. G. Ponterotto, J. M. Casas, L. A. Suzuki, & C. M. Alexander (Eds.), *Handbook of multicultural counseling* (2nd ed., pp. 425–455). Thousand Oaks, CA: Sage.

Ivey, A. (1977). Cultural expertise: Toward systematic outcome criteria in counseling and psychological education. *The Personnel & Guidance Journal,* 55, 296–302.

Jackson, A. P., & Meadows, F. B. (1991). Getting to the bottom to understand the top. *Journal of Counseling & Development,* 70, 72–76.

Lee, C. C. (2008). *Elements of culturally competent counseling* (ACAPCD-24). Alexandria, VA: American Counseling Association.

Leong, F. T. L. (1996). Toward an integrative model for cross-cultural counseling and psychotherapy. *Applied and Preventive Psychology: Current Scientific Perspectives,* 5, 189–209.

Leong, F. T. L., & Blustein, D. L. (2000). Toward a global vision of counseling psychology. *The Counseling Psychologist,* 28, 5–9.

Liu, W. M., Ali, S. R., Soleck, G., Hopps, J., Dunston, K., & Pickett, T., Jr. (2004). Using social class in counseling psychology research. *Journal of Counseling Psychology,* 51, 3–18.

Locke, D. (1990). A not so provincial view of multicultural counseling. *Counselor Education & Supervision,* 30, 18–25.

National Association of Social Workers (NASW). (1999). *Code of ethics*. Washington, DC: Author.

Nelson-Jones, R. (2002). Diverse goals for multicultural counseling and therapy. *Counseling Psychology Quarterly, 15*(2), 133–143.

Nwachuku, U., & Ivey, A. (1991). Culture-specific counseling: An alternative training model. *Journal of Counseling & Development, 70*, 106–111.

Mountain Dreamer, O. (1995). *Dreams of desire*. Toronto: Mountain Dreaming.

Pedersen, P., Crethar, H. C., & Carlson, J. (2008). *Inclusive cultural empathy: Making relationships central in counseling and psychotherapy*. Washington, DC: American Psychological Association.

Pedersen, P. (1990). The multicultural perspective as a fourth force in counseling. *Journal of Mental Health Counseling, 12*(1), 93–95.

Perez, R. M., DeBord, K. A., & Bieschke, K. J. (Eds.). (2000). *Handbook of counseling and psychotherapy with lesbian, gay, and bisexual clients*. Washington, DC: American Psychological Association.

Phillips, J. C., Ingram, K. M., Smith, N. G., & Mindes, E. J. (2003). Methodological and content review of lesbian-, gay-, and bisexual-related articles in counseling journals: 1990–1999. *The Counseling Psychologist, 31*, 25–62.

Ponterotto, J. G., Fuertes, J. N., & Chen, E. C. (2000). Models of multicultural counseling. In S. D. Brown & R. W. Lent (Eds.), *Handbook of counseling psychology* (3rd ed., pp. 639–669). New York: John Wiley.

Ridley, C. R. (1995). *Overcoming unintentional racism in counseling and therapy: A practitioner's guide to intentional intervention*. Thousand Oaks, CA: Sage.

Ridley, C. R., Mendoza, D. W., Kanitz, B. E., Angermeier, L., & Zenk, R. (1994). Cultural sensitivity in multicultural counseling: A perceptual schema model. *Journal of Counseling Psychology, 41*, 125–136.

Robinson, D. T., & Morris, J. R. (2000). Multicultural counseling: Historical context and current training considerations. *The Western Journal of Black Studies, 24*(4), 239.

Russo, N. F., Olmedo, E. L., Stapp, J., & Fulcher, R. (1981). Women and minorities in psychology. *American Psychologist, 36*, 1315–1363.

Smart, J. F., & Smart, D. W. (2006). Models of disability: Implications for the counseling profession. *Journal of Counseling & Development, 84*, 29–40.

Sue, D. W., Bernier, J. E., Durran, A., Feinberg, L., Pedersen, P., Smith, E. J., et al. (1982). Position paper: Cross-cultural counseling competencies. *Counseling Psychologist, 10*, 45–52.

Sue, D. W., & Sue, D. (2008). *Counseling the culturally diverse: Theory and practice* (5th ed.). New York: John Wiley.

Sue, S., & Zane, N. (1987). The role of culture and cultural techniques in psychotherapy: A critique and reformulation. *American Psychologist, 42*, 37–45.

Sue, D. W. (1978). Eliminating cultural oppression in counseling: Towards a general theory. *Journal of Counseling Psychology, 25*(5), 419–428.

Toporek, R. L., Gerstein, L. H., Fouad, N. A., Roysircar, G., & Israel, T. (Eds.). (2006). *Handbook for social justice in counseling psychology: Leadership, vision, and action*. Thousand Oaks, CA: Sage.

Torres-Rivera, E., Phan, L. T., Maddux, C., Wilbur, M. P., & Garrett, M. T. (2001). Process versus content: Integrating personal awareness and counseling skills to meet the multicultural challenge of the twenty-first century. *Counselor Education and Supervision, 41*, 28–40.

Trevino, J. G. (1996). Worldview and change in cross-cultural counseling. *Counseling Psychologist, 24*, 198–215.

U. S. Census Bureau. (2004). U.S. Interim projections by age, sex, race, and Hispanic origin. Retrieved October 28, 2010, from http://www.census.gov/population/www/projections/usinterimproj/natprojtab01a.pdf

Vereen, L. G., Hill, N. R., & McNeal, D. T. (2008). Perceptions of multicultural counseling competency: Integration of the curriculur and the practical. *Journal of Mental Health Counseling, 30*(3), 226–236.

Vontress, C. (1988). An existential approach to cross-cultural counseling. *Journal of Multicultural Counseling & Development, 16*, 73–83.

Weinrach, S. G., & Thomas, K. T. (1998). Diversity sensitive counseling today: A postmodern clash of values. *Journal of Counseling & Development, 76*(2), 115–123.

Witko, T. M. (Ed.). (2006). *Mental health care for urban Indians: Clinical insights from Native practitioners*. Washington, DC: American Psychological Association.

Worthington, R. L., Soth-McNett, A. M., & Moreno, M. V. (2007). Multicultural counseling competencies research: A 20-year content analysis. *Journal of Counseling Psychology, 54*(4), 351–361.

CHAPTER 2

Culture

That we are living more and more in the midst of an enormous collage seems everywhere apparent. It is not just the evening news where assassinations in India, bombings in Lebanon, coups in Africa, and shootings in Central America are set amidst local disasters hardly more legible and followed on by grave discussions of Japanese ways of doing business, Persian forms of passion, or Arab styles of negotiation. It is also an enormous explosion of translation, good, bad, and indifferent, from and to languages—Tamil, Indonesian, Hebrew, and Urdu—previously regarded as marginal and recondite; the migration of cuisines, costumes, furnishings, and decor (caftans in San Francisco, Colonel Sanders in Jogjakarta, and barstools in Kyoto); and the appearance of gamelan themes in avant-grade jazz, Indio myths in Latino novels, and magazine images in African painting.

But most of all, it is that the person we encounter in the grocery is as likely, or nearly, to come from Korea as from Iowa, in the post office from Algeria as from the Auvergne, in the bank from Bombay as from Liverpool. Even rural settings, where alikeness is likely to be more entrenched[,] are not immune; Mexican farmers in the Southwest, Vietnamese fisherman along the Gulf Coast, Iranian physicians in the Midwest.

To live in a collage one must in the first place render oneself capable of sorting out its elements, determining what they are (which usually involves determining where they come from and what they amounted to when they were there) and how, practically, they relate to one another, without at the same time blurring one's own sense of one's own location and one's own identity within it. Less figuratively, "understanding" in the sense of comprehension, perception, and insight needs to be distinguished from "understanding" in the sense of agreement of opinion, union of sentiment, or commonality of commitment; we must learn to grasp what we cannot embrace.

—Clifford Geertz (2000, pp. 85–87)

We see the world not as it is but as we are (Covey, 1990). This perspective is the essence of the cultural approach. All of us have been raised within a particular culture and society, and our upbringing has shaped the ways in which we view the world, make sense of it, and respond to it. Depending on our cultural upbringing, we may differ in small ways or profound ways from each other. One way to think about the pervasiveness and power of culture is to imagine it as a house we grow up in. Because the layout of the rooms is intimately familiar to us, we do not know what our lives would be like if the windows and doors or the very walls were different. We grow up looking out over apartment buildings and we understand the world as such, unlike someone who grows up looking out at mountaintops. To understand the term *multicultural*, one first needs to understand the construct of *culture*. A *construct* is a category or concept that serves as a building block in theory—the metaphorical use of the term is derived from the physical construction of a foundation. In this chapter, we examine the construct of culture; explore its impact; discuss the psychological implications of various cultural frameworks in the context of cultural worldviews, immigration, acculturation, and language; and consider culture-specific illnesses and interventions.

DEFINING CULTURE

Ask anyone what culture is and you may get a different answer from each person you ask. You also may find there are some who do not know what culture is, may have never really thought about it, and might even tell you that they themselves do not have a culture. Ironically, it is not that the person does not have a culture, but that his or her definition of culture may be limited in ways that do not address who that person is culturally. Culture is still there affecting everything that person thinks, feels, does, and says.

Like other constructs we will explore in this book, *culture* has come to have somewhat different definitions in different fields. Before we consider the definition of the word that is generally agreed upon in the field of multicultural counseling, let us consider the derivation and other uses of the term.

An original meaning of the word was *husbandry*, with the verb *cultivate* deriving from *culture*, and one can still see this meaning in references to "cultured pearls" or "tissue cultures" (Fernando, 2002). One of the standard dictionary definitions of the word *culture* pertains to manners, etiquette, and breadth of knowledge about the arts and literature. In this sense, a cultured person is one who may engage in articulate conversations about the distinctions between Brueghel the elder and younger, cabernet sauvignon versus merlot, Alvin Ailey and the Joffrey Ballet, or the magical realism of Salman Rushdie versus that of Jorge Luis Borges. Such a definition of culture implies a formal learning and education, and an array of knowledge that is part of that learning. Notice how exclusionary such a definition of culture is—how many of you could read the above description and say to yourselves with confidence that you knew all these references and could carry on such conversations? Also, notice that little of such knowledge is immediately useful for the everyday business of living. So, if one uses *culture* as a synonym for particular kinds of "civilization," one implies that those with the most culture will have the most luxury to focus on activities unrelated to survival. Such an elitist definition of *culture* implies formal learning and education, and an array of knowledge that is part of that learning resulting in a degree of sophistication that makes one very "cultured." Indeed, the word *culture* derives from the German word *Kultur*, referring to one's degree of sophistication. Notice, if you will, how exclusionary such a definition of culture is and, even more importantly, how, based on an exclusionary definition also infused with privilege, one's culture, from this perspective, also lends status and power over those who are less "cultured."

Some people think that culture is something that characterizes other people from other lands. From this perspective, kimonos are cultural dress, but jeans are not; tamales are cultural food, but hamburgers are ordinary, or normative, food. Here, culture consists of the exotic elements that distinguish certain people from the norm. The authors have frequently noticed that some of the graduate students who come to our multicultural counseling courses with this understanding of culture often believe that they have no culture—because they do not recognize that the ways in which they prepare food, entertain, celebrate, grieve, worship, and arrange their living is cultural. In many ways, this way of viewing the world is about designating ourselves and those like us as "normal," whereas those who are different from us are placed in the margins of our normal world.

In the popular media, the term *culture* is sometimes used interchangeably with *race* or *ethnicity*. Consider, for example, the phrase *Black culture*. It implies that all Black people have a common culture by virtue of their racial membership, regardless of whether they are African Americans, Nigerians, Jamaicans, Haitians, or Brazilians. Although there are many cultural dynamics that are associated with being a Black person in the United States, it is also important to distinguish aspects of race versus culture. For instance, a 50-year-old Jamaican American bus driver in New York City and a 20-year-old Nigerian American college student in Michigan share the same racial grouping, but will have distinguishably different cultural beliefs and values. They also belong to different ethnic groups. **Race** is a construct that classifies persons by shared genetic history and/or physical characteristics such as skin color, whereas **ethnicity** is a common sociocultural heritage that includes similarities of religion, history, and common ancestry. Thus, members of ethnic groups share physical features of race as well as cultural origins. However, it is important to be able to distinguish race and ethnicity from nationality (e.g., a person who is Venezuelan may be White, Indian, Japanese, and so on, or any racial combination). Given the similarities and differences among these terms, it is easy to see why they get used interchangeably. An understanding of the differences in these concepts and their implications for counseling enable us as counselors to better understand the multiple influences on our clients' cultural identities.

Much of the confusion about culture comes from its broad and varied conceptualizations even within the social sciences. Berry, Poortinga, Segall, and Dasen (1992) describe six general categories of the discourse on culture: (1) descriptive uses that highlight the different activities associated; (2) historical contexts that focus on the heritages and traditions associated; (3) normative uses that refer to the rules and norms associated with a culture; (4) psychological descriptions that look at approaches to learning, problem solving, and notions of mental health and illness; (5) structural definitions that focus on the social and organizational elements of a culture; and, finally, (6) genetic descriptions that reference the origins of a culture.

REFLECTION QUESTIONS 2.1

- What is your definition of culture?
- How do you identify your own culture?
- If, as many Americans do, you can count more than one cultural origin in your heritage, what are the primary cultural frameworks you hold?

Culture as Defined in Multicultural Counseling

Researchers and practitioners in the area of multicultural counseling have recognized the need for a workable set of cultural standards and competencies in counseling and supervision to be implemented in both the therapeutic and training processes (Arredondo et al., 1996; D'Andrea & Daniels, 1991; DeLucia-Waack, 1996; Holcomb-McCoy & Myers, 1999; Locke, 1993; Ponterotto, Alexander, & Grieger, 1995). In order to set those standards, leaders in the field need to agree on its definition of culture. Kroeber and Kluckhohn (1952) defined *culture* as "patterns of and for behavior acquired and transmitted by symbols, constituting the distinct achievements of human groups, including their embodiments in artifacts" (p. 81). Goodenough (1981) defines culture as a pattern of assumptions that determines how we see the world (i.e., our *worldview*); culture is therefore, according to Deloria (1988), the expression of the essence of a people. According to Monaghan and Just (2000), culture has to do with those aspects of human cognition and activity that we learn as members of society. The notion that culture is learned is significant, though the learning does not necessarily take place explicitly. As a species, human beings have a uniquely protracted period of infantile and juvenile dependence that allows for a transmission and absorption of ways of knowing and doing that are unique to the society in which we grow up.

For our purposes, we will define **culture** as a total way of life held in common by a group of people who share similarities in speech, behavior, ideology, livelihood, technology, values, and social customs. Notice that *culture* itself is an abstract term, and what are concrete and observable to us are the outcomes of culture, which are noticeable primarily in differences across human beings of the ways we act, think, and behave (Berry et al., 1992). For example, we see the ways in which people in some cultures greet one another by shaking hands firmly, whereas in other cultures they bow their heads, and in yet others they put both hands together. Thus, although we see the ways in which culture is manifested in customary behaviors, we do not see culture itself.

REFLECTION QUESTIONS 2.2

Pause for a moment to consider your own background and upbringing. What did you learn about

- when and how eye contact should be maintained?
- what it means to get older and what kind of value is placed on the aging process?
- how much and what kind of privacy are most valued?
- how much space is appropriate between people in various kinds of situations?
- when, how, and with whom it is or is not appropriate to touch?
- when, how, and with whom is it appropriate to display affection?
- what kind of discipline is appropriate?
- what kind of nonverbal cues are used to communicate what unspoken meanings, reactions, or expectations?
- what is considered beautiful, and why?
- what roles should and should not be played by females and males?

Biological Versus Cultural Behavior

It may seem difficult to distinguish our culture-based behavior from our biologically based behavior. That is because, just like all animal species, humans behave in response to basic biological needs: We eat because we need nourishment; we sleep because we need rest; and we build elaborate shelters to protect ourselves from the elements. Many other animal species build elaborate shelters—beavers build dams of wood and mud across streams, prairie dogs dig networks of tunnels, and bluebirds build nests of intricately woven grasses and pine needles. However, whereas individual members of all other animal species build the same kind of shelter—all bluebirds build grass and pine needle nests—members of the human species build many different kinds of homes. Thus, you might say that the only biological component of living in your home is the simple fact that you live in a home. Everything else about your home is culture-based: the shape and style of it, the materials from which it is built, its proximity to other homes, and whether it is stationary or portable. As a simple exercise, try making a list of other aspects of homes, and you will see that most, if not all, of them are culture-based. You can also try this exercise with other areas of human life—such as sleeping, eating, sexual relations, and having children—and you will soon have lists of simple biological behaviors from which extend labyrinths of culture-based behaviors.

Of course, as noted earlier, we don't actually see culture in our everyday lives. You may feel like a completely natural, completely free agent navigating through life as opposed to an artificial entity resulting from cultural interventions and adjustments. But consider the way you look. How would your hair look without the effects of shampoo, comb, or brush? Would it look differently if you had been born in your grandparent's generation? If you do compare yourself with your ancestors, you might find that their skin is more weather-beaten than yours because of the milder soaps you use. Your clothes, your shoes, the chair you sit in, the floor it stands on, and the building that houses you are all culture. In essence, culture is the de facto human environment that we are born into. The founder of structuralist anthropology, Claude Lévi-Strauss, framed the structures of culture as follows:

> Culture is neither natural nor artificial. It stems from neither genetics nor rational thought, for it is made up of rules of conduct, which were not invented and whose function is generally not understood by the people who obey them. Some of these rules are residues of traditions acquired in the different types of social structure through which ... each human group has passed. Other rules have been consciously accepted or modified for the sake of specific goals. Yet there is no doubt that, between the instincts inherited from our genotype and the rules inspired by reason, the mass of unconscious rules remains more important and more effective; because reason itself ... is a product rather than a cause of cultural evolution. (Lévi-Strauss, 1985, p. 34)

Levels of Culture

In descending order of magnitude, Van der Elst and Bohannan (1999) describe different levels of culture. *Species culture* is the one that all human beings share (i.e., every infant, born undamaged, learns to speak the local language and to acquire the local ways of knowing and behaving). *Societal culture* is the cultural profile based on an interacting collective of people who see themselves as a social unit. When we speak of Hopi, Viking, Mayan, or Tibetan culture, we acknowledge that these groups demonstrated characteristic combinations of values, languages, kinship patterns, artifacts, and traits in their unique application of species culture. In much of this chapter, we discuss this level of culture. Within societies, however, every family raises children in a slightly different manner: Food preferences, vocabulary, jokes, expressions, discipline practices, or memories were specific to your parents, siblings, and self. This *familial culture* is the power of kinship systems and continues to organize our lives beyond our families of origin. *Associational cultures* (e.g., churches, Boy Scouts, Rotary Club, or Internet-based social-networking sites like Facebook or My Space) are examples of organizations that are not kinship based, but are enduring associations that have cultural aspects that also impose expectations and make demands for consent and performance on their members. Finally, *individual cultures* are the characteristic assemblage of habits and one's own unique integration of values, beliefs, expectations, and life experiences as well as biological limits. This last level is the one we live with, which is in turn influenced and shaped by all the other levels of culture.

Everyday Impact of Culture

If we basically define *culture* as a pattern of assumptions that determine how we see the world, then it becomes more obvious that culture is an all-encompassing concept that affects every area of every person's life. Yet, ironically, it is not necessarily something we are likely to think about on a daily basis. As one person cleverly put it, the fish never really knows what water is until it is out of the water. In other words, to truly understand both our own culture and that of others, we have to be able to step out of our all-too-familiar frame of reference and recognize contrasting points of view. In order to do this, we have to be aware of the core components of culture and how they differ from person to person, group to group, and society to society.

For example, the different ways in which people deal with the basic needs of all human beings are culturally based: *How* we eat and *what* we eat are as culturally influenced as *when* we eat. For instance, food preferences as well as food taboos are cultural in origin. Perhaps a billion people on the planet are revolted by the thought of eating the flesh of any animal, whereas others will eat almost nothing else. If you were raised to eat meat and dairy products separately, you may always feel a twinge of discomfort if you change your diet. Although the human species is omnivorous, as individuals we are not. How you eat is determined by your culture: All societies expect their adults to use eating tools of some sort, whether spoon, knife, and fork; fork and spoon; chopsticks; or something different. The habit in North America of switching knife and fork from hand to hand as needed and laying down the knife after use would be considered very strange in Western Europe, where you never put down the fork in your left hand, and only put down the knife in your right hand to pick up your water glass (van der Elst & Bohannan, 1999).

Another natural behavior that is culturally constructed is the elimination of waste products from your body. Although babies do that at will, all adults in a culture do it in culturally specified ways. For instance, in Western societies, whereas the bathroom at home is used by both sexes, public restrooms are gender specific. In nomadic societies in the desert, forest, or tundra, people may well eliminate a few paces away from the group—a practice that would feel as strange to a Westerner as relieving yourself in a corner of your living room.

Culture does not simply influence the expression of biological drives, but also extends to the ways one perceives life. For instance, although all persons with normal vision can see colors through the specialized cells of rods and cones in one's retinae, what colors you see are culturally influenced by the color vocabulary available to you. In English, the elementary colors are violet, indigo, blue, green, yellow, orange, and red, whereas in another language the colors may be divided into dark, light, and red, with green and blue not even a category (van der Elst & Bohannan, 1999). Do you expect to see green grass or blue sky? A Navajo painter in the Southwest might well depict blue grass and green sky, because that's how the landscape looks when the sky turns turquoise at sundown. In another example, we might say in English, "It is raining," because the language predisposes us to think of events in the world as direct effects of specific causes. Indonesians would say, "Ada hujan" (there is rain), because to their way of thinking—that is to say, in their *worldview*—things and events flow together (Monaghan & Just, 2000).

So, as we reflect on the opening quote in this chapter, the collage becomes not a single reality, but many realities based on who is looking at the collage, if indeed it is a collage, and what he or she sees at any given point in time. More than that, the collage becomes, in some ways, what we choose and cherish, and upon which we act and react.

 REFLECTION QUESTIONS 2.3

- How does your culture influence your perception of "problems" and avenues for change when it comes to human nature and experiences in life?
- How might your culture influence your goals in counseling, your assessment of the client, and the methods you use?

CULTURAL WORLDVIEW

If culture is a shared way of life, the "glue" that binds together the people in a culture is a **cultural worldview**, a common system of beliefs, perceptions, attitudes, and values. The importance of worldviews to counseling is that beliefs about health and illness, and loci of control, responsibility, and meaning, shape perceptions of helping, how and where and when to seek help, and who to accept help from. The acceptance of counseling and its credibility to members of a culture is directly related to the cultural beliefs that those members hold and the degree to which the counselor can provide services that are sensitive to and congruent with those beliefs. In Chapter 3, we will consider *worldview* in terms of how individuals view themselves (i.e., their *personal identity*), others, and their environment, and how that, in turn, influences the way individuals think and behave. However, the discussion of culture in this chapter would not be complete without a brief discussion of cultural worldview as it influences behaviors in a cultural context (Brinson & Kottler, 1995). Case Study 2.1 depicts the ways in which treatment will be successful based on the cultural worldview and meaning made by the client.

Castillo (1997) describes the necessity of acknowledging the subjective experience of illness through noticing the ways in which cultural constructs give illness meaning. First, a symptom needs to be identified as an indicator of illness, focusing on a particular sensation, thought, emotion, or behavior as significant. For instance, in Greek culture, for a widow to grieve for 5 years after the death of her husband is considered normative, whereas it would be considered symptomatic of depression in the United States. Second, the illness has cultural significance placed on it that then structures the

CASE STUDY **2.1**

The Case of Mr. Sinha

Mr. Sinha was a 45-year-old South Asian man who was married with four children. He presented as being in great distress and listed symptoms of loss of energy, fatigue, low self-esteem, pervasive guilt, loss of appetite, and loss of sleep—in many ways, a laundry list of symptoms of depression. However, Mr. Sinha understood himself to be suffering from *dhat* syndrome, where excessive loss of semen, considered an essential element of the physical body, results in symptoms of fatigue, weakness, headaches, anxiety, loss of appetite, and suicidal feelings. He felt that daily masturbation and regular sexual intercourse with his wife were the reasons that he was depressed. Diagnosing and treating Mr. Sinha for depression may well lead to a poor outcome for him. Singh (1985) reported that 64% of patients who had these symptoms and were diagnosed as depressed and given anti-depressant treatment did not return after the first visit. A folk cure that was recommended to Mr. Sinha was to maintain sexual abstinence for 2 weeks at a time and begin meditation. Mr. Sinha reported great success with this strategy, feeling a return of energy and elevated mood.

Case Discussion

Thinking About This Case

1. As you consider how Mr. Sinha presented himself, how might you begin the conversation to understand the context of his issues?

2. What might be some drawbacks to diagnosing Mr. Sinha with depression without any consideration of cultural factors?

In the above case study, notice that the treatment fits the client's understanding of the meaning of his illness. However, a European American man, Mr. Johnson, who presents with the same symptoms as the client above will not share the construct of his illness as *dhat* and will have as poor an outcome if sexual abstinence is prescribed because that is not how he explains his illness. Notice here that it is important that a culturally specific approach takes into consideration the cultural identity and meaning ascribed by the client, rather than simply assigning a treatment by the numbers or based on the symptoms. In such a case, the appropriateness of the intervention and its effectiveness were founded on a thorough assessment and knowledge of the cultural context of the ailment, and were responsive to the meanings that Mr. Sinha had. Diagnosing Mr. Sinha with depression might have been accurate but not functional in a cultural context. The often recommended course of antidepressants and cognitive-behavioral therapy that might well follow such a diagnosis would probably not be as successful with Mr. Sinha.

Source: Adapted from Castillo (1997, pp. 28–32).

---

person's experience of the illness. For instance, in some Latin American cultures, a syndrome named *susto* appears to meet the criteria for anxiety disorder; it is characterized by anxiety, physical weakness, restlessness, and apathy, and is believed to result from being frightened to such an extent that the soul is separated from the body (Rubel, O'Nell, & Collado, 1985). The cultural significance placed by the surrounding society on this condition is based on the retrieval of the person's soul. The person suffering from *susto* experiences her condition, not as an anxiety disorder, but as a trauma. Such a client may well be helped much more by a visit to a folk healer than by a complete reliance on psychotropic medication for her anxiety. Cultures provide explanations for illness in terms of causation, onset, effects, course, and appropriate treatment, and it behooves the counselor to take such explanations into consideration in assessing and treating clients.

CULTURAL IDENTITY

Culture provides a necessary context in which we are socialized into each of our respective worldviews, and through which develop our own **cultural identity,** or association with our culture of origin and all of the meanings, perceptions, and expectations associated with every dimension of a person's life within that culture. Our cultural identities also serve as an invaluable frame of reference for every choice that we make, and help guide us in unfamiliar contexts as well as those we know very well. In Chapter 3, we will consider how our personal identities—that is, how we define ourselves as individuals in the context of our culture—may be very similar or very different from our cultural identities. As we move through life, we are confronted with situations that force us to further solidify what we already know and think about ourselves and the world we live in, or to question and rethink what we believed to be true about ourselves, others, and life in general. By both learning and choosing how to view the world, we also learn and choose how to define ourselves in relation to the many worlds in which we may find ourselves.

Enculturation and Acculturation

Enculturation denotes the processes by which a person is socialized into his or her primary culture, whereas **acculturation** occurs as a person responds to the influence of the dominant or second culture. Transmission of primary cultural knowledge, awareness, and values occurs from a number of sources, including one's families, peers, and "own-group" institutions (Organista, Marín, & Chun, 2010). In a society like the c, where European American culture is dominant, these enculturation experiences are often in conflict with the dominant culture's influences and messages. African Americans, who are generational offspring of enslaved Africans, have maintained a subculture within the European American–dominated society that retains defined characteristics of its own. Alternatively, some recent immigrants, for instance first-generation Iranian Americans, were brought up in a country where their own cultural group was the larger society and then moved to the United States, where their culture is a nondominant subgroup in U.S. society. If a person has a successful enculturation experience, he or she can function effectively within his or her cultural group of origin. The degree to which one is enculturated may affect the manner in which one responds to acculturation. The pressure of acculturation may reverse or change the degree of enculturation (Organista et al., 2010).

Levels of acculturation

Marín (1992) developed a psychosocial definition of *acculturation* as a process of attitudinal and behavioral change, undergone willingly or unwillingly, by individuals who reside in multicultural societies or who come into contact with a new culture through immigration, colonization, or other political changes. The three levels of attitudinal and behavioral learning start with the *superficial* one, which consists of learning the facts and history of the dominant culture and forgetting facts about one's culture of origin. At the *intermediate* level, changes take place in the more central behaviors in a person's life such as language preferences and use; the ethnicity of one's friends, neighbors, and spouse; and the preferences for names given to children. The third level of *significance* involves changes that take place in the individual's beliefs, values, and norms that describe the person's worldview and interaction patterns (Marín, 1992).

Modes of acculturation

The four modes of acculturation are theorized to be assimilation, separation, marginalization, and integration, with each mode associated with a different set of stressors regarding social and psychological issues (Organista et al., 2010). **Assimilation** denotes a shift toward the dominant culture together with a rejection of one's culture of origin, with a goal of complete absorption and acceptance by the dominant culture. Such cases run the risk of rejection by families and communities as well as lack of acceptance by the dominant culture, and may therefore experience high levels of anxiety and low self-esteem (LaFromboise, Coleman, & Gerton, 1993). In contrast, the **separation** mode describes those who retain their cultural values and identity while rejecting those of the dominant culture. These individuals may be effective in their own communities, but may not be able to negotiate the dominant culture and powerful systems, often turning to indigenous social supports and health care (Koss-Chioino, 2000). **Marginalization** involves a rejection of both the culture of origin and the dominant culture; such individuals have difficulty with social functioning and acceptance, and may lack a sense of cultural identity and self-efficacy. Finally, the *integration* mode, also referred to as **biculturalism**, involves a flexible balancing of some dominant-culture attitudes and practices with retention of culture-of-origin practices and identity. These individuals have a wider behavioral repertoire that is effective across varying cultural contexts, brings a sense of belonging to both cultures, and maintains an integrated cultural identity (Sam & Berry, 2006).

Dealing with life's many pressures and opportunities gives clients an interesting challenge to achieve a meaningful sense of personal and cultural identity through **bicultural competence,** defined as an individual's ability to effectively utilize "dual modes of social behavior that are appropriately employed in different situations" (LaFromboise & Rowe, 1983, p. 592). In order to be culturally competent, according to LaFromboise et al. (1993), an individual must do the following:

> (a) possess a strong personal identity, (b) have knowledge of and facility with the beliefs and values of the culture, (c) display sensitivity to the affective processes of the culture, (d) communicate clearly in the language of the given cultural group, (e) perform socially sanctioned behavior, (f) maintain active social relations within the cultural group, and (g) negotiate the institutional structures of that culture. (p. 396)

Thus, the biculturally competent individual possesses a high degree of resiliency through a strong sense of him or herself in one or more cultural contexts. Understanding the experience of the biculturally competent individual becomes important in understanding what it means to cross-cultural boundaries, and how to best work with others who also must cross these boundaries successfully.

Overall, it is important to remember that our cultural identities are not one-dimensional. Many other factors and dynamics intersect and influence our cultural experience. Ethnic and racial identity development describes the process by which individuals become aware of, ascribe meaning to, and integrate racial and cultural information into their overall self-concept (Aponte & Johnson, 2000). Acculturation and ethnic and racial identity are complex and multidimensional processes that are considered central to understanding the mental health needs of ALANA populations (Aponte & Johnson, 2000). These constructs interact with and are influenced by factors such as socioeconomic status; residence in terms of both length of time in the United States and the ethnic density of the surrounding community; racism and oppression; worldview, language usage, and religious and spiritual beliefs; as well as gender, familial, and social support structures (Aponte & Johnson, 2000). Sam and Berry (2006) provide a framework for examining the interactive effects of acculturation status and ethnic identity in terms of beliefs about psychological issues, symptoms experienced, as well as help seeking, expectations, and treatment outcomes.

Immigration

The term *migration* is used to describe the movement of people across as well as within nations. *Immigration* is the influx of people into the nation, whereas *emigration* refers to the departure of a nation's people (Al-Issa & Tousignant, 1997). According to the U.S. Department of Homeland Security (Rytina and Saeger, 2005), 1 in 11 Americans is born in another country, and 3,000 immigrants arrive every day, with both legal and illegal immigration adding approximately 1 million people to the population every year. The population of New York City is currently judged to be over 40% first-generation immigrants. Changing laws and policies, unstable economic and political conditions in various parts of the world, regional conflicts, and interethnic marriages are some of the reasons for this increased immigration (Mahalingam, 2006).

Sojourners, refugees, and immigrants experience unique stresses, and this behooves counselors to be aware of the additional impact of their experiences in multicultural counseling. **Sojourners** are persons who arrive in a country intending to stay for a temporary period, and in turn this affects how they make adaptations to the host country. **Refugees** may adapt through necessity but because they are exiled from their country of origin with very limited choices, there may be a great deal of resistance and grief. Finally, **immigrants** may have some sort of choice in coming to the new country, but such choices have little to do with the psychological readiness to abandon the culture of origin or embrace the host culture. Premigration experiences give rise to the migration and shape the experience of the migration, whereas postmigration experiences are shaped by what came before (the culture of origin) and the fit or lack thereof between the host culture and the immigrant's culture of origin. The nature of the migration may be stressful if it is involuntary.

The case of refugees is particularly important. Since the second World War, there has been a rise in refugees due to increasing situations of political instability; communal and interethnic conflicts; wars; genocide; natural disasters such as flood, drought, earthquake, or fire; social disasters of poverty, famine, deportation, resettlement, and the forced removal of populations; as well as religious and social persecution leading to an estimated current refugee population of 26 million (Bemak & Chung, 2002). For many refugees, overlaying the premigration trauma that necessitated their departure from the home culture is the migration experience, which often consists of escapes, dangerous and traumatic journeys, existence in refugee camps, and being at the mercy of foreign bureaucracies that refugees are ill-equipped to navigate. Refugees are, therefore, at risk for a higher incidence of mental illness than the general population (Blackwell, 2005). Developing the psychoeducational multilevel model (MLM) for counseling refugees, Bemak and Chung describe a process consisting of a set of skills and awareness that a counselor must possess, including knowledge of the distinctive refugee experience. Figure 2.1 provides an overview of the model. Notice that the four levels may be implemented concurrently and that although the levels are separated, the interaction is essential for the successful achievement of goals. Interventions can be cognitive, affective, and behavioral as long as they are inclusive of the client's cultural foundations and experiences.

Because so much of U.S. society originated through immigration, it is important for counselors to assess the generational status and country of origin of all their clients. Children who are born here become more assimilated to mainstream U.S. society than their immigrant parents. These second-generation immigrants, whose parents were the original immigrants, may have issues of cross-generational cultural conflict. Family constituency and

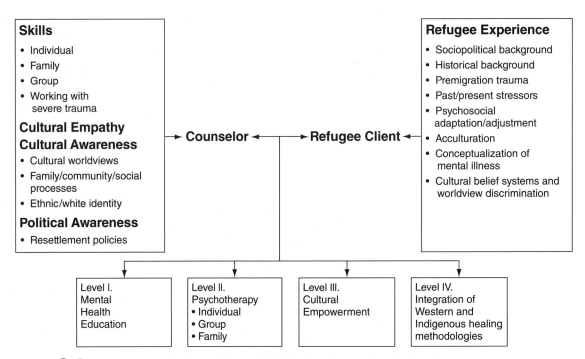

FIGURE **2.1** Overview of Multilevel Model (MLM) for Counseling Refugees

kinship networks are also factors here because some immigrant communities are very small and tightly woven, whereas others are spread out.

Language

Language is a central feature of human identity, defining self and others in terms of identities and places in society. Within human society, meaning is continually being made, and speech is one of the most important ways in which humans create and share such meaning. The evocative use of the term *mother tongue* to describe the first language learned signifies the importance of language in defining an individual's origins. Culture is the medium through which language emerges in its particular shape and form. Languages exist in the contexts of the culture in which they arose and often are structured based on the worldview of the originating culture. Language users define contexts, social structures, and their relationship to discourse through the various forms available to them such as passive or active voice, and personal or formal voice, by using various affective keys (Besnier, 1990).

Research appears to support the notion that the language people speak is a guide to the language in which they think (Bonvillain, 2008). Although human languages may be able to express a great range of thoughts and emotions, cultural norms and rules may structure the speaking form used and its expressiveness. These norms are mediated by variables of gender and class, which have been demonstrated to have an effect on the spoken form and language usage (Bonvillain, 2008).

Much of the literature about linguistics in mental health delivery states that the impediment for multilingual clients is the inability of clinicians to understand their communication accurately (Constantino & Malgady, 1998). Although new forms of counseling such as art therapy, play therapy, and dance therapy have incorporated many aspects of nonverbal communication, the primary dimension in which counselor and client have traditionally communicated is through the domain of speech. *Talk therapy* focuses within the oral mode, and language is its medium. It relies on the assumptions that both counselor and client share not only a common language within which they can communicate but also a common understanding of the constructs within that language. Given how central language is to cultural self-constructions, when the client's primary language is not one understood by the counselor, the counselor must make greater effort to accurately understand the client's worldview (Speicher, 2000).

One important point about the use of language is its role in forming a relational bridge between the self and other. As such, it contains within it a representation of both the self who is speaking and the other who is spoken to (Pérez Foster, 1996). In describing home and identity, although the immigrant or exile may have left behind the geographical place of origin, he or she still has language as a portable signifier of culture and place (McCarty & Zepeda, 1999). Akhtar (1999) describes the immigrant's journey, moving through speaking only the language of the home country to using a new language to true bilingualism, as a difficult one. One can trace the immigrant's development of mastery of the new language through its appearance in spontaneous humor, dreams, and talking during sleep. Kristeva (1988) describes this linguistic splitting of the self between the new and the old as

> that language of once-upon-a-time that fades and won't make up its mind to leave you forever.... You learn to use another instrument, like expressing yourself in algebra or on the violin.... You have the impression that the new language is your resurrection: a new skin, a new sex. But the illusion is torn apart when you listen to yourself.... Thus, between two languages, your element is silence. (pp. 20, in Amati Mehler et al., 1993, pp. 264–265)

A final issue in this discussion is to clarify that language and culture do not always reflect each other. In other words, a multicultural person is not automatically multilingual, nor is a multilingual person automatically multicultural. There are many English-speaking African Americans and Native Americans as well as Asians and Latinos in the United States who are multicultural but monolingual. *Sociolinguistics* is the study of variation within the use of a particular language (Fishman, 1999), and this is strongly influenced by ethnic identity. African Americans who are descendants of those Africans enslaved and brought to the United States have had their original West African languages of origin erased, and are primarily English language speakers. However, they have been shown to have particular forms of English speech and usage that consist of distinct dialects (Fishman, 1999). In such cases, the nature of the language usage and emphases, as well as dialects, speed, and slang, may be the ways in which individuals strive to diversify the language to reflect unique perspectives (Javier, Vasquez, & Marcos, 1998).

THE ROLE OF CULTURE IN A MULTICULTURAL SOCIETY

As the opening chapter quote from Clifford Geertz described, increasingly the separations we used to see between cultures are becoming blurred as human beings who originated from different cultures now live in the same neighborhoods. There are now few isolated cultures in the world, and increasingly we come in contact with each other. After all, *Baywatch* (seemingly a quintessential American depiction) was one of the most popular television shows watched around the world with the advent of cable television. The increasing contact has developed the notion of cultural relativism. If we believe that the content of our culture is the historical experience of people that shapes our perceptions of the world around us, it stands to reason that no one cultural worldview is superior to another or that it is the normative measure against all others. So cultures can be judged only in relation to each other, and the meaning of a belief or behavior can be understood only relative to its own cultural context. Does this mean that all behaviors are entitled to a claim of cultural distinctiveness that requires respect? How do we allow for cultural relativism and yet act against practices that we see as oppressive to a segment of society? The following discussion might help to clarify these issues.

As one begins to explore the considerable variation in child-rearing beliefs and behaviors cross-culturally, it becomes clear that there is no universal standard for child rearing, or for child abuse and neglect. When a child is sick, a Vietnamese custom is to rub hot coins along the child's body, often forcefully enough to leave bruises. There have been instances where a child with such bruises has been reported and the family has been investigated for child abuse. In another case, an East African mother had cut the faces of her two young sons with a razor blade and rubbed charcoal into the lacerations. The boys were removed from her care and placed into foster care. She was prosecuted for child abuse. However, the mother was a member of a tribe that traditionally practices facial scarring. Her actions were an attempt to assert the cultural identity of her children where, without such markings, her boys would be unable to participate as adults in their culture. A failure to assure one's children of such scars would thus be viewed as neglectful or abusive within the cultural context of her tribe (Gardiner, Mutter, & Kosmizki, 1998). If we fail to allow for a cultural perspective in defining child abuse and neglect, we find ourselves in the position in which our own set of cultural beliefs and practices are presumed to be preferable, and in fact superior, to another. How might one explain to these Vietnamese and East African mothers that the pain and discomfort a European American mother might inflict on her children in orthodontic work is more legitimate and indicative of maternal care? At the same time, we cannot take the stance of accepting the inhumane treatment of children in the name of cultural sensitivity. This is a continuing dilemma for helpers who work cross-culturally. One way to resolve it is to first understand if the behavior has a function and meaning that are culturally based, and address the behavior in its multicultural context without taking on a superior moral position. So, although one must acknowledge that a behavior has function and meaning in the culture of origin, it must be assessed to see if it is appropriate and functional in the new culture. Without judging the value of the behavior in the culture of origin, a counselor can then work with a client to see if a balance can be maintained whereby those same meanings can be met in another way in the new culture that would be more acceptable.

REFLECTION QUESTIONS 2.4

Pause for a moment, and reflect on what you consider to be your most deeply held beliefs. Try to make a brief list of those beliefs that you hold most precious, then answer the following questions:

- Why do you believe what you believe, and from where do these beliefs come?
- Have any of your most deeply held beliefs ever been challenged?
- Have any of your beliefs changed over time in any way? What caused them to change, and why?
- Do any of your most deeply held beliefs conflict with those of the people closest to you, and if so, how have you reconciled this conflict in beliefs?

CULTURE AND EFFECTIVE COUNSELING

This section focuses on some of the disorders and syndromes that have been characterized as culturally specific in the field as well as provides a brief description of some therapies that have evolved that are distinct from what we consider to be counseling in their epistemology, assessment, and interventions.

Culture-Bound Syndromes

Ideas about wellness and illness vary across cultures. In Western cultures, the mind is regarded as distinct from the body, so that mental illness resides in the mind, and even the term *psychosomatic* implies an unreal physical condition rather than any true integration between the mind and body. In the Chinese culture, illness is caused by an imbalance of the two complementary aspects of life energy, the yin and yang. African cultures often perceive health as a more social rather than simply biological concept, where healthy living is woven into the social fabric of living harmoniously with others (Lambo, 1961). In Tibetan thought, on the other hand, enlightenment and insanity are both focused on the recognition of transience and how this is accepted and comprehended or denied and repressed (Clifford, 1981). Regardless of the various perspectives, the Western model has dominance in the two major texts of psychological disorders, *The Diagnostic and Statistical Manual of Mental Disorders* (DSM-IV-TR; American Psychiatric Association, 2000) and *The International Classification of Disorders* (ICD-10; World Health Organization, 1993). One way to mark this is that those disorders that can be classified by the mind–body split take their place in these texts' normative and standard depictions of disorders. Those illnesses that cannot be so labeled, and that take place outside European and European American culture, are placed in the category of "culture-bound syndromes" in the DSM-IV-TR appendix and "culture-specific disorders" in the annex of the ICD-10. Table 2.1 describes a selection of the **culture-bound syndromes** depicted in the DSM-IV-TR. According to Canion and Alegria (2008), the Western model essentially subscribes to a universalistic model of psychopathology, where core disorders are considered to be universal but the variance among subgroups could lie in the manifestation of symptoms or the degree to which a behavior is considered abnormal. To address the criticisms, in the DSM-IV-TR, modifications were made to incorporate information on the ways culture, gender, or the developmental level of the individual influenced the clinical manifestations of the various disorders, adding guidelines for the in-depth assessment of the individual's cultural background, such as the cultural expression of the disorder, psychosocial functioning, cultural context, and cultural differences between the clinician and client (Matsumoto & Juang, 2004).

Canion and Alegria (2008) offer recommendations to clinicians to assist them in assessing the extent to which cultural background and context affect the manifestation of symptoms and the possible existence of culture-bound syndromes. Some of these include assessing what is considered pathological behavior versus what is considered normal in the environment; decoding what kinds of behavioral labels and terminology are used in the culture to

TABLE **2.1**
A Selection of Culture-Bound Syndromes

Syndrome	Cultural Origin	Description
Amok or *mata elap*	Malaysia	A dissociative episode characterized by a period of brooding followed by an outburst of violent, aggressive, or homicidal behavior directed at people and objects. The episode tends to be precipitated by a perceived insult or slight and seems to be prevalent only among males. The episode is often accompanied by persecutory ideas, automatism, amnesia for the period of the episode, exhaustion, and a return to the premorbid state following the episode. Some instances of *amok* may occur during a brief psychotic episode or constitute the onset or exacerbation of a chronic psychotic process. Similar to *cafard* or *cathard* (Polynesia), *mal de pelea* (Puerto Rico), *iich'aa* (Navaho), and syndromes found in Laos, Papua New Guinea, and the Philippines.
Boufée deliriante	West Africa and Haiti	Sudden outburst of agitated and aggressive behavior, marked confusion, and psychomotor excitement. It may sometimes be accompanied by visual and auditory hallucinations or paranoid ideation.
Brain fag or *brain fog*	West Africa	A condition experienced primarily by high school or university male students. Symptoms include difficulties in concentrating, remembering, and thinking. Students often state that their brains are "fatigued." Additional symptoms center around the head and neck and include pain, pressure, tightness, blurring of vision, heat, or burning. *Brain tiredness* or fatigue from "too much thinking" is an idiom of distress in many cultures.
Falling out or *blacking out*	Southern United States and Caribbean	Episodes characterized by sudden collapse, either without warning or preceded by feelings of dizziness or "swimming" in the head. The individual's eyes are usually open, but the person claims to be unable to see. The person usually hears and understands what is occurring around him or her, but feels powerless to move.
Ghost sickness	American Indian groups	A preoccupation with death and the deceased, sometimes associated with witchcraft. Symptoms may include bad dreams, weakness, feelings of danger, loss of appetite, fainting, dizziness, fear, anxiety, hallucinations, loss of consciousness, confusion, feelings of futility, and a sense of suffocation.
Hwa-byung or *wool-hwa-bung*	Korea	*Anger syndrome*: Symptoms are attributed to the suppression of anger and include insomnia, fatigue, panic, fear of impending death, dysphoric affect, indigestion, anorexia, dyspnea, palpitations, generalized aches and pains, and a feeling of a mass in the epigastrium.
Koro	Malaysia	An episode of sudden and intense anxiety that the penis (or, in the rare female cases, the vulva and nipples) will recede into the body and possibly cause death. Syndrome occurs throughout South and East Asia under different names: *suo yang* (China), *jinjinia bemar* (Assam), and *rok-joo* (Thailand). It has been identified in isolated cases in the United States and Europe, as well as among diasporic ethnic Chinese or Southeast Asians.

(continued)

TABLE **2.1** (*continued*)

Syndrome	Cultural Origin	Description
Latah	Malaysia and Indonesia	Hypersensitivity to sudden fright, often with echopraxia, echolalia, command obedience, and dissociative or trancelike behavior. The Malaysian syndrome is more frequent in middle-aged women.
Locura	Latin America	A severe form of chronic psychosis, attributed to an inherited vulnerability, the effect of multiple life difficulties, or a combination of the two. Symptoms include incoherence, agitation, auditory and visual hallucinations, an inability to follow rules of social interaction, unpredictability, and possible violence.
Pibloktoq or *Arctic hysteria*	Greenland Eskimos	An abrupt dissociative episode accompanied by extreme excitement of up to 30 minutes' duration and frequently followed by convulsive seizures and coma lasting up to 12 hours. The individual may be withdrawn or mildly irritable for a period of hours or days before the attack and will typically report having complete amnesia during the attack. During the attack, the individual may tear off his or her clothing, break furniture, shout obscenities, eat feces, flee from protective shelters, or perform other irrational or dangerous acts. The syndrome is found throughout the Arctic with local names.
Qi-gong psychotic reaction	China	An acute, time-limited episode characterized by dissociative, paranoid, or other psychotic or nonpsychotic symptoms that occur after participating in the Chinese folk health-enhancing practice of qi-gong. Especially vulnerable are individuals who become overly involved in the practice.
Sangue dormido	Portuguese Cape Verdeans	Literally, "sleeping blood." Symptoms include pain, numbness, tremor, paralysis, convulsions, stroke, blindness, heart attack, infection, and miscarriage.
Shinkeishitsu	Japan	Syndrome marked by obsessions, perfectionism, ambivalence, social withdrawal, neurasthenia, and hypochondriasis.
Zar	Ethiopia, Somalia, Egypt, Sudan, Iran, and elsewhere in North Africa and the Middle East	An experience of spirit possession. Symptoms may include dissociative episodes with laughing, shouting, hitting the head against a wall, singing, or weeping. Individuals may show apathy and withdrawal, refusing to eat or carry out daily tasks, or may develop a long-term relationship with the possessing spirit. Such behavior is not necessarily considered pathological locally.

describe behavior; developing trust and facilitating disclosure by using self and position, as well as exploring the client's social position in the culture and using assessment question in ways that indicate the desire to understand accurately across cultures rather than a deficit in attention; and, finally, before deciding that something is worthy of a psychiatric diagnosis, evaluating whether the behaviors cause distress or conflict in the culture or are adaptive to the culture.

Diagnostic assessment can be especially challenging when a clinician from one ethnic or cultural group uses the DSM-IV-TR classification to evaluate an individual from a different ethnic or cultural group. A clinician who is unfamiliar with the nuances of an individual's cultural frame of reference may incorrectly judge as psychopathology those normal variations in behavior, belief, or experience that are particular to the individual's culture. For example, certain religious practices or beliefs (e.g., hearing or seeing a deceased relative during bereavement) may be misdiagnosed as manifestations of a psychotic disorder. Applying personality disorder criteria across cultural settings may be especially difficult because of the wide cultural variations in concepts of self, styles of communication, and coping mechanisms.

Even though certain disorders such as schizophrenia are seen as universal across cultures (World Health Organization, 1995), there are often distinct differences in onset, course, symptoms, and, therefore, effective treatment (Kleinman, 1988). In the United States, acute psychotic symptoms are associated with schizophrenia, which, according to the DSM-IV-TR, is a disorder with a poor prognosis, or chance for recovery. On the other hand, in many non-Western societies such as India, Jamaica, Bali, Tanzania, and Nigeria, it is more common for people to present psychotic reactions with a short duration (days or weeks) and have a complete recovery (Sartorius, 1986). There are also significant cross-cultural differences in the presentation of depressive moods. Generally in non-Western societies, depression is expressed with somatic (physical) symptoms, less verbalization of depressive mood, fewer guilt feelings, more projection, lesser severity, and shorter duration (Al-Issa, 1995). Interesting claims have been made to explain *somatization,* or the expression of psychological problems as physical problems, among non-Western depressive clients. Al-Issa suggested that practitioners of the traditional medicine of non-Western countries emphasize somatopsychic aspects of diseases more than its psychological dimensions.

It is also important to understand the impacts of somatic symptoms in collectivist societies. In such cultures, somatic symptoms can play the role of an adaptive social function by getting more attention from a client's support network. Cross-cultural differences in emotional expression also offer useful insights for understanding somatization among non-Western countries. For instance, a World Health Organization study (1973), in Marsella (1988) reported that there are no equivalent words for *depression* in Chinese or Yoruba. In fact, many non-Indo-European languages do not differentiate between certain emotions as compared with other languages (Leff, 1988). In these languages, distress might be expressed in different ways than the Western counselor is accustomed to listen for. A number of culturally salient somatic languages are employed to express depressed mood or anxiety in many cultures; examples include headaches, dizziness, and a lack of energy in Chinese culture, and a crawling sensation in the body and increasing bodily heat in Nigerian culture (Matsumoto & Juang, 2004).

Culture can impact the symptom manifestation of disorders as well as their prevalence and etiology. For instance, *taijinkyoufu-syo* (fear of interpersonal interactions) is a culture-bound syndrome in Japan, which may be similar to a social phobia in DSM-IV-TR. Whereas clients with social phobia in the United States are concerned with being embarrassed or rejected by others, Japanese clients presenting with *taijinkyoufu-syo* experience intense fear that their body, its parts, or its functions are displeasing, embarrassing, or offensive to other people in appearance, odor, facial expression, or movements (American Psychiatric Association, 2000). The intense anxiety involved in both disorders is manifested in culturally appropriate ways in each society. Thus, in collectivist Japanese society, anxiety is generated by the possibility of causing harm and discomfort to others, whereas in individualistic U.S. society, clients are concerned with the negative impact posed by others on themselves. If the culturally specific manifestation of anxiety were dismissed, a counselor working with a Japanese client with *taijinkyoufu-syo* symptoms might diagnose him or her as having body dysmorphic disorder (BDD) because the fear of a body part being offensive can seem exaggerated or delusional.

Culturally Based Treatments

Although Western treatments have typically focused on internal causes of illness, using for example a psychodynamic approach that places both the cause and cure of a disorder within the individual, or a physical treatment such as antipsychotic medications to address the hearing of voices, some recent approaches have developed such as family systems therapies that take the family context and interactive patterns into account. Herbal remedies are an example of a non-Western physical treatment, though they tend to be used very differently. For instance, Ayurvedic herbal remedies are not used to target a specific condition, but rather to rebalance the body to restore natural rhythms. The herbs may be orally ingested as pills or tinctures, burned for inhalation, or massaged on the body in oils; the method is as important as the ingredient.

In the Chinese method of acupuncture, needles are inserted at carefully selected points along the body to rebalance those aspects of the body's yin and yang that have become disordered. Acupuncture has become increasingly popular in the West for pain relief and anesthesia.

Two psychological approaches, *Morita therapy* and *Naikan therapy*, were developed in accordance with Japanese cultural traditions. Morita is a highly structured form of therapy that involves two stages: The first stage is complete bed rest, followed by a gradual adaptation to reality through working in groups. The client maintains a written diary that is reviewed and corrected for cognitive flaws by the Morita therapist during the process. The therapy aims at modifying the self-perpetuating cycle of unrealistic expectations and selective focus on subjective discomfort through cultivating more self-enhancing and productive attitudes (Sansone, 2005). In Naikan therapy, an interviewer leads clients through a meditative process in which they examine the past and observe themselves. In both therapies, the basic purpose is to begin to accept things as they are, exemplified by the Japanese word *sunao*, indicating a harmonious self in relation to others (Sato, 2001).

Removing unwanted influences, spirits, or conflicts through exorcism is practiced throughout the world, though the method and purpose vary greatly. Often the indigenous healer performs a formal, ritualized ceremony. Sacred formulas may be recited, tobacco used to aid in sucking out an intrusive object, or various symbolic sacrifices and temptations made to draw out the unwanted spirit. Among the Navajo, curing rites or "sings" are ceremonies that are used for psychopathology, to prevent sickness or injury, or to alleviate guilt or anxiety. The myth-based recitations such as the Blessing Way, Life Way, Enemy Way, and so on are carried out by the shamans, focus on the designated client and extended family, and can go on for as long as 9 days (Dana, 1998). The Sioux may use sweat lodges and vision quests for healing purposes. Among Afro-Caribbeans and Latinos, healers known as *curanderos(as)*, *santeros(as)*, or *espiritistos(as)* (Koss-Chioino, 2000) may use plants, herbs, and rituals to cure ailments.

NTU therapy is a counseling approach used with African American populations (McLean & Marini, 2003) based on the Afrocentric model of Nguzo Saba. The word, "NTU," comes from the Bantu peoples of Central Africa and describes the spiritual essence that comprises all material phenomena. Spiritually based, the NTU approach assists in healing by rediscovering natural alignment with the client and his or her relationships. The stages include harmony, awareness, alignment, actualization, and synthesis, and Nguzo Saba works within the guidelines of the seven principles of Kwanzaa, which include the following:

- *Umoja* (Unity): To strive for and to maintain unity in the family, community, nation, and race.
- *Kujichagulia* (Self-Determination): To define ourselves, name ourselves, create for ourselves, and speak for ourselves.
- *Ujima* (Collective Work and Responsibility): To build and maintain our community together and make our brothers' and sisters' problems our problems, and to solve them together.
- *Ujamaa* (Cooperative Economics): To build and maintain our own stores, shops, and other businesses and to profit from them together.
- *Nia* (Purpose): To make our collective vocation the building and developing of our community in order to restore our people to their traditional greatness.
- *Kuumba* (Creativity): To do always as much as we can, in the way we can, in order to leave our community more beautiful and beneficial than we inherited it.
- *Imani* (Faith): To believe with all our heart in our people, our parents, our teachers, our leaders, and the righteousness and victory of our struggle.

What does all this mean for a counselor who is working in an agency or school environment with clients who are traditional in their cultural adaptation? Case Study 2.2 is an example of how one counselor integrated counseling with indigenous healing approaches to achieve a successful resolution for his client.

CASE STUDY **2.2**

The Case of Mai

The Hmong are a seminomadic people of Southeast Asia. Mai, a 26-year-old Hmong woman, who was a first-generation immigrant, presented at a community agency with symptoms of depression. She had been brought by her husband, who was concerned about her listlessness, general fatigue, and sadness. In conversations with Mai, the counselor learned that this condition had lasted about 7 months and dated from the birth of her child. She had bad dreams that left her unable to sleep, and she felt unable to care for her infant. Although it was possible to assign a diagnosis of postpartum depression to Mai at this point, the counselor decided that further exploration was needed to better understand Mai's condition. She reported that the birth had been traumatic because she had been admitted to the hospital and the doctor had decided an emergency caesarian was medically necessary.

After the initial meeting with Mai, the counselor consulted with some cultural sources in the Hmong community. He learned that a central belief among the Hmong is that each person has three souls. A soul is able to wander off occasionally, and it usually is able to return to its body. Ill health occurs when a soul leaves the body because it is frightened away for various reasons and is unable to find its way home. In their next meeting, the counselor brought this topic up with Mai, and she began to reveal her deep-seated belief that under the general anesthetic, while she was unconscious, one of her souls—whose duty is to take care of her well-being—left her body and was unable to reenter her body. Because she was moved out of the operating theatre and gained her consciousness in a recovery room, she believed that her soul was left in that operating theatre. She felt sure that the departure of this soul was the main cause of her ill health and her inability to care for her son.

In subsequent sessions, the counselor continued to explore other aspects of Mai's acculturation and adaptation to the United States, her relationship with her husband, and the impact of her infant child. He also consulted again with his cultural resource in the Hmong community. In order to regain her health, Mai needed to undergo a soul-calling ceremony, and it had to be performed at the theatre in which the caesarean was done and where the soul was still waiting to be

called back. With Mai's permission, the main details of her ordeal were relayed to an elder who knew how to conduct the soul-calling ritual. With further assistance from Mai's obstetrician, the hospital gave permission to perform the ceremony while the operating room was not in use. The soul-calling ceremony required various ingredients, including incense, an egg, a bowl of raw rice, and a live chicken. On completion of the ceremony, Mai reported feeling much better because she was sure her soul had come back to her. Although counseling continued for several weeks after, the focus changed to behavioral assignments to take on an increasingly active caretaking role with her infant and reestablish her relationship with her husband.

Case Discussion
Thinking About This Case
1. What process allowed the counselor to gain knowledge about Mai's cultural explanation of her condition?
2. Without integrating culture, what might have been the typical approaches that the counselor may have taken to Mai?

Notice that the counselor in this case was not Hmong, nor was he conversant with Hmong culture. But he knew that he needed to consult with community leaders and research Hmong cultural information to better understand his client and serve her effectively. Rather than confining his counseling to standard agency procedures, he chose instead a process that included a high degree of advocacy, negotiation, and consultation. Although the ritual was a significant element in his work with Mai, he also used the trust and relief experienced from the ritual's success to explore other elements in ongoing work with Mai. In addition, he used his resources and networks outside the Hmong community to facilitate the procedure of the ritual.

If culture had not been integrated with the treatment process, the counselor may well have referred Mai for a psychiatric referral for medication for postpartum depression, and tried to treat her accordingly. There is a high likelihood that this approach would have been ineffective given the conflict with her core beliefs of how she understood her ailment.

TOOLS FOR CULTURALLY COMPETENT COUNSELING

By focusing on competent multicultural practice with a clear understanding of culture, we are better able to approach clients from a variety of backgrounds and experiences with effective interventions. These interventions must be based, however, on a solid understanding of the client's view of the world and his or her subsequent needs in the therapeutic context.

The first tool we will review is a mnemonic framework that uses the easily remembered acronym ETHNIC. It is for providers working with clients who are traditional in their cultural adaptation (Levin et al., 2000).

EXAMPLE **2.1**
ETHNIC: A Framework for Culturally Competent Practice

Explanation Question clients to find out what they think is the explanation for their problem: What do you think may be the reason you have this problem? What do friends, family, and others say about it? Do you know anyone else who has had or who now has this kind of problem? Have you heard about it, read about it, or seen it on TV, on the radio, or in a newspaper? (If clients cannot offer an explanation, ask what most concerns them about their problems.)

Treatments Ask clients what they think about treatment: What kinds of remedies or other treatments have you tried for this problem? Is there anything you eat, drink, or do (or avoid) on a regular basis to stay healthy? Tell me about it. What kind of treatment are you seeking from me?

Healers Ask clients about healers in their culture: Have you sought any advice from alternative or folk healers, friends, or other people who are not counselors for help with your problems? Tell me about it.

Negotiation Try to find options that will be mutually acceptable to you and your client and that incorporate the client's beliefs, rather than contradicting them: For instance, encouraging a client to both pray to her ancestors for advice while helping her hear her own inner thoughts about her decision and see if she is getting congruent messages.

Intervention Determine an intervention with your client that may incorporate alternate treatments, spirituality, and healers as well as other cultural practices (e.g., ritual cleansings, and foods eaten or avoided): For instance, a client may attend a sweat lodge and consult with a tribal shaman to clarify his life direction.

Collaboration Collaborate with the client, family members, other health care members, healers, and community resources: Since clients live in a contextual web of relationships, it is helpful to incorporate these relationships to assist the effectiveness of counseling rather than ignore them. A counselor may well, with the client's permission, see if the pastor of the local church the client attends would be a resource to the client; or invite the *padrino* (godfather) of a Latino client into counseling to help the relationship between the client and his parents.

CASE STUDY **2.3**

The Case of Kyung-Sil Choi

Kyung-Sil Choi was born in South Korea in 1996. Orphaned at birth, she was adopted by Americans Bill and Coleen O'Hara and was brought to the United States at the age of 6 months. She was renamed Maureen and was raised in Bill and Coleen's South Boston neighborhood, where their large extended Irish American family had lived for several generations. Maureen flourished throughout her preschool years. She was made much of by her family, learned Irish jigs along with her many cousins at family *céili*, marched in the St. Patrick's Day parades, and attended St. Augustine's Church and made regular confessions to Father Kelly. At age 5, Maureen announced proudly to her admiring family, "I am 100% Irish!" Her parents laughed heartily and passed her back and forth for hugs and kisses.

When Maureen entered kindergarten, one of the first questions her classmates asked her was "Where are you from?" Noticing that Maureen just stared back at her classmates, unable to answer, the teacher intervened: "Class, Maureen is from a far-away land called Korea." She took the opportunity to show the class where the United States and Korea are on the big globe in their classroom. Then the well-meaning teacher turned to Maureen with a big smile and added, "Oh, and Maureen, you can bring in a Korean picture when we have our Diversity Day celebration."

Case Discussion

Thinking About This Case

1. What are Maureen's race, ethnicity and culture? Are they the same or different?
2. Are there ways in which Maureen might have been influenced by Korean culture even though she came to the U.S. as an infant?
3. What do you think might be the effect of this classroom incident on Maureen? How might Maureen's parents have better prepared her for such an inevitable situation?
4. As Maureen matures, she may become curious about her cultural origins. Discuss ways in which a high school counselor might help a teenager like Maureen deal with these feelings and desires.

5. Discuss how the story of Maureen, which is not at all uncommon in the United States today, illustrates the pitfalls for counselors of pigeonholing individuals by their apparent race.

This is complicated, because although we might label Maureen's race as *Asian* because of the visual identifiers that her teacher and other schoolmates used to label her as foreign, she is also culturally immersed in Irish American norms and values. Yet, due to that interaction between the external and internal perceptions of self, Maureen cannot be just "100% Irish." After all, the family that raised her is not 100% Irish, either: Their culture has been influenced and shaped by the American experience, so that now there are distinct differences between Irish and Irish American cultures. In addition, research has shown that cultural influences are transmitted very early, and some can be felt even in the womb (van der Elst & Bohannan, 1999). For instance, the fetus is often able to "hear" the biological mother's voice and patterns of speech and connect to them on subliminal levels. Aspects such as language abilities or type of eye contact can be formed very early. So, there are ways in which Maureen might well respond to stimuli in ways that are culturally more akin to Korean culture, even though her conscious memory does not include anything Korean.

In any case, this first school experience is probably going to be merely the first in a long series of being pigeonholed and perceived differently by others than Maureen perceives herself. At some point, she may well ask her parents for more information about her origins, wish to visit Korea, or try to learn more about Korean culture and language, scrutinizing herself for evidence of familiarity of place and belonging. Depending on how her adoptive family reacts to her quest, by either supporting it or being threatened by it, she may in turn align herself differently. It is difficult as an adolescent to be developmentally searching for identity and not be shaken when others consign conflicting identities. Some process of resolution must be undertaken, and counseling may well be helpful to assist this process.

REFLECTION EXERCISE **2.1**

Cultural Genogram

To begin to map out your own cultural heritage, it can be helpful to complete a cultural genogram. A genogram is a map of relationships between individuals connected through kinship across generations. Essentially, the more we know about our families, the more we know about ourselves. A cultural genogram goes further, beyond the links in family, to explore how constructs of social identity such as culture, gender, religion, class, and sexual orientation impact the familial messages and values that got passed down. It can help you identify the influences on you and your unique heritage (Hardy & Laszloffy, 1995).

1. Start by developing a map of your family. In most cases, you can go back three generations, but you will need to do what makes sense in the context of your family.
2. Define your culture of origin. This refers to the major group(s) from which you descended; in most cases this will mean the first generation to come to the United States, but for Native Americans it may mean their tribal affiliation. Use symbols and colors to depict the various heritages, adding in a mix of colors to depict intercultural heritages.
3. Identify the major constructs and beliefs that came down from these cultures. These are essentially messages about life aspects such as work, relationship, communication, the expression of emotion, the value of education, and so on.
4. Examine your genogram, and see how all these messages and influences may have shaped how you view the world.

OPENING THE DIALOGUE ON CULTURE

With all of the topics discussed in this chapter, you are now challenged to think through how you would utilize this information in session with any number of clients from a variety of cultural backgrounds and worldviews. The questions for reflection offered to you throughout this chapter also serve as excellent process questions for opening the dialogue with clients on culture. Some of these questions are listed here to assist you in terms of opening that dialogue.

Values and Beliefs

- What do you value, why do you believe what you believe, and from where do these values and beliefs come?
- Have any of your most deeply held values and beliefs ever been challenged, and if so, how? How did you reconcile or deal with these challenges?

- Have any of your values and beliefs changed over time in any way? What caused them to change, and why?
- Do any of your most deeply held values and beliefs conflict with those of the people closest to you, and if so, how have you reconciled this conflict?

Learning About the Client's Culture

- How do you identify your own culture?
- Because you are the expert on your own culture, help me learn more about you by responding to the following in the context of your culture:
  - When and how eye contact should be maintained?
  - What it means to get older, and what kind of value is placed on the aging process?
  - How much and what kind of privacy is most valued?
  - How much space is appropriate between people in various kinds of situations?
  - When, how, and whom it is or is not appropriate to touch?
  - When, how, and with whom it is appropriate to display affection?
  - What kind of discipline is appropriate?
  - What kind of nonverbal cues are used to communicate what unspoken meanings, reactions, or expectations?
  - What is considered beautiful and why?
  - What roles should and should not be played by females and males?

Culture and Counseling

- If you can count more than one cultural origin in your heritage, what are the primary cultural frameworks you hold, and how might this affect what you are bringing to counseling in terms of both struggles and resources?
- How does your culture influence your perception of "problems" and avenues for change when it comes to human nature and experiences in life?
- How might your culture influence your goals in counseling, your perception of your life and struggles at this point, and ways for reaching comfortable means of resolution for you?

CONCLUSION AND IMPLICATIONS

Historically, the counseling profession has mirrored the dominant cultural value of assimilation using mainstream cultural understanding and interventions (Aponte & Wohl, 2000). The continually changing demographic profile of the United States, coupled with the increasing need for culturally relevant counseling services around the globe, highlights the need for practitioners to have an understanding of culture, and become sensitized to its salience in counseling. Understanding the universal and culture-specific characteristics in our beliefs becomes increasingly important to

allow us to deal dynamically and flexibly with those around us. If we truly see the world not as it is but as we are, then the importance for counselors to see our clients as they see themselves, not as we see them, cannot be overstated.

In this chapter, we have examined and defined the concept of culture as a pattern of assumptions that determines how we see the world, what the world means to us, and how we will act or react in this world. Furthermore, we have explored the impact of culture, and discussed the psychological implications of various cultural frameworks in the context of language, migration, enculturation, acculturation, culture-specific illnesses and interventions, and cultural worldviews. The collage is ever present in both depth and breadth; it is waiting to be understood, appreciated, changed, and enriched in life and in the therapeutic process with all of its opportunity for growth. So many worlds await us on the continual journey, and in order to better understand how to move in and out of worlds for the betterment of our clients, we must better understand worldviews and personal identities as they relate to the counseling process and the human experience.

GLOSSARY

Acculturation: The process by which a person responds to the influence of the dominant culture or a second culture.

Assimilation: A shift toward the dominant culture together with a rejection of one's culture of origin, with a goal of complete absorption and acceptance by the dominant culture.

Bicultural competence: An individual's ability to effectively utilize "dual modes of social behavior that are appropriately employed in different situations" (LaFromboise & Rowe, 1983, p. 592).

Biculturalism: A flexible balancing of some dominant-culture attitudes and practices with retention of culture-of-origin practices and identity.

Cultural identity: The embodiment of the cultural norms, beliefs, values, and worldview and one's sense of affiliation and belonging to a group identity.

Cultural worldview: The commonly shared system of beliefs, perceptions, attitudes, and values in a culture.

Culture: A total way of life held in common by a group of people who share similarities in speech, behavior, ideology, livelihood, technology, values, and social customs.

Culture-bound syndrome: A combination of psychiatric and somatic symptoms that are considered to be a recognizable disorder only within a specific society or culture.

Enculturation: The process by which a person is socialized into his or her primary culture, receiving primary cultural knowledge, awareness, and values.

Ethnicity: A common sociocultural heritage that includes similarities of religion, history, and common ancestry.

Immigrant: A person who leaves one country to settle permanently in another.

Marginalization: A rejection of both the culture of origin and the dominant culture; such individuals have difficulty with social functioning and acceptance, and may lack a sense of cultural identity and self-efficacy.

Race: A construct that classifies persons by shared genetic history and/or physical characteristics such as skin color.

Refugee: One who comes to a new country unable or unwilling to return to his or her home country due to war, famine, political instability, or persecution due to race, religion, political opinion, or membership in a particular social group.

Separation: A mode that describes those who retain their cultural values and identity while rejecting those of the dominant culture.

Sojourner: A temporary resident who holds on to one's culture of origin and may make only surface adaptations to the host culture.

REFERENCES

Akhtar, S. (1999). *Immigration and identity: turmoil, treatment, and transformation.* Northvale, NJ: Jason Aronson.

Al-Issa, I. (Ed.). (1995). *Handbook of culture and mental illness: An international perspective* (pp. 3–64). Madison, CT: International Universities Press.

Al-Issa, I., & Tousignant, M. (1997). *Ethnicity, immigration, and psychopathology* (Plenum Series on Stress and Coping). New York: Plenum Press.

American Psychiatric Association. (2000). *Diagnostic and statistical manual of mental disorders* (4th ed., text rev.). Washington, DC: Author.

Aponte, J. F., & Johnson, L. R. (2000). The impact of culture on the intervention and treatment of ethnic populations. In J. A. Aponte & J. Wohl (Eds.), *Psychological intervention and cultural diversity.* Needham Heights, MA: Allyn & Bacon.

Aponte, J., & Wohl, J. (Eds.). (2000). *Psychological intervention and cultural diversity.* Needham Heights, MA: Allyn & Bacon.

Arredondo, P., Toperek, R., Brown, S. P., Jones, J., Locke, D. C., Sanchez, J., et al. (1996). Operationalization of multicultural counseling competencies. *Journal of Multicultural Counseling and Development, 24,* 42–78.

Bemak, F., & Chung, R. C. (2002). Counseling and psychotherapy with refugees. In. P. Pedersen, J. G. Draguns, W. J. Lonner, & J. E. Trimble (Eds.), *Counseling across cultures* (5th ed., pp. 209–232). Thousand Oaks, CA: Sage.

Berry, J. W., Poortinga, Y. H., Segall, M. H., & Dasen, P. R. (1992). *Cross-cultural psychology: Research and applications.* NY: Cambridge University Press.

Berry, J. W., & Kim, U. (1988). Acculturation and mental health. In P. R. Dasen, J. W. Berry, & N. Sartorius (Eds.), *Health and cross-cultural psychology: Towards applications* (pp. 207–236). Newbury Park, CA: Sage.

Besnier, N. (1990). Language and affect. *Annual Review of Anthropology, 19,* 419–451.

Blackwell, D. (2005). *Counseling and psychotherapy with refugees.* London: Jessica Kingsley.

Bonvillain, N. (2008). *Language, culture, and communication: The meaning of messages.* Upper Saddle River, NJ: Pearson Prentice Hall.

Brinson, J. A. & Kottler, J. (1995). International students in counseling: Some alternative models. *Journal of College Student Psychotherapy, 9*(3), 57–70.

Canion, G., & Alegria, M. (2008). Psychiatric diagnosis: Is it universal or relative to culture? *Journal of Child Psychology and Psychiatry, 49*(3), 237–250.

Castillo, R. J. (1997). *Culture and mental illness: A client-centered approach.* Pacific Grove, CA: Brooks/Cole.

Clifford, S. H. (1981). Toward a new era in psychotherapy. *Academic Psychology Bulletin, 3*(2), 209–216.

Constantino, G., & Malgady, R. (1998). Overcoming cultural and linguistic bias in diagnostic evaluation and psychological assessment of Hispanic patients. In R. Javier & W. Herron (Eds.). *Personality development and psychotherapy in our diverse society: A sourcebook* (pp. 465–486). Northvale, NJ: Jason Aronson.

Covey, S. (1990). *The seven habits of highly effective people: Powerful lessons in personal change.* New York: Free Press.

Dana, R. H. (1998). *Understanding cultural identity in intervention and assessment* (Multicultural Aspects of Counseling Series 9). Thousand Oaks, CA: Sage.

D'Andrea, M., & Daniels, J. (1991). Exploring the different levels of multicultural counseling training in counselor education. *Journal of Counseling and Development, 70,* 78–85.

Deloria, V., Jr. (1988). *Custer died for your sins: An Indian manifesto.* Norman: University of Oklahoma.

DeLucia-Waack, J. (Ed.). (1996). *Multicultural counseling competencies: Implications for training and practice.* Alexandria, VA: American Counseling Association.

Rytina, N. F. & Saeger, C. (2005). Naturalizations in the United States. Annual Flow Report of the Department of Homeland Security. Retrieved November 2, 2010 from http://www.dhs.gov/xlibrary/assets/statistics/publications/NaturalizationFlowReport2004.pdf

Fernando, S. (2002). *Mental health, race and culture* (2nd ed.). Hampshire, UK: Palgrave.

Fishman, J. (1999). Sociolinguistics. In J. A. Fishman (Ed.), *Handbook of language and ethnic identity* (pp. 152–163). Oxford: Oxford University Press.

Gardiner, H. W., Mutter, J. D., & Kosmizki, C. (1998). *Lives across cultures: Cross cultural human development.* Boston: Allyn & Bacon.

Geertz, C. (2000). *Available light: Anthropological reflections on philosophical topics.* Princeton, NJ: Princeton University Press.

Goodenough, W. H. (1981). *Culture, language, and society.* Menlo Park, CA: Benjamin Cummings.

Hardy, K. V., & Laszloffy, T. A. (1995). The cultural genogram: Key to training culturally competent family therapists. *Journal of Marital and Family Therapy, 21*(3), 227–237.

Holcomb-McCoy, C. C., & Myers, J. E. (1999). Multicultural competence and counselor training: A national survey. *Journal of Counseling and Development, 77,* 294–302.

Javier, R., Vasquez, C., & Marcos, L. (1998). Common errors by interpreters in communicating with linguistically diverse patients. In R. Javier & W. Herron (Eds.), *Personality development and psychotherapy in our diverse society: A sourcebook* (pp. 521–534). Northvale, NJ: Jason Aronson.

Kleinman, A. (1988). *Rethinking psychiatry.* New York: Free Press.

Koss-Chioino, J. D. (2000). Traditional and folk approaches among ethnic minorities. In J. F. Aponte & J. Wohl (Eds.), *Psychological intervention and cultural diversity* (pp. 149–166). Needham Heights, MA: Allyn & Bacon.

Kristeva, J, (1988) "Toccata et fugue pour l'étranger" in *Etrangers à nous-mêmes,* France: Librairie Arthème Fayard, 9-60. In J. Amati-Mehler

S. Argentieri, J. Canestri, S. Argentieri (1993). *Babel of the unconscious: Mother tongue and foreign languages in the psychoanalytic dimension* (pp 264–265). Portland, OR: International Universities Press.

Kroeber, A. & Kluckhohn, C. (1952). *Culture*. New York: Meridian Books.

LaFromboise, T., Coleman, H. L. K., & Gerton, J. (1993). Psychological impact of biculturalism: Evidence and theory. *Psychological Bulletin, 114*, 395–412.

LaFromboise, T. D., & Rowe, W. (1983). Skills training for bicultural competence: Rationale and application. *Journal of Counseling Psychology, 30*, 589–595.

Lambo, T. A. (1961). A form of social psychiatry in Africa. *World Mental Health, 13*(4), 190–203.

Leff, J. (1988). *Psychiatry around the globe*. London: Gaskell.

Levi-Strauss, C. (1985). *The view from afar*. Translated by J. Neugroschel and P. Hoss. Chicago: University of Chicago Press.

Levin, S. J., Like, R. C., & Gottlieb, J. E. (2000). Appendix: Useful clinical interviewing mnemonics. *Patient Care. Special Issue: Caring for Diverse Populations: Breaking Down Barriers, 34*(9), 188–189.

Locke, D. C. (1993). Diversity in the practice of mental health counseling. *Journal of Mental Health Counseling, 15*, 228–231.

Mahalingam, R. (Ed.). (2006). *Cultural psychology of immigrants*. Mahwah, NJ: Lawrence Erlbaum.

Marín, G. (1992). Issues in the measurement of acculturation among Hispanics. In K. E. Geisinger (Ed.), *Psychological testing of Hispanics* (pp. 235–251). Washington, DC: American Psychological Association.

Marsella, A. J. (1988). Cross-cultural research on severe mental disorders: Issues and findings. *Acta Psychiatrica Scandinavica, 78*(344), 7–22.

Matsumoto, D., & Juang, L. (2004). *Culture and psychology* (3rd ed.). Belmont, CA: Wadsworth.

McCarty, T. L., & Zepeda, O. (1999). Amerindians. In J. A. Fishman (Ed.), *Handbook of language and ethnic identity* (pp. 197–210). Oxford: Oxford University Press.

McLean, R., & Marini, I. (2003). Counseling issues and approaches working with families of African American gay male members with HIV/AIDS. *Journal of Family Psychotherapy, 14*(1), 9–21.

Monaghan, J., & Just, P. (2000). *Social and cultural anthropology: A very short introduction*. Oxford: Oxford University Press.

Organista, P. B., Marín, G., & Chun, K. M. (2010). *The psychology of ethnic groups in the United States*. Thousand Oaks, CA: Sage.

Pérez Foster, R. (1996). Assessing the psychodynamic function of language in the bilingual patient. In R. Pérez Foster, M. Moskowitz, & R. Javier (Eds.), *Reaching across boundaries of culture and class* (pp. 243–263). Northvale, NJ: Jason Aronson.

Ponterotto, J. G., Alexander, C. M., & Grieger, I. (1995). A multicultural competency checklist for counseling training programs. *Journal of Multicultural Counseling and Development, 23*, 11–20.

Rubel, A. J., O'Nell, C. W., & Collado, R. (1985). The folk illness called susto. In R. C. Simons & C. C. Hughes (Eds.), *The culture-bound syndromes: Folk illnesses of psychiatric and anthropological interest* (pp. 333–350). Dordrecht, the Netherlands: Reidel.

Sam, D. L., & Berry, J. W. (2006). *The Cambridge handbook of acculturation psychology*. Cambridge: Cambridge University Press.

Sansone, D. (2005). Morita therapy and constructive living: Choice theory and reality therapy's Eastern family. *International Journal of Reality Therapy, 25*(1), 26–29.

Sartorius, A. (1986). Early manifestation and first contact incidence of schizophrenia. *Psychological Medicine, 16*, 909–928.

Sato, T. (2001). Autonomy and relatedness in psychopathology and treatment: A cross-cultural formulation. *Genetic, Social, and General Psychology Monographs, 127*(1), 89–97.

Singh, G. (1985). Dhat syndrome revisited. *Indian Journal of Psychiatry, 27*, 119–121.

Speicher, M. (2000). Cultural and personal dimensions in human life. *Clinical Social Work Journal, 28*(4), 441–447.

Van der Elst, D., & Bohannan, P. (1999). *Culture as given, culture as choice*. Prospect Heights, IL: Waveland Press.

World Health Organization. (1993). *The international statistical classification of diseases and related health problems* (10th rev.). Geneva: Author.

World Health Organization. (1995). *Schizophrenia: Epidemiology of mental disorders and psychosocial problems*. Geneva: Author.

CHAPTER 3

Worldview and Identity

I am a red man. If the Great Spirit had desired me to be a white man, he would have made me so in the first place. He put in your heart certain wishes and plans, in my heart he put other and different desires. Each man is good in His sight. It is not necessary for eagles to be crows.

—Sitting Bull, Lakota chief (cited in Deloria, 1994, p. 198)

Sitting Bull understood that "red men" and "white men" look at the world in different ways. Throughout American history, the differences in the ways that different groups of people look at the world—and our inability to grasp that there are ways to look at the world other than our own—have hindered our ability to live in peace with one another. For most of us, our view of the world is something we take for granted because what is true for us must be true for others as well, right? Keep that question in mind as you read this chapter.

DEFINING WORLDVIEW AND PERSONAL IDENTITY

In this chapter, we present a brief history of the origins of worldview and its relationship to other important constructs such as race, class, and gender. In addition, a number of studies are described that illustrate the similarities and differences of worldviews among various ethnic groups. We explore a model of personal identity that demonstrates the scope of an individual's identity and how it is influenced by sociopolitical and historical contexts, thus shaping worldview. Finally, case illustrations will help to highlight issues to consider when counseling clients.

We define **cultural worldview** as the system of beliefs, perceptions, attitudes, and values held in common by the individuals in a culture. In this chapter, we focus on **individual worldview**, which is the unique way in which each of us sees, interprets, and ascribes meaning to the world. Our individual worldviews are based on our cultural worldview and unique life experiences. Take, for example, Chahaya, a 50-year-old man who was brought up in a small village in Indonesia and immigrated to the United States at the age of 21. Compare this man's worldview with the worldview of his brother Santoso, who has never left his culture of origin, and you will find both common and uncommon elements. They might share certain aspects of their cultural heritage like the foods they eat, traditional practices, or the language; however, because Chahaya left the village, he has had unique experiences that shape his individual worldview.

The notion that there are differences between cultural and individual worldviews is widely endorsed by multicultural scholars and empirically supported by the research. For example, Sue and Sue (2008) point out that the spiritual and religious traditions of many Asian cultures value humans as basically good and stress harmony between humans and nature. However, in an exploratory study in which Sodowsky, Maguire, Johnson, Kohles, Ngumba, et al. (1994) assessed worldviews in a diverse sample of students, they found that the mainland Chinese and Taiwanese students endorsed some values that appear contrary to their traditional cultural beliefs. In survey responses similar to the responses of White American students, many Asian students indicated they believed that human nature is primarily evil and endorsed human control over nature.

Worldview is one of the most important concepts in multicultural counseling because it involves the way individuals view themselves, others, and their environment, and how that, in turn, influences the way that individuals think and behave (Ibrahim, Roysircar-Sodowsky, & Ohnishi, 2001; Josephson & Peteet, 2004). A definition that captures the overall complexity of the concept of worldview in the psychological literature was offered by Lonner and Ibrahim (2002):

> The notion of **worldview** pertains to how an individual sees the world from moral, social, ethical, and philosophical perspectives. A person's worldview is the source of his or her values, beliefs, and assumptions. These are derived from cultural, social, religious, and ethnic and/or racial perspectives, and are among the benefits and consequences of the socialization and enculturation of the individual. (p. 358)

Lonner and Ibrahim also note that although a group of people might have a similar worldview, the way in which each individual reacts to stressful situations is influenced by the construction of his or her cultural and personal identities. In the previous chapter, we defined **cultural identity** as our association with our culture of origin and all of the meanings, perceptions, and expectations associated with life within that culture. In this chapter, we introduce the concept of **personal identity**, by which we mean the way in which we define ourselves as individuals in the context of our culture (both our culture of origin and our present culture) and as individuals influenced by our unique personal experiences.

WORLDVIEW

Every day, we interact with family, friends, partners, strangers, acquaintances, coworkers, and clients who may have very similar or very different views of the world than we do. It is safe to say that human nature is such that we tend to gravitate toward those who share a worldview similar to ours. There is something comforting about knowing that someone understands the world as we do and, therefore, also understands us to some extent. There can be something disconcerting about knowing that someone sees the world very differently than we do, especially if that person's view somehow threatens what we hold to be true and valuable in life.

In many ways, worldview is about placing ourselves and those like us at the center of our "normal" world, whereas those who are different from us are placed in the margins. **Ethnocentrism,** or the belief that one's worldview is normative, real, and universal, is pervasive in most societies. Bennett (1986) described a useful stage model of ethnocentrism. This stage model starts with *denial of other worldviews*, which usually results from isolation and lack of encounter with other worldviews. It is followed by the *stage of defense*, which uses a stance of denigration through negative stereotyping and a feeling of superiority toward other worldviews. For example, European Americans might acknowledge that Latin Americans view the world differently, but stereotyping the Latin American worldview as guided by **machismo** (male dominance) denigrates it and suggests that it need not be taken seriously as a competing view of reality. Finally, the *stage of minimization of differences* trivializes other worldviews by rendering differences as unimportant. In contrast, the stage of **ethnorelativism** includes moving through acceptance, including acknowledgment of differences in values and behaviors; in the stage of adaptation, one learns to relate and communicate across those differences; and, finally, in the stage of integration, one transcends an original indigenous culture and can respond from multiple cultural vantages.

Fortunately, most individuals are capable of developing their capacity for seeing, understanding, and valuing multiple views of the world, even those that stand in stark contrast to their own. As counselors faced with the challenge of working with clients whose views of the world may run the whole gambit, we are also faced with the challenge of keeping our eyes, minds, and hearts open to multiple truths and ways of seeing, believing, and approaching life. One of the underlying keys to effective multicultural counseling is a continual and intentional effort to understand the evolving worldview of our clients in relation to our own. Counseling is, indeed, an opportunity for both counselor and client to further enhance the many learning opportunities that life is already providing on a regular basis; when done well, counseling can provide some of the most powerful critical incidents of all for clients as well as counselors. The culturally competent counselor considers the complexities of a client's worldview and seeks to understand how it influences the client's perceptions and behaviors.

Worldviews and Value Orientations

In their early studies of cultural worldviews, Kluckhohn and Strodtbeck (1961) began to recognize particular areas of difference in cultural values. They noticed, for example, that people from different cultures value *time* in different ways. In some cultures, time is precise and definite; people schedule their lives around the time on the clock. In other cultures, time is variable; the pace of people's lives varies with the seasons and the weather. Kluckhohn and Strodtbeck eventually identified five areas of value differences in cultural worldviews. Essentially, these areas of value difference center on (a) a view of humans as good, bad, or both; (b) the relationship between humans and nature, characterized as mastery over, harmony with, or subjugation of nature; (c) time orientation that is focused on the past, present, or future; (d) relationships with other people described as individualistic, collateral (relationships beyond nuclear family that includes grandparents, cousins, uncles, aunts, etc.), or lineal (relationships that extend beyond immediate family and tied to genealogy and ancestry), and (e) human activity orientation as action and personal achievement focused (i.e., *doing*), personal growth and development focused (i.e., *being in becoming*), or carefree and spontaneous (i.e., *being*).

Of course, within the broad framework of cultural value orientations, there is a wide range of *within-group* variations in value orientations that are influenced by such factors as generational status, gender, class, geographic location, degree of acculturation, and adherence to traditions in a given culture. Nonetheless, for general comparison purposes, these value orientations have been used to illustrate differences among the four largest ethnic groups (Native Americans, Asian Americans, African Americans, and Latinos) and to compare them with European Americans, the dominant cultural group in the United States (Dana, 1993; Sue & Sue, 2008).

For example, whereas European American society promotes individual achievement, in the worldview of many Native Americans, achievement is only possible in the context of tribal group affiliation or family (Garrett & Garrett, 1994). The dominant U.S. culture values a rigid time orientation, whereas many Latino cultural worldviews are based on a more fluid sense of time (Santiago-Rivera, Arredondo, & Gallardo-Cooper, 2002). Likewise, Sue and Sue (2008) noted that whereas the dominant U.S. culture stresses individualism in relationships, Japanese and Chinese American cultures can be considered lineal in that their affiliation with others is linked to past generations.

Kluckhohn and Strodtbeck's (1961) values framework also influenced renowned scholars, such as Derald Wing Sue, whose conceptualizations of the worldview construct are widely known and used in the counseling profession (e.g., Sue, 1978). We will next look at Sue's construct of worldview as he defined it in terms of locus of control and responsibility. Then we will consider other concepts of worldview.

Locus of Control and Responsibility

Derald Wing Sue first introduced the worldview construct in a landmark article entitled "World Views and Counseling," which was published in 1978 in the *Personnel and Guidance Journal*. He defined *worldview* as a set of values that influence attitudes, beliefs, and behaviors, and he argued that every individual's worldview is influenced by culture and race, as well as sociopolitical and historical forces.

Locus of Control	Locus of Responsibility: Internal	Locus of Responsibility: External
Internal	Quadrant 1 *Internal* locus of control and *internal* locus of responsibility	Quadrant 4 *Internal* locus of control and *external* locus of responsibility
External	Quadrant 2 *External* locus of control and *internal* locus of responsibility	Quadrant 3 *External* locus of control and *external* locus of responsibility

FIGURE **3.1** Sue's Categories of Worldview

Sue proposed that worldviews can best be understood by organizing them into four broad categories. As shown in Figure 3.1, Sue's four categories are formed by the intersection of two *psychological orientations*, or dimensions: **locus of control** (the degree to which an individual has the ability to master his or her environment) and **locus of responsibility** (the degree to which the individual can take ownership for his or her actions and life circumstances). According to Sue's model, these two dimensions operate independently, but when they intersect, four quadrants are formed: Quadrant 1 is internal locus of control and internal locus of responsibility, quadrant 2 is locus of control and internal locus of responsibility, quadrant 3 is external locus of control and external locus of responsibility, and quadrant 4 is internal locus of control and external locus of responsibility. Each quadrant of Sue's model incorporates a unique set of values that have been influenced by culture, race, and sociopolitical and historical forces and that in turn influence each individual's attitudes, beliefs, and behaviors.

Individuals who fall into quadrant 1 (internal locus and internal locus of responsibility) value success, attribute their successes to themselves, and believe in independence, power, and control over all aspects of life. Sue suggested that most middle-class European Americans fall into this quadrant.

Individuals who fall into quadrant 2 (external locus of control and internal locus of responsibility) believe that they have little control over their environments and lives while simultaneously holding the belief that everything that is wrong in their lives is their own fault. These individuals may hold negative beliefs about themselves and members of their own cultural and ethnic groups, deny that they are discriminated against, and reject their own cultural heritage while placing greater value on U.S. majority culture and society. In quadrant 2 we find, for example, Blacks who wish they were White, women who accept that women are by definition inferior to men, gays who desperately want to be heterosexual, and disabled individuals who believe that their disabilities make them deserving of the discrimination levied against them.

Individuals in quadrant 3 (external locus of control and external locus of responsibility) neither despise nor blame themselves for the inequality and injustices they suffer, but see poverty, inequality, discrimination, and segregation as just the way the world is. They view the causes of such things as powerful and external, and thus not amenable to change. Individuals in this quadrant tend to accept the circumstances of their lives and believe that it is futile to try to change them.

Finally, individuals in quadrant 4 (internal locus of control and external locus of responsibility) fully understand the societal context of the barriers that they face but see themselves as agents of change. Sue refers to individuals in this quadrant as having racial pride, political consciousness, and a strong sense of personal efficacy. We (the authors) would expand this definition to include individuals with pride in their gender, their sexual orientation, and/or their sense of self-worth regardless of their abilities and physical attractiveness.

Sue cautions that his four worldview categories should not be considered discrete or static. Besides the considerable variation found within each category, individuals may possess a combination of more than one worldview. A particular Latina American, for example, may fall into quadrant 2 in her relationships with men, but quadrant 4 in her role as an activist for racial equality.

In a comprehensive review of the literature on worldview, Koltko-Rivera (2004) noted that the concept is quite complex and continues to evolve. He proposes a new conceptualization that incorporates many of the aspects and dimensions introduced by other scholars. For example, his framework consists of a variety of broad dimensions such as human nature, will, truth, and world and life that relate to one's culture, emotions, behaviors, and cognitions. (For a detailed review of his model, see Koltko-Rivera, 2004.)

Individualism and **collectivism** value orientations are considered part of a worldview. According to Hofstede (2001), who completed a large multinational investigation of cultural attitudes, *individualism* refers to societies where individuals are only loosely connected, and people are expected to be independent and look after themselves and perhaps their immediate families. *Collectivism* characterizes societies where people are a part of cohesive groups from birth onward, and are protected by the group in exchange for loyalty and effort on behalf of the group. Societies tend to fall along a continuum from radical individualism, of which mainstream U.S. society is an example, to extreme collectivism, of which China is an example. Hofstede (2001) also identified other relevant dimensions that influence cultural behaviors. For instance, *power distance* relates to the extent that people within a culture expect that power will be distributed unequally, which in turn impacts the degree of hierarchical structure in a society.

Race, Culture, and Worldview

Because culture and worldview are foundational constructs, they are linked to other important characteristics and attributes of individuals and the groups to which they belong. For instance, race is intimately related to culture and worldview. As we know, different racial groups have different cultures specific to their distinct histories, geographies, physical appearances, and languages, to name a few. As Kambon (1992) noted, each culture construes a worldview that is based on their lived experiences and social realities. For example, Gaines, Larbie, Patel, Pereira, and Sereke-Melake (2005) found that individuals of African descent reported a stronger collectivistic worldview compared to individuals of European descent, and that the collectivistic worldview has served to help buffer the deleterious effects of racism and discrimination faced by African Americans (Stephenson, 2004).

Gender and Worldview

Gender roles are learned in early stages of development, and reinforced in a variety of ways, such as through family, religion, laws and policies, and the culture of a given society (Hansen, Gama, & Harkins, 2001). Likewise, gender differences occur at an early age through differing socialization. Therefore, one can clearly see that gender is a central part of an individual's identity and is significant in the formation of an individual's worldview. According to Ibrahim, a person's gender and cultural background intersect to create and define reality (1999). Thus, although we learn to be men and women from our cultures, we also experience our cultures differently depending on the gender role we have. For instance, a young girl in an Arab culture learns that being a woman includes being modest, nurturing, and intimately related with other women through connections with men. By living day-to-day in accordance with her gender role, she experiences life in her culture differently from her brother.

The notion that there are gender differences in worldview has been empirically supported. For instance, D'Rozario (1996) compared the attitudes of a sample of Singaporean international college students with a sample of American college students and found, not surprisingly, that there were distinct differences between the two groups in their beliefs about human nature and social relationships. Interestingly, however, in *both* groups more men than women endorsed lineality and individualism. More recently, Madson and Trafimow (2001) found that in a sample of 317 college students, women endorsed higher collectivistic characteristics to describe themselves (e.g., interdependence and friendships) than did the men in the sample.

REFLECTION QUESTIONS 3.1

- What is your own worldview, and how does it shape your personal identity?
- Where did your worldview originate, and how is it changing?
- How might your worldview affect the way you approach counseling?
- How does the choice of counseling as your profession affect your worldview?
- How might a client's worldview affect diagnosis and treatment outcomes?

WORLDVIEW AND EFFECTIVE COUNSELING

To become culturally competent, counselors must consider the complexities involved in conceptualizing a client's worldview, and how it influences perceptions and behaviors. Equally important, counselors are urged to explore how their worldview influences their own counseling practice. As we discuss worldview and its relation to cultural and personal identities, we do so to better understand how to most effectively work with a whole host of clients who hold varying worldviews that need to be understood, valued, supported, advocated for, and, in some instances, challenged for the betterment of the client in his or her continual evolution as a person.

Farah Ibrahim proposed a theoretical framework for counseling that places worldview and cultural identity at the core of an individual's life (Ibrahim et al., 2001). Ibrahim et al. argued that worldview

> can be a key variable in understanding a client's cultural assumptions and how they influence his or her cognitive structures and affective structures and reactions. Worldview is the mediating variable that provides an explanatory principle used by mental health professionals in defining a problem and its severity that confront the client. (p. 426)

Understanding a Client's Worldview in Context

From Ibrahim's perspective, worldview should be a central theme in all aspects of counseling, from diagnosis and treatment planning to counseling outcomes. Additionally, Ibrahim and her colleagues underscore the notion that other important factors such as personal identity, socioeconomic background (e.g., education, income, and geographic residence), level of acculturation, gender, religious affiliation, sexual orientation, age, and language background must be considered in relation to worldview. As shown in Example 3.1, Lonner and Ibrahim (2002) outlined a set of questions that, in many respects, provides the context with which to understand the client's worldview.

Assessing a Client's Worldview

Acknowledging the importance of understanding client's worldviews in clinical practice, Ibrahim and her colleagues developed a practical assessment tool for counselors, the Scale to Assess World View (SAWV) (Ibrahim & Kahn, 1984; Ibrahim & Owen, 1994). The SAWV contains 45 questions, and respondents' answers to the questions reveal various aspects of their worldviews. In analyzing a client's responses, the counselor looks for the following general themes that will help to characterize the client's worldview:

- *Optimistic*: Beliefs associated with humans being good, and with a quest for harmony with nature and spiritual well-being, including the belief that nature is powerful.
- *Traditional*: Beliefs that social relationships are mostly lineal-hierarchical, time is primarily a future orientation, and humans have control and power over the natural world.

EXAMPLE **3.1**
Contextual Factors in Understanding Cultural Identity and Worldview

1. How is gender conceptualized, and what is its impact, in the client's primary group?
2. What is the sociopolitical history of the group to which the client belongs, and how does he or she relate to this history?
3. What is the client's generational status (e.g., third-generation Japanese American, or second-generation Chinese Canadian)?
4. What is the history of migration in the client's group?
5. Was the migration of the client's group a free choice, or was it forced (e.g., as for slaves or war refugees)?
6. What is the status of the client's religious and/or spiritual beliefs, and what, if anything, does that imply in the current setting?
7. What is the client's age? What does this mean to the client in terms of his or her primary cultural group and in the larger society?
8. What is the client's stage of life, and what does it mean in his or her primary group?
9. What languages does the client speak? Does the client understand these languages well?
10. What is the client's sexual orientation? How does his or her own cultural group relate to that orientation? How does the larger society feel about the client's orientation?
11. What is the client's ability or disability status? How is this perceived within the client's primary cultural group and in the larger social system?

Source: From W. Lonner & F. Ibrahim, "Appraisal and assessment in cross-cultural counseling," in P. B. Pedersen, J. G. Draguns, W. J. Lonner, & J. E. Trimble (Eds.), *Counseling Across Cultures*. Copyright © 2002 by Sage. Reprinted with permission.

- *Here and now*: Beliefs that focus on the present with a spontaneous way of being.
- *Pessimistic*: Beliefs associated with viewing nature as powerful, relationships as collateral, and humans as essentially bad.

In a more expanded conceptualization of worldview Koltko-Rivera (2000) developed the Worldview Assessment Instrument (WAI), consisting of 54 items that measure a variety of areas such as locus of control (beliefs about causality), relationship to group (collectivism), relationship to authority (democratic idealism), and agency (beliefs about free will) (cited in Coll, 2008).

Essentially, assessing a client's worldview provides a more complete picture of his or her frame of reference and subjective reality. It can help to understand the client's basic beliefs and assumptions, and how the client

The Case of Ya Ting

Ya Ting is a 23-year-old woman who recently came to the United States from Hong Kong to pursue graduate studies. She was very enthusiastic and confident about attending graduate school, and her parents were very proud that she had been admitted into a top university. This was her first time in the United States. The first few weeks were filled with excitement as she learned her way around campus, met new classmates, and attended classes. However, as the weeks passed, Ya Ting realized that her English skills were not as strong as she once thought and she began struggling in her courses. She spent an inordinate number of hours reading and taking copious notes. Over time she has been socializing less with her classmates and spending more time alone trying to keep up with schoolwork. Currently, Ya Ting is losing weight and not sleeping well. She has begun to feel overwhelmed and has approached her academic advisor. She presents her concerns as feeling "bad because I am having problems with my English." The advisor suggests that she drop a course. However, she refuses to do so, stating that "dropping a class would put me behind my classmates and my parents don't want this to happen." The advisor also suggests that she see a counselor for help; however, Ya Ting responds by saying, "I don't want to see a counselor for personal concerns—what I need is help with English."

Case Discussion
Thinking About This Case
1. What would you need to know as a counselor in order to be of assistance to this client?
2. How would you go about finding out what you need to know in a way that is culturally responsive to her needs and experiences?

At first glance, we might see an obvious resistance on the part of this client to seeking help from a counselor for personal difficulties related to her academic struggles. To what reason we attribute this resistance, however, completely depends on the client's values, beliefs, expectations, and perceptions about her current situation. As we have discussed so far in this chapter, the client's worldview—influenced by any number of dimensions such age, ability and attractiveness, ethnicity and race, gender, language and nationality, religion and spirituality, sexual orientation, and socioeconomic class—could serve either as a mediating factor or as a limiting factor in helping her function well in her current environment. The client identifies language as her primary concern—the barrier keeping her from achieving her goal of succeeding in classes. But is there more to the picture than that? Her weight loss and sleep problems suggest anxiety and stress. What theoretical approach and method of intervention do you think would work best with this client? A solution-focused approach that respects her priorities, while exploring her expectations and assumptions, may be helpful here.

approaches problems. Equally important, counselors can use such measures to assess their own worldviews and compare them with their clients' worldviews. By engaging in this process, counselors can determine the extent to which aspects of worldview are shared, and work toward finding what Ibrahim et al. (2001) call "common ground" with a client.

Effecting Change in Worldview

If counseling, in essence, is about changing lives, then we must consider what effects counseling has on clients' worldviews. Debates about the so-called mutability of the worldview construct center on whether life-altering events that have a profound impact on an individual can change his or her worldview or whether only superficial aspects of worldview change while core values and beliefs remain the same (Ibrahim & Kahn, 1984; Koltko-Rivera, 2004). Take, for example, the man who emigrated from Indonesia. As he underwent the acculturation process in the United States, his worldview did simultaneously undergo change. But was it profound change or superficial change? The very nature of how acculturation has been conceptualized—as a process of psychological and behavioral change that occurs as a consequence of exposure to a new culture (Marín, 1992)—leads one to conclude that worldview must undergo some transformation. What remains to be learned by researchers is the degree of transformation. The answer has significant bearing on how counselors approach their work with clients in terms of treatment focus and the use of interventions intended to be both therapeutic and culturally responsive. Counselors might ask, "How do I know if my interventions are changing maladaptive behaviors or core beliefs—and where do I draw the line?" "How do I know if what I am doing as a counselor is considered an imposition of values or beliefs from the client's cultural frame of reference?" and "How do I know if what I consider to be effective counseling from the point of view of my professional training also matches what the client perceives as effective counseling within his or her cultural context?"

Whether worldview is changeable or not, the question raises obvious ethical issues for the counselor. In psychotherapy, client change should be focused on "changing maladaptive attitudinal responses, perceptions, and behaviors that have been learned and are ineffective coping mechanisms or strategies for the client" (Ibrahim et al., 2001, pp. 448–449). Psychotherapy should not focus on "reconstructing basic beliefs and values that are at the core of a client's cultural and gender identity" (Ibrahim et al., 2001, pp. 448–449). Sometimes, the line is indeed a thin one that must be considered carefully and with much self-reflection as well as feedback from the client.

WORLDVIEW AND COUNSELING THEORIES

Fundamentally, client conceptualization and the development of a treatment plan, including the selection of interventions, are predicated on a sound theoretical framework. There is general agreement that an effective treatment approach is driven by theory for both ethical and good practice reasons. In other words, a theory shapes the definition of the client's problem(s) and directs the counseling process. However, some multicultural counseling experts claim that traditional theories of counseling and therapy are essentially culture bound because they convey a specific philosophy and worldview based on a Euro-American value orientation (e.g., Ivey, 1993; Pedersen, 1997; Sue & Sundberg, 1996). In particular, this argument has been used to partially explain why ethnic groups underutilize counseling services. For instance, Sue, Ivey, and Pedersen (1996) have long maintained that behavioral, cognitive, and psychoanalytic theories came out of the Euro-American tradition and essentially "reflect the values, mores, customs, philosophies, and language of that culture" (p. 5).

This perspective has led scholars to promote the idea that new multicultural counseling theories need to be developed. Corey (2008) argues, however, that current theories can be refined and adapted to be more responsive to the wider range of worldviews among diverse clients. Recognizing that no one theory or approach is equally effective across all cultures, he suggests that an integration of theories may be a solution. Whether or not current theories are inappropriate for working with culturally diverse clients remains a controversial topic. Ironically, what you think of this entire issue and the way it affects your work as a counselor is integrally tied to your personal identity. Therefore, in order to best reflect on this issue and the others raised in this chapter so far, we must further explore the concept of personal identity in terms of what it means for our clients, what it means for us as counselors, and what impact it has on counseling work in general.

PERSONAL IDENTITY

As we move through life, we are confronted with situations that force us to further solidify what we already know and think about ourselves and the world we live in, or to question and rethink what we believed to be true about ourselves, others, and life in general. By both learning and choosing how to view the world, we also learn and choose how to define ourselves in relation to the many worlds in which we find ourselves. Our cultural identities serve as an invaluable frame of reference for every choice that we make, and help guide us in unfamiliar and familiar contexts alike. As such, a discussion of worldview would not be complete without an examination of its relationship to cultural and personal identities as widely recognized concepts that are interrelated (Arredondo, 1999; Arredondo et al., 1996; Arredondo & Perez, 2006; Ibrahim, 1991; Sue & Sue, 2008).

Cultural identity and *personal identity* are terms that frequently appear in the multicultural counseling literature, and are often used interchangeably because, in many respects, their definitions have similar features. For example, Côté and Levine (2002) describe identity from both sociological and psychological standpoints in an attempt to "achieve a multidimensional understanding" of this concept. Specifically, identity consists of three basic parts: (a) *Social identity* is characterized as the individual's position in a given social setting, and this part of an individual's identity is largely influenced by prescribed social roles and cultural elements that, according to Côté and Levine, shape the individual; (b) *personal identity* is the individual's identity influenced by unique personal experiences, and this aspect of identity is "idiosyncratic" and referred to as a person's "individuality"; and (c) *ego identity* is that part of the self (i.e., personal agency) responsible for the control of thoughts, feelings, and behaviors. Heavily influenced by Erik Erikson's identity development theory, Côté and Levine proposed that an individual's ego strength depends on the type and quality of social interactions.

Conceptually, their framework has several elements that parallel personal and cultural identity as described by multicultural counseling and cross-cultural psychology scholars. For example, as we saw earlier, Lonner and Ibrahim (2002) define *cultural identity* as "how an individual defines him- or herself from a cultural perspective.... [It] subsumes gender identity and has implications for the meaning attached to it by the client, the client's cultural group, and the larger society" (p. 359). In essence, a client's cultural identity involves a variety of dimensions that could be considered part of a "social identity" such as generational status, sociopolitical history, perceptions of the client's cultural group, as well as qualities specific to the

REFLECTION EXERCISE **3.1**

Describing the Components of Your Personal Identity

If we were to ask you to describe yourself as a person in terms of all of the following components of personal identity, what would you say? In this exercise, try as best you can to fill in the table. Then answer the questions about your personal identity, the integrated whole that defines who you are as a person. Later, as you read this section of the chapter, you may find it illuminating to refer back to the way you described your own identity.

Dimensions of Personal and Cultural Identity	Self-Description
Ability	
Attractiveness	
Age	
Ethnicity	
Race	
Gender	
Generational status and history	
Language	
Nationality	
Religion and/or spirituality	
Sexual orientation	
Socioeconomic class	

1. Did you find that some of these components were more important than others in your description of your cultural identity?
2. Which components were you easily able to describe? Which were more difficult?
3. Can you recall the many experiences and influences that helped to shape each component for you? What were some of the most significant experiences you have had so far that influenced your definition of your cultural identity?
4. Which of the components listed above do you think were chosen for you as opposed to being chosen by you?
5. Have any of the components changed over time, and if so, how?

individual that can be considered "personal identity" such as language, gender, life stage, and abilities.

Personal identity is associated with every dimension of a person's life, including such factors as age, ability, ethnicity, race, gender, language, religion spirituality, sexual orientation, and socioeconomic class. The meanings associated with every one of these components dictate how we think, feel, act, react, and navigate our way through this very complex set of experiences called life. We have already established that individual worldview and identity are in some ways similar and in other ways different from cultural worldview and identity. In addition, some of the components of our identity are ones that we are able to choose or change, some are not, and some are changed for us by the circumstances of our lives.

In the context of developing multicultural competencies in the profession, other perspectives and frameworks have been introduced that help advance our understanding of the complexity of worldview and its relationship to other factors. One such framework is the personal dimensions of identity (PDI) model (Arredondo & Glauner, 1992). This model is often cited as a useful way of viewing clients holistically and individually, as well as gaining an appreciation for the influence of external forces that shape their worldview and behaviors (Munley et al., 2002).

The PDI has three dimensions that interact. As can be seen in Figure 3.2, dimension A consists of a variety of factors such as age, race, gender, ethnicity, and cultural background that are primarily "fixed" and visible characteristics of the individual. Essentially, we are born with these characteristics. Arredondo and Glauner (1992) include social class as part of this dimension while acknowledging that it may be quite possible to be born into a given social class group and then move to another social class status, depending on life circumstances. They note that social class status operates in different

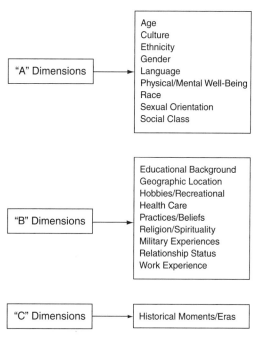

FIGURE **3.2** Personal Dimensions Model

REFLECTION EXERCISE **3.2**

Considering the A, B, and C Dimensions of Your Personal Identity

According to the PDI model, the components that you listed in Reflection Exercise 3.1 would be considered the dimension A factors of your personal identity. Now take a moment to list your dimension B factors (income, where you live, education, etc.). In what ways are your dimension B factors shaped by your A factors?

- Identify some of the dimension C events that have taken place in your lifetime and have meaningful historical context, such as living in the new millennium, the post–September 11 world, the war with Iraq, and so on.
- How have your dimension B factors been shaped by these events?
- Reflect on how dimension B of your identity might have been different if you were living during other eras, such as the Great Depression of the 1930s or in the 17th century.

ways depending on the country of birth, socioeconomic structure of its society, and economic means of the family. Sometimes social class status is not based on socioeconomic indicators, but rather on perceptions based on ethnic background, mode of dress, and gender. Dimension A has features that, according to Arredondo et al. (1996), "readily engender stereotypes, assumptions, and judgments, both positively and negatively," about people (p. 4).

Dimension C is conceptualized as eras or events that have historical and sociopolitical significance. Dimension B includes education, place of residency, income, citizenship, and marital status, which are considered consequences of dimensions A and C. For instance, an individual's age, ethnicity, race, and social class in relation to historical, sociopolitical, and economic contexts will affect dimensions in the B group such as income, where he or she lives (geographic location), and educational attainment. Other factors in B are less influenced by dimensions A and C; however, one can see the relationships among them and argue that many of them are overlooked in the assessment, diagnosis, and treatment processes.

Despite its heuristic value, the PDI has not received wider research attention; however, it has been applied to clinical work. For instance, Rotter and Casado (1998) creatively applied PDI factors in working with Latino clients. Specifically, using the dimensions as a framework, counselors are able to obtain a more complete client picture by incorporating the dimensions into the assessment process, which in turn helps direct treatment at various stages of therapy.

One of the ongoing criticisms of psychology research centers on the underrepresentation of oppressed groups in sample selection, as well as the inadequate effort given to identifying and reporting variables such as cultural

The Case of Alexandra

Alexandra is a 48-year-old female of Puerto Rican heritage who was born on the island of Puerto Rico but raised in the Bronx, New York City. Her parents met and were married in Puerto Rico. Subsequently, they immigrated to the United States in the mid-1950s a year after Alexandra was born. The first few years were a hardship for the family. They knew very little English and had a difficult time adjusting to the long winters, and the father could not get steady employment. Alexandra's mother worked as a seamstress. Over time the parents were able to buy a modest house and hold steady jobs. They also helped to pay for Alexandra's college education. The family had many friends in their neighborhood. Alexandra was raised in a strict but loving home. For example, her father would not allow her to date until she was 16 years old or stay out past 11 p.m. He was watchful of Alexandra's friends and wanted her to have only Latino friends. Having experienced overt discrimination when the family first arrived in this country, he did not trust *Americanos* (Americans). The parents were devoted Catholics and went to church regularly on Sundays. At the age of 19, Alexandra married Enrique, who is also Puerto Rican, right after completing a 2-year degree, and a year later they had their first child (a boy). A few years later, they had their second child (a girl). Enrique also obtained a 2-year degree and worked as a sales rep for a large clothing store. Alexandra was employed as a teacher's aide for many years, then went back to school after the children were older to obtain a teaching degree. She is currently employed as a social studies teacher, enjoys her job, and is proud of her accomplishments. She believes that it is necessary for her to do her best at everything because "Americans have a poor image of Puerto Ricans." One of their children is attending a 4-year college and living at home, and the other joined the Army and is stationed overseas.

Alexandra and Enrique were happily married for 20 years; however, within the last 2 years Alexandra's mother suddenly passed away, Enrique lost his job and was increasingly irritable. More recently, Enrique confessed that he was having an affair and wanted a divorce. He agreed to move out of the house upon Alexandra's request. Alexandra is showing signs of depression such as significant weight gain, sleepless

nights, constant crying, and low energy level. She frequently misses work. The school principal has brought this to her attention, recommending that she see a counselor to help "sort out her problems." Embarrassed and distraught about her job performance, mental state, and family crisis, Alexandra agrees to see a counselor.

Case Discussion
Thinking About This Case

1. What is her generational status?
2. What is her age? What is her life stage and its significance?
3. What is the history of migration to the United States?
4. Was migration a choice?
5. What are her religion and religious background, and what role do these have in her life?
6. What is the sociopolitical history of her reference group?

The PDI helps to obtain a conceptual understanding of how Alexandra's age, gender, ethnicity, cultural background, language abilities, and social class influence a number of the B dimensions. For example, her parents were financially able to help her afford a college education, but also believed that it was their duty to do so. What other B dimensions are present in this case? For example, Alexandra has a teaching degree and a professional career. She reports being proud of her accomplishments and enjoys her current job, yet feels embarrassed about her current performance. With the recent turn of events (e.g., loss of her mother-in-law, and marital problems), Alexandra is showing clear signs of distress. Identifying sources of support is critical. It is important to note the influence of religion. She married fairly young by today's standards. For instance, her religious beliefs may heavily influence her attitudes about marriage, and Enrique's affair and desire for a divorce. In addition, Alexandra was born in the 1950s during a time of racial unrest and most likely witnessed the civil rights movements in this country. It would be important to explore these C dimensions with her to determine how they influenced her values and beliefs, as well as her relationships with non-Latinos.

background and socioeconomic status that, if one views research from a worldview perspective, influence outcomes (e.g., Fisher, 1993; Graham, 1992). To address some of these issues, Munley et al. (2002) examined over 400 published works in nine major American Psychological Association journals to determine the extent to which participants were described using PDI dimensions. Not surprisingly, Munley and colleagues found that of the factors listed in dimension A, most of these studies reported age, gender, and racial and ethnic backgrounds; a very small percentage assessed social class, language, and physical disabilities; and even fewer reported sexual orientation. Of the factors listed in dimension B, education and geographic location were reported by most of these studies. All other factors such as citizenship status, income, religion, and military experience were virtually nonexistent. Likewise, only a handful of studies reported aspects of dimension C (historic eras and events). One could argue that the main reason for the lack of attention given to the multitude of factors outlined in the PDI is that some of these factors are not relevant to the basic research questions posed in these various studies. Although this may be the case, one could argue that the generalizability of research findings will remain an issue. Undeniably, general descriptors such as race, gender, ethnicity, and social class are important to consider in research; however, their treatment in the literature often promotes stereotyping rather than reduces it. As such, it behooves us to examine how these factors intersect with other dimensions such as those outlined in Arredondo and Glauner's (1992) framework in order to increase our understanding of individual differences.

RACIAL AND ETHNIC IDENTITY

Racial and ethnic identity and its development among various ethnic and cultural groups in the United States are areas that have received considerable attention in cross-cultural psychology and multicultural counseling. This interest spans well over 3 decades and continues to stimulate extensive research resulting in the development of a variety of theoretical frameworks (e.g., Bernal & Knight, 1993; Cross, 1971, 1995, 2001; Helms, 1990, 1995; Phinney, 1989, 1990). Furthermore, racial identity development theory is a critical part of understanding the significance of race in understanding individual and group-based identity development.

Before presenting these varied approaches, it is important to further discuss the concepts of *ethnic identity* and *racial identity* as defined and studied. It is common to see in the literature that these terms are used synonymously. However, Janet Helms (1996), a pioneer in racial identity theory, is probably one of the few scholars who make a distinction between race and ethnicity. She views models of *racial identity* and its development as those that center on responses to the experiences of oppression in contemporary society, whereas models of *ethnic identity* and its development have a cultural focus (e.g., customs, beliefs, and values). Similarly, Maurianne Adams (2001) emphasized that **ethnicity** refers to the beliefs, customs, traditions, values, and language shared by a group of people that differ from those of other groups.

Interestingly, the focus of her conceptualization of ethnicity is based on culture and not on physical characteristics that, as noted earlier, are central in the construction of race. Furthermore, Phinney (1996) argued that ethnicity encompasses both culture and race. Although these distinctions have merit, our preference is to consider both given the plethora of research on identity development among culturally different minority groups.

There is considerable agreement, whether one prefers the term *racial identity* or *ethnic identity*, that it is an important aspect of overall psychological functioning, and involves an ongoing process of self-examination and reflection (Bernal & Knight, 1993; Parham, 2002). Finally, both racial and ethnic identities have been conceptualized as complex multidimensional and developmental phenomena. Within the psychological literature, a number of models have emerged that are based on different theories, some of which are called *racial identity* and others *ethnic identity* (e.g., Fischer & Moradi, 2001). Likewise, models that focus on *biracial identity* (e.g., Kerwin & Ponterotto, 1995) and *multiracial identity* (Wijeyesinghe & Jackson, 2001) have also surfaced in recent years. The overall purpose of the following section is to provide conceptual understanding of a number of these models, including an overview of their theoretical foundations with the intent of offering a general perspective. For further reading, refer to the monograph series in which ethnic identity development is described in greater detail specific to a particular group (e.g., African Americans or Native Americans).

REFLECTION QUESTIONS 3.2

- How do you define your personal identity?
- How do you define your racial identity?
- How do you define your ethnic identity?
- How do others define you in terms of your personal, racial, and ethnic identity?
- How do you reconcile any discrepancies between how you define yourself personally, racially, and/or ethnically, and how others define you?

RACIAL IDENTITY DEVELOPMENT THEORIES

Cross's Nigrescence Model of Black Identity Formation

In the 1970s, William Cross, a pioneer in racial identity formation among African Americans and Blacks, developed one of the most widely used frameworks that, in many respects, is the prototype for many of the current models. At the time, the civil rights movement, particularly the Black power movement, greatly influenced his conceptualization of the **theory of Nigrescence** and the stages of **Black identity formation** (Cross, 1971, 1995). In the early years of the theory's evolution, the main premise was that Blacks undergo a "conversion process" in which the individual's racial identity formation is characterized by a movement through stages. Since the 1970s, Cross has refined and expanded Nigrescence theory to reflect a broader conceptualization of Black identity consisting of not only an individual's self-concept but also different types of identities that are developed through what he calls the "socialization and re-socialization experiences" occurring throughout the life cycle. The theory also describes ways in which Black identity is continually challenged and enhanced in different social contexts (Cross & Vandiver, 2001; Vandiver, Cross, Worrell, & Fhagen-Smith, 2002). Briefly described, this is the revised four-stage model:

1. *Preencounter stage,* in which Blacks deny their culture and value the dominant society (White culture); this may stem from negative stereotypes about Blacks and/or negative views about being Black. The two identities in this stage are *assimilation,* described as "pro-American and race is not important" (Vandiver et al., p. 72), and *anti-Black,* in which there is self-hatred and "miseducation" about African Americans.

2. *Encounter stage,* in which a situation or a series of situations occurs that pushes the individual to question and reexamine old ways of thinking and behaving. In this stage, there is a search for Black identity coupled with feelings of guilt and anger with the dominant society.

3. *Immersion/emersion stage,* in which there is a full commitment to Black culture. This stage is characterized as two separate identities: *anti-White* and *intense Black involvement.* The individual with an *anti-White* identity may have little tolerance for White society and moves away from the values held by the dominant culture. An *intense Black involvement* identity is described as an exaggerated immersion into Black culture.

4. *Internalization stage,* where there is a new sense of security and self-confidence with being Black, and in which an individual strives to resolve conflicts with the dominant culture. In this stage, the individual advocates for change in Black communities by becoming actively involved. Cokley (2002) noted that this stage is characterized by two identities: *Black nationalism,* which embraces an Afrocentric worldview, and *multiculturalist inclusive identity,* in which an individual incorporates other identities, such as gender and sexual orientation.

Helms's Models of Racial Identity Development

Janet Helms, another pioneer in racial identity development, elaborated on Cross's Negro-to-Black conversion, and borrowed from Atkinson, Morten, and Sue's (1989) 5-stage racial/cultural identity development model (R/CID) to formulate theories on (a) Black identity development, (b) White identity development, and (c) People of Color identity development (Helms, 1990, 1995). The basic premise of these theories is that individuals go through a process in which they achieve a sense of self that is more internalized, integrative, and satisfying. Thompson and Carter (1997) referred to it as striving for "racial self-actualization" (p. 17). In order for this transformation to occur, individuals must encounter experiences that challenge racism and oppression (e.g., racist acts, attitudes, beliefs, and behaviors), undergo self-reflection about their meaning and impact, and work toward eliminating racism in its various forms (e.g., institutional and cultural) (Thompson & Carter, 1997). Interestingly, Helms (1995) conceptualized the People of Color racial identity theory to include

Asian Americans and Pacific Islanders, Latinos and Hispanics, and Native Americans and notes that People of Color must "recognize and overcome the psychological manifestations of internalized racism" (p. 189).

In many respects, Helms's model of identity development for People of Color parallels her model for Blacks. Essentially, individuals undergo a transformation process of racial identity formation described as statuses. Briefly outlined, these statuses are as follows:

1. *Preencounter* for Blacks and *conformity* for People of Color, which involves devaluing their ethnic or racial group membership, blaming their group for its position in society (e.g., lack of political power and poor socioeconomic status), lacking awareness of racial issues in society, and viewing Whites as superior.
2. *Encounter* for Blacks and *dissonance* for People of Color, where individuals experience events that force them to face the realization that they are not equal to Whites. This realization may create confusion, and as Helms notes it can cause so much anxiety that the individual copes by repressing experiences.
3. *Immersion/emersion* status is characterized by a complete immersion in the culture of origin and a rejection of Whites. Anger toward Whites and "hypervigilance" on any issue concerning racial differences may be apparent during this time.
4. *Internalization*, the final stage (for both Blacks and People of Color), is characterized as a complete acceptance of a new and integrated identity associated with a broader understanding of and action toward combating oppression and racism (Helms, 1995; Thompson & Carter, 1997).

To help illustrate these stages, the life of a prominent African American leader, Malcolm X, is presented in Example 3.2 to further explore the impact of racism and the concept of racial identity development.

Multidimensional Model of Racial Identity (MMRI)

Sellers, Smith, Shelton, Rowley, and Chavous (1998) set out to reconceptualize African American racial identity by proposing an alternative framework that is called the multidimensional model of racial identity (MMRI). As stated by Sellers et al. (1998), African American racial identity is defined as "the significance and qualitative meaning that individuals attribute to their membership within the Black racial group within their self-concepts" (p. 23). Essentially, the MMRI proposes the following:

1. There are aspects of identity that remain constant while external forces cause other components of identity to change.
2. Racial identity is only one of multiple identities in which its relative importance and saliency can be examined contextually.
3. The emphasis is on the individual's perception of his or her racial identity, as well as the personal meaning of being Black.

It is important to note that it is not a development model as compared to Cross's Nigrescence model (1971, 1995) or Helm's Black racial identity

EXAMPLE **3.2**
The Life of Malcolm X

Malcolm X was born Malcolm Little in 1925 in Omaha, Nebraska, the son of Louise and Earl Little. His father was a Baptist preacher active in Marcus Garvey's Universal Negro Improvement Association. Malcolm, along with his siblings, experienced dramatic confrontations with racism throughout his childhood. Hooded Klansmen burned their home in Lansing, Michigan; Earl Little was killed under mysterious circumstances; welfare agencies split up the children and eventually committed Louise Little to a state mental institution; and Malcolm X was forced to live in a detention home run by a racist white couple. By the eighth grade, he left school; moved to Boston, Massachusetts, to live with his half-sister Ella; and discovered the underground world of African American hipsters.

Malcolm's entry into the masculine culture of the zoot suit, the "conked" (straightened) hair, and the lindy hop coincided with the outbreak of World War II, rising black militancy, and outbreaks of race riots in Detroit, Michigan, and other cities. Malcolm X dodged the draft, and his primary source of income derived from petty hustling, drug dealing, pimping, gambling, and viciously exploiting women. In 1946, his luck ran out; he was arrested for burglary and sentenced to 10 years in prison.

In prison, Malcolm began studying the teachings of the Lost-Found Nation of Islam, the black Muslim group founded by Wallace D. Fard and led by Elijah Muhammad (Elijah Poole). Submitting to the discipline and guidance of the Nation, he became a voracious reader of the Qu'ran and the Bible. He also immersed himself in works of literature and history at the prison library. This can be framed as his movement from the *encounter* to *immersion* stages in racial identity development. However, it is less clear at what point in his life he experienced a "preencounter stage". Perhaps it was earlier in his life. Nonetheless, his remarkable transformation can be seen during the later years.

Upon his release in 1952 he renamed himself Malcolm X, symbolically repudiating the "white man's name" because African American family names are often the names of the slave owners who held their ancestors as property. As a devoted follower of Elijah Muhammad, Malcolm X rose quickly within the Nation's ranks, and through national speaking engagements, through television appearances, and by establishing *Muhammad Speaks*—the Nation's first nationally distributed newspaper—he put the Nation of Islam on the map. His sharp criticisms of civil rights leaders for advocating integration into White society instead of building Black institutions and defending themselves from racist violence generated opposition from both conservatives and liberals.

(continued)

Example **1.2** (*continued*)

He began developing an independent Pan-Africanist and, in some respects, Third World political perspective during the 1950s, when anticolonial wars and decolonization were pressing public issues. As early as 1954, Malcolm X gave a speech comparing the situation in Vietnam with that of the Mau Mau Rebellion in colonial Kenya, framing both of these movements as uprisings of the "darker races" creating a "tidal wave" against U.S. and European imperialism. He toured Egypt, Sudan, Nigeria, and Ghana in 1959. This period marks his *internalization* stage.

His increasing differences with the philosophies of the Nation's leadership, and particularly with Elijah Muhammad, erupted into an open schism after he learned Muhammad planned to have him assassinated. On March 8, 1964, he announced his resignation and formed the Muslim Mosque, Inc., an Islamic movement devoted to working in the political sphere and cooperating with civil rights leaders. That same year, he made his pilgrimage to Mecca and took a second tour of several African and Arab nations. The trip proved life altering, as Malcolm met "blonde-haired, blue-eyed men I could call my brothers." He renamed himself El-Hajj Malik El-Shabazz, adopted from Sunni Islam, and returned to the United States with a new outlook on integration. This time, instead of just preaching to African Americans, he had a message for all races. He publicly acknowledged that Whites were no longer devils, though he still remained a Black Nationalist and staunch believer in Black self-determination and self-organization. He had entered the *internalization–commitment* stage of racial development. However, his enemies did not allow his work to continue. At a speaking engagement in the Manhattan's Audubon Ballroom on February 21, 1965, three gunmen from the Nation of Islam rushed onstage and shot Malcolm X 15 times at close range. In his short life of 39 years, he publicly demonstrated an astounding journey of transformation that continues to serve as an inspiration to many.

framework. However, the MMRI's major contribution is its attempt to examine the extent to which racial identity influences behavior in the context of specific situations.

Helms's Model of White Racial Attitudes Toward People of Color

For Whites, Helms proposed a model in which racial attitudes toward Blacks and other ethnic groups are central themes. Briefly, the stages are as follows:

1. *Contact,* where there is a lack of awareness or complete denial that racial differences exist, possibly out of fear or discomfort.
2. *Disintegration,* in which there is a state of confusion resulting from knowing that one belongs to a White racial group that perhaps has a history of discriminating against other ethnic groups. There may be attempts to go to extremes such as deliberately seeking out Blacks or completely isolating oneself from Blacks.

3. *Reintegration,* where there is a sense of superiority over other racial groups, promoting stereotypes, and avoiding places where there are People of Color.
4. *Pseudo-independence,* in which there is a superficial acceptance of members of other racial groups, and the beginning of self-awareness about one's "privileged status as White."
5. *Immersion-emersion,* where there is a deeper understanding about what it means to be White. Similar to Black racial identity development, Whites may become hypervigilant.
6. *Autonomy,* the final stage, is a complete acceptance of both the strengths and weaknesses of White society, including culture and group member-ship. The individual no longer feels threatened, is comfortable with being White, and works toward eliminating oppression (Helms, 1995; Thompson & Carter, 1997).

ETHNIC IDENTITY DEVELOPMENT THEORIES

Beyond models of racial identity development, there are models describing eth-nic identity, and its development in specific groups such as Asian Americans, Hispanics and Latinos, and Native Americans and American Indians also appears in the literature. Some of these models are guided by social identity theory, focusing on a sense of belonging to a group that helps bolster a posi-tive self-concept and sense of self (e.g., Horse, 2001; Sellers et al., 1998), whereas others center on a process that is similar to ego identity formation in which individuals achieve an identity by experiencing a crisis that leads to role exploration followed by making commitments (e.g., Erikson, 1968; Phinney, 1989, 1992).

An often cited **ethnic identity development model** for adolescents is prof-fered by Jean Phinney (1992), who proposed a 3-stage process in which an in-dividual moves from complete acceptance of the cultural values, beliefs, and behaviors of the dominant culture (*unexamined ethnic identity*) to exploration of his or her ethnicity (*ethnic identity search*) and, finally, to an achieved iden-tity (*ethnic identity achievement*) characterized by positive feelings toward oneself and others. Phinney (1993) also noted that individuals may continue to achieve higher levels of ethnic consciousness beyond the stages outlined in her model. It is important to note that this model is "multiethnic" in the sense that it can be applied to African American, Latino and Hispanic, Asian American, and White youth.

Specific models of ethnic identity development for Asian Americans, Latinos and Hispanics, and Native Americans and American Indians are fairly new, and many of them are less defined, partly because of the enormous variability within these various groups. Scholars contend that it is virtually impossible to capture the multiplicity of factors that may contribute to the identity of such diverse eth-nic groups. Nonetheless, progress has been made in identifying different aspects and stages of the identity formation processes for these heterogeneous ethnic and cultural groups.

Asian Americans

Asian American identity development is also multidimensional, and such factors as generational status, acculturation, and different aspects of the family (e.g., functioning, relationships, and roles) need to be considered (Sodowsky, Kwan, & Pannu, 1995). The study of Asian American identity is a relatively new phenomenon; however, a model developed in the 1980s and still relevant today is proffered by Jean Kim (2001), who describes a 5-stage development process mirroring aspects of both ego identity development theory and Janet Helms's theory of racial identity.

Stage 1, *ethnic awareness*, begins before the individual enters the school system. The process of achieving awareness of Asian heritage is closely tied to one's degree of exposure to the culture and similar others. Accordingly, the family protects and shields the child from external forces and serves as the main referent group. In stage 2, *White identification*, the individual begins to experience being different as he or she comes into contact with Whites, gradually adopting their values and behaviors, and acquiring a sense of alienation from other Asians. This stage is also characterized as a time when a negative self-concept emerges as a result of experiencing racism. In the third stage, *awakening to social political consciousness*, the individual begins to gain greater awareness of political and social forces that lead to oppression in White society. There is a shift toward accepting "minority status," but the individual does not internalize perceptions of inferiority. Stage 4, *redirection to an Asian consciousness*, is characterized as shifting from identifying as a minority to identifying as an Asian American with a heightened sense of pride. The individual is immersed in Asian culture and may harbor feelings of anger and resentment toward Whites. Finally, in *incorporation* (stage 5), there is an integration of various identities (social and racial) with an emergence of a more meaningful personal identity as Asian.

Jewish

Few models of Jewish identity appear in the psychological literature; however, there is a growing interest in examining its role in family life (Semans & Fish, 2000) and parenting practices (Davey, Fish, Askew, & Robila, 2003), and the extent to which it is related to cultural practices, interpersonal relationships, and Jewish community involvement (Kivisto & Nefzger, 1993). An early model proposed by Zak (1973) provides a framework that conceptualizes Jewish American identity as involving two distinct aspects: (a) the importance and degree to which the individual affiliates with and is sensitive to Jewish issues, and feels what Zak calls a sense of "interdependence of Jews in the world" (p. 893); and (b) the extent to which there is a sense of belongingness, interdependence, and sensitivity toward all Americans. Clearly, more attention should be given to identifying key factors that contribute to Jewish ethnic identity.

Latinos and Hispanics

The creation of theories about the development of Latino ethnic identity remains an elusive and challenging task because of the population's heterogeneity in terms of national origin, traditions, and migration histories, as well as the blending of many cultures and ancestors. Nonetheless, there have been attempts to conceptualize Latino ethnic identity, keeping in mind the diversity within the population.

For Latinos and Hispanics, one of the most salient factors to consider is **acculturation**, defined as the process of attitudinal and behavioral learning and change that takes place as individuals come into contact with a culture that is different from their culture of origin (Marín, 1992). The acculturation process influences the degree to which individuals adhere to traditional values, beliefs customs, and language preference and use, as well as the degree to which they adopt the values, customs, and beliefs of the new culture. Consequently, one can appreciate the significance that acculturation has on Latino identity when viewed from this perspective.

Latino ethnic identity development can be framed as fluid and continuous rather than as a linear, stage-related process. In fact, Ferdman and Gallegos (2001) see it as a complex interplay of a number of dimensions that involve the degree to which a Latino individual affiliates with his or her ethnic group, how he or she self-identifies, and how non-Latinos perceive the group as a whole. He also describes his framework as one involving different "orientations" rather than as a linear model of development.

Specifically, a *Latino-integrated* orientation is described as a blending of a variety of social identities such as gender, class, and work and profession. Latinos with such an orientation have a broader appreciation for and a balanced view of the group as a whole, and are aware of the group's negative and positive characteristics, including a heightened awareness of the complexity of U.S. society and culture. Ferdman and Gallegos (2001) further elaborate that a *Latino-identified* orientation is characterized as a preference for a "pan-Latino identity" (p. 51), in which there is a strong affiliation with Latinos as a racial group, often attributing only positive characteristics. There is an awareness of institutional barriers, discrimination, and racism, as well as their impact on Latinos. On the other hand, the *subgroup-identified* orientation focuses solely on an affiliation with the individual's country of origin group, such as Puerto Ricans, Mexicans, or Dominicans. There is a sense of collective consciousness, but it is primarily directed at the Latino subgroup, which may be perceived as being "better than" the other Latino groups.

According to Ferdman and Gallegos (2001), Latinos who have this type of orientation focus on their culture and ethnicity. The *Latino as "other"* orientation is described as affiliating with the larger minority group and is not Latino centered. Individuals with this orientation have little knowledge about their own culture and heritage, self-identify as not White or non-White but "other," and are sensitive to how the group is perceived by others. The *undifferentiated* orientation refers to the acceptance of the dominant culture with little or no interest in affiliating with other Latinos. Interestingly, individuals with this orientation view themselves as no different from others. This sameness quality is reflected in easily accepting the dominant culture's norms. Finally, in the *White-identified* orientation, individuals see themselves as White and have the ideals associated with being in a position of power and privilege in society.

The preference is to be and act White with a dichotomous view of race (i.e., one is either Black or White). Ferdman's model is dynamic such that specific experiences, as well as historical and major life events, can propel someone to reexamine his or her identity.

Native American

In conceptualizing Native American identity, one must consider tribal membership, and specific customs and traditions that define *Indianness* as elaborated by Choney, Berryhill-Paake, and Robbins (1995). Furthermore, Choney et al. (1995) conceptualize a model of *personal identity* among Indian people in the context of an expanded view of acculturation involving cognitive, behavioral, affective, and social-environmental domains across five levels: traditional, transitional, bicultural, assimilated, and marginal. From a different angle, Native American identity has been viewed as "native consciousness" influenced by a variety of factors including the degree to which the individual is anchored in tribal traditions and native language (Horse, 2001).

Biracial and Multiracial Identity

With the rapid increase in the number of biracial and multiracial individuals, there has been more attention given to their unique challenges and experiences. Not until the 2000 U.S. Census have we been able to, with some accuracy, identify the size of this population, which was about 7 million people in 2000 (U.S. Bureau of the Census, 2001). Because biracial and multiracial individuals are of mixed heritage and internalize more than one culture, there has been increased attention given to their identity development. As such, **biracial identity** *and* **multiracial identity development** models have surfaced in recent years.

A "biracial" individual is the first generation in his or her family whose parents are of different races and cultural backgrounds. For example, the individual might have an African American father and a White mother, or an Asian mother and a White father. Kerwin and Ponterotto (1995) noted that the underlying premise of most of these models is that biracial individuals struggle with finding acceptance among individuals like themselves, and are often confronted with the pressure of choosing between races (e.g., Asian or Black, or White or Black). Poston (1990) argued that the biracial individual must strive to integrate more than one culture and racial identity into his or her sense of self. In addition, these models tend to be conceptualized as life span developmental stages in which children become aware that they are different through contact with peers and other groups, struggle to be accepted throughout their adolescent years, and as young adults may immerse themselves in one culture and reject the other. Finally, in adulthood, there is an ongoing attempt to achieve an integration of cultures. In support of this position, Suzuki-Crumly and Hyers (2004) found that biracial individuals self-identify as bicultural, that is, identify with both of their cultures (i.e., Black and White, or Asian and White).

Although the frameworks just described increase our understanding of identity development among biracial individuals, they appear to be limited.

Wijeyesinghe and Jackson (2001) noted that such models imply that all biracial groups (e.g., African American–European, Asian–White, or Asian–African American) are lumped together into one group, and assume that their experiences in the realm of identity development are the same. In response to this, he developed a framework that takes into account a broader range of racial identities as well as the multitude of contributing factors that make up what he prefers to call *multiracial identity*. The Factor Model of Multiracial Identity (FMMI) consists of an individual's (a) racial ancestry; (b) socialization and childhood experiences; (c) exposure to and connection with cultural background; (d) physical characteristics; (e) variety of social, historical, economic and political contexts; (f) spiritual beliefs; and (g) social identities such as gender, profession, work, and class.

In recent years, there has been a growing acknowledgment that multiracial identity development is more than just two (or more) races. In fact, Henriksen and Paladino (2009) argue that we must move beyond the boundaries of "race" and consider other dimensions that all interact with and influence one's identity development. In their Multiple Heritage Identity Development model (MHID), ethnicity, gender, sexual orientation, national origin, religion and spirituality, indigenous heritage, and language are central aspects. The model involves a series of developmental periods that identify movement toward a racial identity for multiple-heritage individuals.

In summary, ethnicity and race shape our beliefs and behaviors, and are integral parts of an individual's personality. These diverse models and perspectives provide valuable insight into the complexity of identity development among different cultural and ethnic groups.

In addition to the important roles of racial and ethnic identities in counseling clients, counselors must also examine their own identities and their effect on the counseling relationship and process, as illustrated in Case Study 3.3.

Case Study 3.3 clearly illustrates several important points. First, the counselor is at a different level of awareness and understanding about racial and ethnic issues compared to the client. Interestingly, she has experience working with a diverse clientele yet had little experience discussing issues of race and ethnicity with a White client. Therefore, the counselor needed to carefully monitor her own behaviors and attitudes toward the client. Second, the client was unaware of how her biases were affecting her well-being. Finally, the counselor was willing to take the risk of challenging the client on this issue, resulting in heightened client self-understanding.

OPENING THE DIALOGUE ON WORLDVIEW, PERSONAL AND CULTURAL IDENTITIES, AND RACIAL AND ETHNIC IDENTITIES

With all of the topics discussed in this chapter, you are now challenged to think through how you would utilize this information in session with any number of clients from a variety of cultural backgrounds and worldviews. Questions for reflection offered to you throughout this chapter also serve as excellent process questions for opening the dialogue with clients on worldview

CASE STUDY **3.3**

The Case of a 40-Year-Old White American Lesbian

The client is a 40-year-old White American lesbian who is also an evangelical and devout Christian. She is a social worker who works part-time in several different agencies (including a Jewish mental health agency), seeing a variety of clients in a large urban area. Her clientele is often racially and economically diverse.

The client has addressed several significant issues in therapy, including her relationship with her family of origin, her social isolation and increasing distrust of people, her intense emotionality and its impact on her work and social relationships, as well as career and body image concerns. Whenever under duress, this client focuses her anger and intolerance on individuals or groups that are racially or religiously different from her. On several occasions in therapy, the client expressed frustration or anger with Jews and Blacks because of specific work-related concerns. At times she presented a hypersensitivity and slight paranoia about their perceptions of her and their behavior (which often seemed to fit racial and religious stereotypes).

The counselor, who is a White American female, has a small private practice in a large urban city with a diverse client population. She has had extensive training in the area of multicultural counseling. She is often bothered and offended by some of the client's remarks. The counselor, who often confronts such prejudice and intolerance in other life settings, was unsure how to address the client's behavior within the session in a therapeutic fashion. When the client was challenged, she often became defensive and described herself as having no bias. Over time, she was willing to admit that she had become increasingly intolerant and focused her energy on other people who had nothing to do with her unhappiness. The counselor had rarely worked with racial or racial identity issues within a White–White dyad, and although she could assess and

understand her client's level of racial identity, she sometimes had to monitor her emotional reaction within the session so it would not get in the way.

Case Discussion
Thinking About This Case
As you read this case, address the following questions:

1. As the counselor, how will you conceptualize your role in addressing racial and ethnic identity in counseling?
2. How might you address the client's biases?
3. How might the situation be different with a White–Person of Color dyad? How does the counselor's racial and ethnic identity interweave with the client's?

According to Reynolds and Baluch (2001), the counselor, who is White, had significant training in multicultural counseling, yet has limited experience addressing racial issues and racial identity with clients who are also White. In this case, the counselor is well aware of the client's stereotypical attitudes toward other racial-ethnic and cultural groups and wants to address this in counseling, but is somewhat unsure how to do it in an effective manner. One of the challenges for counselors in situations like this is to remain open and empathic while attempting to address racial concerns. Likewise, counselors need to explore their own attitudes and beliefs toward other groups, as well as closely monitor their own emotional reactions.

Source: From A. L. Reynolds & S. Baluch, "Racial Identity Theories in Counseling: A Literature Review and Evaluation," in C. L. Wijeyesinghe & B. W. Jackson III (Eds.), 2001, *New Perspectives on Racial Identity Development: A Theoretical and Practical Anthology*. Copyright © 2001 by New York University Press. Reprinted with permission.

and personal and cultural identities. Some of these questions are listed here to assist you in terms of opening the dialogue with your clients:

- What is your worldview, and how does it shape your personal identity? Following are some specific examples of areas that can be explored:
  - What is your ability or disability status? How is this perceived within your primary cultural group and in society?
  - How old are you, and what does this mean to you in terms of your life, your group affiliation, your experience within society, your

presenting issue(s) in counseling, and your relationship with me as your counselor?

- What do you consider your life stage at this point, and what does that mean for you?
- What is your race or ethnicity, how important is that to you in terms of counseling, and what you are dealing with in this process? How might my race or ethnicity affect you in this process?
- What is the sociopolitical history of the group to which you belong, and how do you relate to this history? Again, how does this influence what you are dealing with now, if at all?
- How do you conceptualize gender, and what is its impact on your life?
- What is your generational status (e.g., third-generation Japanese American, or second-generation Chinese Canadian)?
- What is the history of migration for your cultural group? Was the migration of your group a free choice, or was it forced (e.g., as for slaves or war refugees)?
- What language(s) do you speak? What do you consider to be your nationality, and how does that influence your view of the world?
- What are some of your religious and/or spiritual beliefs, and what, if anything, does that imply in the current setting?
- What is your sexual orientation, and how does your own cultural group relate to that orientation? How does the larger society feel about your orientation?
- What do you consider your socioeconomic class to be, and how does that influence your life?

Use the following chart with your client to better describe his or her personal and cultural identities, and to see how any of these dimensions relate to the presenting issue(s):

Dimensions of Personal and Cultural Identity	Self-Description
Ability	
Attractiveness	
Age	
Ethnicity	
Race	
Gender	
Generational status and history	
Language	
Nationality	
Religion and/or spirituality	
Sexual orientation	
Socioeconomic class	

- Which dimensions were you easily able to describe? Which were more difficult?
- Which of the dimensions listed above do you think were chosen for you as opposed to being chosen by you?
- Are some of these dimensions more important than others in your description of your cultural identity; and if so, which ones and why?
- Can you recall the many experiences and influences that helped to shape each dimension for you? What were some of the most significant experiences you have had so far that influenced your definition of your cultural identity?
- Have any of the dimensions changed over time; and if so, how?
- Based on the dimensions you have described to me, where did your worldview originate, and how is it changing now?
- How might your worldview affect the way you approach this process of participating in counseling?
- How might your worldview affect what you would consider appropriate treatment goals?
- What else might be important for me to know about you to be of the most help?

CONCLUSION AND IMPLICATIONS

Culturally competent counselors are aware of how racial and ethnic identity is intimately related to life experiences and overall psychological well-being and mental health functioning. For instance, a strong affiliation with one's ethnic group (achieved racial and ethnic identity) has been associated with positive self-esteem (e.g., Phinney & Chavira, 1992), higher levels of academic achievement (Beale Spencer, Noll, Stoltzfus, & Harpalani, 2001), and perceived self-efficacy (Phillips Smith, Walker, Fields, Brookins, & Seay, 1999) among minority youth. On the flip side, there is a growing body of literature suggesting that certain stages of ethnic identity development are associated with adverse mental health. For example, the preencounter stage as outlined by Helms and Cross has been linked to higher levels of depressive symptoms (e.g., Munford, 1994; Pyant & Yanico, 1991).

The scant literature suggests that there are benefits of examining its saliency and relevance in counseling clients. For instance, it should be considered as part of the overall assessment of client concerns to determine if, indeed, it is central to the individual's well-being. The counselor might ask, "How is the client's sense of self influenced by his or her environment, and how does this relate to the presenting problem?" and "How salient is racial identity for the client?" Awareness of the pervasiveness of racism as well as the multitude of barriers that ethnic minorities face, the individual's

"ethnic self" is most likely to play an important role in the individual's life. As such, incorporating the assessment of racial and ethnic identity early on in the counseling process may facilitate the development of treatment interventions that lead to a stronger working therapeutic alliance and promote positive outcomes (Thompson & Carter, 1997). (For an excellent review of measures of racial and ethnic identity, refer to Fischer & Moradi, 2001.)

In this chapter, we have presented a brief history of the origins of worldview and its relationship to the dimensions of cultural identity, including age, ability and attractiveness, ethnicity and race, gender, language and nationality, religion and spirituality, sexual orientation, and socioeconomic class. In addition, a number of studies and specific examples were described that illustrate the similarities and differences of worldviews among various ethnic groups. We also explored several models of identity that demonstrate how it is influenced by sociopolitical and historical contexts as well as the phenomenological experience of the here and now. Finally, case illustrations were provided to help highlight issues for consideration when counseling clients from a variety of worldviews and differing cultural identities. As we have explored the concept of worldview and its relation to cultural identity, we have done so to better understand how to most effectively work with a whole host of clients who hold varying worldviews that need to be understood, valued, supported, advocated for, and, in some instances, challenged for the betterment of the client in his or her continual evolution as a person.

As noted, earlier multiculturalism sought to understand individuals in their unique context, but among the many factors to consider, worldview is one of the most important constructs. Its centrality is based on the notion that it is the source of an individual's values,

beliefs, and assumptions that come from cultural, social, and ethnic backgrounds, as well as unique lived experiences. Likewise, counselors are challenged to continually be in a process of awareness and self-reflection in order to recognize how their own worldview influences their counseling practice. We have presented various models and perspectives to assist you in conceptualizing clients, including ways to incorporate them in diagnostic and treatment plans.

GLOSSARY

Acculturation: The process of adaptation from one's country of origin to a new country of residence. Defined by Marín (1992) as the process of attitudinal and behavioral learning and change after coming in contact with a different culture.

Asian American identity development: A model proposed by Kim (2001) that describes Asian American identity development in five stages: (a) ethnic awareness, (b) White identification, (c) awakening to social political consciousness, (d) redirection to an Asian consciousness, and (e) incorporation.

Biracial identity development: A process of accepting and integrating more than one culture and racial identity into one's sense of self.

Black identity formation: A process of Black identity development conceptualized by Cross (1971, 1995; Cross & Vandiver, 2001) as consisting of four stages: (a) preencounter, (b) encounter, (c) immersion and emersion, and (d) internalization.

Collectivism: An orientation emphasizing group cohesiveness and group goals rather than individual goals. The group is considered more important than the individual.

Cultural identity: Affiliation with the culture of origin (e.g., cultural values, beliefs, practices, and language).

Cultural worldview: A system of beliefs, perceptions, attitudes, and values held in common by the individual in a culture.

Ethnic identity development model: A model developed by Phinney (1992) for adolescents in which an individual moves from complete acceptance of cultural values, beliefs, and behaviors of the dominant culture to an identity based on one's ethnicity (beliefs, customs, traditions and values of one's culture of origin).

Achieving an ethnic identity is characterized by positive feelings of self and others. The stages in Phinney's model are (a) unexamined ethnic identity, (b) ethnic identity search, and (c) ethnic identity achievement.

Ethnicity: The beliefs, customs, traditions, values, and language shared by a group of people.

Ethnocentrism: The belief that one's worldview is normative and universal.

Ethnorelativism: The ability to acknowledge and value cultural differences.

Identity development for People of Color: A model of racial identity development for Asian Americans and Pacific Islanders, Latinos, and Native Americans proposed by Helms (1990, 1995) in which individuals from these various groups undergo a process of achieving a sense of self that is internalized, integrated, and satisfying. The process involves a series of statuses: (a) conformity, (b) dissonance, (c) immersion and emersion, and (d) internalization.

Individualism: An orientation emphasizing individuality, independence and self-reliance. Individual rather than collective group goals are desired.

Individual worldview: A unique way in which an individual sees, interprets, and ascribes meaning to the world. It is based on a cultural context and unique life experiences.

Latino ethnic identity development: A process of identity development for Latinos characterized by Ferdman and Gallegos (2001) as consisting of orientations rather than stages. They are (a) Latino-integrated, (b) Latino-identified, (c) subgroup-identified, (d) Latino as "other," and (e) undifferentiated.

Locus of control: The degree to which the individual has the ability to master his or her environment.

Locus of responsibility: The degree to which the individual can take ownership for his or her actions and life circumstances.

Machismo: Male chauvinism.

Multidimensional model of racial identity (MMRI): A model of racial identity proposed by Sellers et al. (1998) that focuses on the self-concept and personal meaning of being Black. It is not a development model of ethnic identity, but rather focuses on how racial identity influences behavior in different situations.

Multiple heritage identity development model: A model developed by Henriksen and Paladino (2009) that focuses on multiple identities including race, identity, sexual orientation, national origin, religion, spirituality, language, and indigenous heritage.

Multiracial identity development: Development of a sense of self that incorporates more than one racial and cultural heritage. This term has often been used interchangeably with biracial identity; however, it has included other identities and dimensions such as gender, social class, physical characteristics, and spiritual beliefs as outlined in the factor model of multiracial identity.

Personal dimensions of identity (PDI): A model of identity developed by Arredondo and Glauner (1992) consisting of a variety of dimensions that interact and influence how a person thinks, behaves, and views the world.

Personal identity: The way an individual defines himself or herself in the context of his or her culture of origin and present culture, which is influenced by personal experiences. Personal identity can encompass a wide variety of dimensions such as age, gender, race, ethnicity, social class, sexual orientation, and personal agency.

Racial identity development: Development of an identity based on race and responses to experiences of oppression. Often characterized by movement in stages in which individuals achieve a sense of racial identity that is more internalized, integrated, and satisfying.

Theory of Nigrescence: A framework developed by Cross (1971, 1995) in which African Americans and Blacks undergo a process of identity formation. The theory also proposes that Black identity is continuously challenged by the dominant society and different social contexts.

White racial attitudes toward People of Color: A framework developed by Helms (1995) in which Whites undergo a process of attitudinal change toward people of color (e.g., African Americans, Asian Americans, Latinos, and Native Americans). It consists of stages: (a) contact, (b) disintegration, (c) reintegration, (d) pseudo-independence, (e) immersion and emersion, and (f) autonomy.

Worldview: How an individual sees himself or herself, others, and his or her environment. Lonner and Ibrahim (2002) define it as the way in which an individual perceives his or her world from philosophical, moral, ethical, social, and moral contexts.

REFERENCES

Adams, M. (2001). Cross processes of racial identity development. In C. Wijeyesinghe & B. W. Jackson III (Eds.), *New perspectives on racial identity development: A theoretical and practical anthology* (pp. 209–242). New York: New York University Press.

Arredondo, P. (1999). Multicultural counseling as a tool to address oppression and racism. *Journal of Counseling and Development, 77,* 102–108.

Arredondo, P., & Glauner, T. (1992). *Personal dimensions of identity model.* Boston: Empowerment Workshops.

Arredondo, P, & Perez, P. (2006). Historical perspectives on the multicultural guidelines and contemporary applications. *Professional Psychology: Research and Practice, 37,* 1–5.

Arredondo, P., Toporek, R., Brown, S. P., Jones, J., Locke, D., Sanchez, J., et al. (1996). *Operationalization of the multicultural competencies.* Alexandria, VA: Association of Multicultural Counseling and Development of the American Counseling Association.

Atkinson, D. R., Morten, G., & Sue, D. W. (1989). A minority identity development model. In D. R. Atkinson, G. Morten, & D. W. Sue (Eds.), *Counseling American minorities* (pp. 35–52). Dubuque, IA: William C. Brown.

Beale Spenser, M., Noll, E., Stoltzfus, J., & Harpalani, V. (2001). Identity and school adjustment: Revising the "acting white" assumption. *Educational Psychologists, 36,* 21–30.

Bennett, M. J. (1986). A developmental approach to training for intercultural sensitivity, *International Journal of Intercultural Relations, 10,* 179–196.

Bernal, M. E., & Knight, G. P. (1993). *Ethnic identity: Formation and transmission among Hispanics and other minorities.* Albany, NY: State University of New York Press.

Choney, S. K., Berryhill-Paake, E., & Robbins, R. R. (1995). The acculturation of American Indians. In J. G. Ponterotto, J. M. Casas, L.A. Suzuki, L.A., & C. M. Alexander (Eds.), *Handbook of multicultural counseling* (pp. 73–92). Thousand Oaks, CA: Sage.

Cokley, K. O. (2002). Testing Cross's Revised Racial Identity Model: An examination of the relationship between racial identity and internalized racialism. *Journal of Counseling Psychology, 49,* 476–483.

Coll, J. E. (2008). An examination of the relationship between optimism and worldview among university students. *College Student Journal, 42,* 395–401.

Corey, G. (2009). *Theory and practice of counseling and psychotherapy* (8th edition). Belmont, CA: Thomson Brooks/Cole.

Côté, J. E., & Levine, C. G. (2002). *Identity formation: Agency, and culture: A social psychological synthesis.* Mahwah, NJ: Lawrence Erlbaum.

Cross, W. (1971). The Negro- to- Black conversion experience. *Black World, 20,* 13–27.

Cross, W. (1995). The psychology of Nigrescence: Revising the Cross Model. In J. G. Ponterotto, J. M. Casas, L. A. Suzuki, L.A., & C. M. Alexander (Eds.), *Handbook of multicultural counseling* (pp. 93–122). Thousand Oaks, CA: Sage.

Cross, W., & Vandiver, B. J. (2001). Nigrescence theory and measurement: Introducing the Cross Racial Identity Scale (CRIS). In J. G. Ponterotto, J. M. Casas, L. A. Suzuki, L. A., & C. M. Alexander (Eds.), *Handbook of multicultural counseling* (pp. 371–393). Thousand Oaks, CA: Sage.

Dana, R. H. (1993). *Multicultural assessment perspectives for professional psychology.* Needham Heights, MA: Allyn & Bacon.

Davey, M., Stone Fish, L., Askew, J., & Robila, M. (2003). Parenting practices and the transmission of ethnic identity. *Journal of Marital and Family Therapy, 29,* 195–208.

Deloria, V., Jr. (1994). *God is red: A Native view of religion.* Golden, CO: Fulcrum.

D'Rozario, V. A. (1996). Singaporean and Unites States college students' worldview, expectations of counseling, and perceptions of counselor effectiveness based on directive and nondirective counseling style. *Dissertation Abstracts International, 56,* 2564.

Erikson, E. H. (1968). *Identity: Youth and crisis.* New York: Norton.

Fischer, A. R., & Moradi, B. (2001). Racial and ethnic identity: Recent developments and needed directions.

In J. Ponterotto, J. M. Casas, L. A. Suzuki, & C. M. Alexander (Eds.), *Handbook of multicultural counseling* (pp. 341–370). Thousand Oaks, CA: Sage.

Ferdman, B. M., & Gallegos, P. I. (2001). Racial identity development and Latinos in the United States. In C. L. Wijeyesinghe & B. W. Jackson III. (Eds.), *New perspectives on racial identity development: A theoretical and practical anthology* (pp. 32–66). New York: New York University Press.

Fisher, C. B. (1993). Joining science and application: Ethical challenges for researchers and practitioners. *Professional Psychology: Research and Practice, 24,* 378–381.

Gaines, S. O., Jr., Larbie, J., Patel, S., Pereira, L., & Sereke-Melake, Z. (2005). Cultural values among African-descended persons in the United Kingdom: Comparisons with European-descended and Asian-descended persons. *Journal of Black Psychology, 31,* 130–151.

Garrett, J. T., & Garrett, M. W. (1994). The path to good medicine: Understanding and counseling Native America Indians. *Journal of Multicultural Counseling and Development, 22,* 134–144.

Graham, S. (1992). "Most of the subjects were White and middle class": Trends in published research on African Americans in selected APA journals, 1970–1989. *American Psychologists, 47,* 629–639.

Hansen, L. S., Gama, E. M. P., & Harkins, A. K. (2001). Revisiting gender issues in multicultural counseling. In P. B. Pedersen, J. G. Draguns, W. J. Lonner, & J. E. Trimble (Eds.), *Counseling across cultures* (pp. 163–184). Thousand Oaks, CA: Sage.

Helms, J. E. (1990). *Black and White racial identity: Theory, research and practice.* Westport, CT: Greenwood.

Helms, J. E. (1995). An update of Helms's White and People of Color Racial Identity Models. In J. G. Ponterotto, J. M. Casas, L. A. Suzuki, L. A., & C. M. Alexander (Eds.), *Handbook of multicultural counseling* (pp. 181–198). Thousand Oaks, CA: Sage.

Helms, J. E. (1996). Toward a methodology for measuring and assessing racial as distinguishing from ethnic identity. In G. R. Sodowsky, & J. C. Impara (Eds.), *Multicultural assessment in counseling and clinical psychology* (pp. 143–192). Lincoln, NE: Buros Institute of Mental Measurement.

Henriksen, R. C., & Paladino, D. A. (2001). *Counseling multiple heritage individuals, couples, and families.* Alexandria, VA: American Counseling Association.

Hofstede, G. (2001). *Culture's consequences: Comparing, values, behaviors, and organizations across nations* (2nd edition). Thousand Oaks, CA: Sage.

Horse, P. G. (2001). Reflections on American Indian identity. In C. L. Wijeyesinghe & B. W. Jackson III. (Eds.), *New perspectives on racial identity development: A theoretical and practical anthology.* (pp. 91–107). New York: New York University Press.

Ibrahim, F. A. (1991). Contribution of cultural worldview to generic counseling and development. *Journal of Counseling and Development, 70*, 13–19.

Ibrahim, F. A. (1999). Transcultural counseling: Existential worldview theory and cultural identity. In J. McFadden (Ed.), *Transcultural counseling* (2nd ed., pp. 23–57). Alexandria, VA: American Counseling Association.

Ibrahim, F. A., & Kahn, H. (1984). *Scale to Assess Worldview© (SAWV)*. Unpublished instrument, Storrs, CT.

Ibrahim, F. A., & Owen, S. V. (1994). Factor analytic structure of the Scale to Assess World View. *Current Psychology: Development, Learning, Personality, Social, 13*, 201–209.

Ibrahim, F. A., Roysircar-Sodowsky, G. R., & Ohnishi, H. (2001). Worldview: Recent developments and needed directions. In J. G. Ponterotto, J. M. Casas, L. A. Suzuki, & C. M. Alexander (Eds.), *Handbook of multicultural counseling* (2nd ed., pp. 425–455). Thousand Oaks, CA: Sage.

Ivey, A. E. (1993). On the need for reconstruction of our present practice of counseling and psychotherapy. *The Counseling Psychologist, 21*, 225–228.

Josephson, A. M., & Peteet, J. R. (Eds.). (2004). *Handbook of spirituality and worldview in clinical practice.* Arlington, VA: American Psychiatric Publishing.

Kambon, K. K. (1992). *The African personality in America: An African-centered framework.* Tallahassee, FL: Nubian Nation.

Kerwin, C., & Ponterotto, J. G. (1995). Biracial identity development: Theory and research. In J. G. Ponterotto, J. M. Casas, L. A. Suzuki, L. A., & C. M. Alexander (Eds.), *Handbook of multicultural counseling* (pp. 199–217). Thousand Oaks, CA: Sage.

Kluckhohn, F. R., & Strodtbeck, F. L. (1961). *Variations in value orientations.* Evanston, IL: Row, Patterson.

Kim, J. (2001). Asian American identity development theory. In C. L. Wijeyesinghe & B. W. Jackson III. (Eds.), *New perspectives on racial identity development: A theoretical and practical anthology* (pp. 67–90). New York: New York University Press.

Kivisto, P., & Nefzger, B. (1993). Symbolic ethnicity and American Jews: The relationship of ethnic identity to behavior and group affiliation. *Social Science Journal, 30*, 1–12.

Koltko-Rivera, M. E. (2000). The Worldview Assessment Instrument (WAI): The development and preliminary validation of an instrument to assess worldview components relevant to counseling and psychotherapy. Doctoral dissertation, New York University. *Dissertation Abstracts International, 61*, 2266B. (UMI Microform No. 996888433)

Koltko-Rivera, M. E. (2004). The psychology of worldviews. *Review of General Psychology, 8*, 3–58.

Lonner, W., & Ibrahim, F. A. (2002). Appraisal and assessment in cross-cultural counseling. In P. B. Pedersen, J. G. Draguns, W. J. Lonner, & J. E. Trimble (Eds.), *Counseling across cultures* (pp. 355–379). Thousand Oaks, CA: Sage.

Madson, L. A., & Trafimow, D. (2001). Gender comparisons in the private, collective, and allocentric selves. *The Journal of Social Psychology, 141*, 551–559.

Marín. G. (1992). Issues in the measurement of acculturation of Hispanics. In K. F. Geisinger (Ed.), *Psychological testing of Hispanics* (pp. 235–251). Washington, DC: American Psychological Association.

Munford, M. B. (1994). Relationship of gender, self-esteem, social class, and racial identity to depression in blacks. *Journal of Black Psychology, 20*, 157–174.

Munley, P., Anderson, M. Z., Baines, A. L., Briggs, D., Dolan, J. P., Jr., & Koyama, M. (2002). Personal dimensions of identity and empirical research in APA journals. *Cultural Diversity and Ethnic Minority Psychology, 8*, 357–365.

Parham, T. A. (2002). *Counseling persons of African descent: raising the bar of practitioner competence.* Thousand Oaks, CA: Sage.

Pedersen, P. B. (1997). *Culture-centered counseling interventions.* Thousand Oaks, CA: Sage.

Phillips Smith, E., Walker, K., Fields, L., Brookins, C. C., & Seay, R. C. (1999). Ethnic identity and its relationship to self-esteem, perceived efficacy and prosocial attitudes in early adolescence. *Journal of Adolescence, 22*, 867–880.

Phinney, J. S. (1989). Stages of ethnic identity in minority adolescents. *Journal of Early Adolescence, 9*, 34–49.

Phinney, J. S. (1990). Ethnic identity in adolescents and adults: Review of research. *Psychological Bulletin, 108*, 499–514.

Phinney, J. S. (1992). The Multigroup Ethnic Identity Measure: A new scale for use with diverse groups. *Journal of Adolescent Research, 13*, 156–176.

Phinney, J. S. (1993). A three-stage model of ethnic identity development in adolescence. In M. E. Bernal & G. P. Knight (Eds.), *Ethnic identity: Formation and transmission among Hispanics and other minorities* (pp. 61–79). Albany, NY: State University of New York Press.

Phinney, J. (1996). Understanding ethnic diversity: The role of ethnic identity. *American Behavioral Scientist, 40*, 143–152.

Phinney, J. S., & Chavira, V. (1992). Ethnic identity and self-esteem: An exploration longitudinal study. *Journal of Adolescence, 15*, 271–281.

Poston, C. W. (1990). The Biracial Identity Model: A needed addition. *Journal of Counseling and Development, 69*, 152–155.

Pyant, C. T., & Yanico, B. J. (1991). Relationship of racial identity and gender-role attitudes to Black women's psychological well-being. *Journal of Counseling Psychology, 38*, 315–322.

Reynolds, A. L., & Baluch, S. (2001). Racial identity theories in counseling: A literature review and evaluation. In C. L. Wijeyesinghe & B. W. Jackson III (Eds.), *New perspectives on racial identity development: A theoretical and practical anthology* (pp. 167–181). New York: New York University Press.

Rotter, J. C., & Casado, M. (1998). Promoting strengths and celebrating culture: Working with Hispanic families. *The Family Journal: Counseling and Therapy for Couples and Families, 6*, 132–136.

Santiago-Rivera, A. L., Arredondo, P., & Gallardo-Cooper, M. (2002). *Counseling Latinos and la familia: A practical guide*. Thousand Oaks, CA: Sage.

Sodowsky, R. G., Kwan, K. L. K., Pannu, R. (1995). Ethnic identity of Asians in the United States. In J. G. Ponterotto, J. M. Casas, L.A. Suzuki, L.A., & C. M. Alexander (Eds.), *Handbook of multicultural counseling* (pp. 123–154). Thousand Oaks, CA: Sage.

Sodowsky, G. R., Maguire, K., Johnson, P., Kohles, R., Ngumba, W. et al. (1994). Worldviews of White America, mainland Chinese, Taiwanese, and African students in a midwestern university: An investigation into between-group differences. *Journal of Cross-Cultural Psychology, 25*, 309–324.

Stephenson, E. (2004). The African diaspora and culture-based coping strategies. In J. L. Chin (Ed.), *The psychology of prejudice and discrimination: Racism in America* (Vol. 1, pp. 95–118). Westport, CT: Praeger/Greenwood.

Sue, D., & Sundberg, N. B. (1996). Research and research hypotheses about effectiveness in intercultural counseling. In P. Pedersen, J. G. Draguns, W. J. Lonner, & J. E. Trimble (Eds.), *Counseling across cultures* (4th ed., pp. 323–352). Thousand Oaks, CA: Sage.

Sue, D. W. (1978). World views and counseling. *Personnel and Guidance Journal, 56*, 458–462.

Sue, D. W., Ivey, A. E., & Pedersen, P. B. (1996). *A theory of multicultural counseling and therapy*. Pacific Grove, CA: Brooks/Cole.

Sue, D. W., & Sue, D. (2008). *Counseling the culturally different: Theory and practice* (5th ed.). New York: John Wiley.

Suzuki-Crumly, J., & Hyers, L. L. (2004). The relationship among ethnic identity, psychological well-being, and intergroup competence: An investigation of two biracial groups. *Cultural Diversity and Ethnic Minority Psychology, 10*, 137–150.

Thompson, C. E., & Carter, R. T. (1997). An overview and elaboration of Helms' Racial Identity Development Theory. In C. E. Thompson, & R.T. Carter (Eds.), *Racial identity theory: Applications to individuals, group, and organizational interventions* (pp. 15–32). Mahwah, NJ: Erlbaum.

Umberson, D. (1993). Sociodemographic position, worldview, and psychological distress. *Social Science Quarterly, 74*, 575–589.

U.S. Bureau of the Census. (2001). *The two or more races population: 2000.* Retrieved from http://www.census.gov/prod/2001pubs/c2kbr01-6.pdf

Vandiver, B. J., Cross, W. E., Worrell, F. C., & Fhagen-Smith, P. E. (2002). Validating the Cross Racial Identity Scale. *Journal of Counseling Psychology, 49*, 71–85.

Wijeyesinghe, C. L., & Jackson, B. W., III. (Eds.). (2001). *New perspectives on racial identity development: A theoretical and practical anthology.* New York: New York University Press.

Wijeyesinghe, C. L. (Ed.). (2001). Racial identity in multiracial people: An alternative paradigm. In C. L. Wijeyesinghe & B. W. Jackson III (Eds.), *New perspectives on racial identity development: A theoretical and practical anthology* (pp. 129–152). New York: New York University Press.

Zak, I. (1973). Dimensions of Jewish American identity. *Psychological Reports, 33*, 891–900.

CHAPTER 4

Oppression, Power, and Privilege

The root of the word "oppression" is the element "press." The press of the crowd; pressed into military service; to press a pair of pants; printing press; press the button. Presses are used to mold things or flatten them or reduce them in bulk, sometimes to reduce them by squeezing out the gasses or liquids in them. Something pressed is something caught between or among forces and barriers which are so related to each other that jointly they restrain, restrict, or prevent the thing's motion or mobility. Mould. Immobilize. Reduce.

The experience of oppressed people is that the living of one's life is confined and shaped by forces and barriers which are not accidental or occasional and hence avoidable, but are systematically related to each other in such a way as to catch one between and among them and restrict or penalize motion in any direction. It is the experience of being caged in; all avenues, in every direction, are blocked or booby-trapped.

Cages. Consider a birdcage. If you look very closely at just one wire in the cage, you cannot see the other wires. If your conception of what is before you is determined by this myopic focus, you could look at that one wire, up and down the length of it, and be unable to see why a bird would not just fly around the wire any time it wanted to go somewhere. Furthermore, even if, one day at a time, you myopically inspected each wire, you still could not see why a bird would have trouble going past the wires to get anywhere. There is no physical property of any one wire, nothing that the closest scrutiny could discover, that will reveal how a bird could be inhibited or harmed by it except in the most accidental way. It is only when you step back, stop looking at the wires one by one, microscopically, and take a macroscopic view of the whole cage, that you can see why the bird does not go anywhere; and then you will see it in a moment. It will require no great subtly of mental powers. It is perfectly obvious that the bird is surrounded by a network of systematically related barriers, no one of which would be the least hindrance to its flight, but which, in their relations to each other, are as confining as the solid walls of a dungeon.

—Marilyn Frye (1995, pp. 81–84)

All of us can remember instances when we have felt inferior, shamed, lacking, or inadequate, or been denied access or opportunity for reasons we felt were unfair. Like the metaphor Frye (1995) uses in the above example, each of the instances you may remember are like the individual wires in the cage. **Oppression** is the experience of a host of such instances interlocking around a person, leading to systematic barriers that constrain and imprison him or her. In this chapter, we will discuss oppression and its related constructs.

Our race, ethnicity, class, gender, sexual orientation, physical and mental ability, age, and religious identities are all simultaneous and intersecting components of our personal identity. In isolation, any one of these identities is incomplete. Think about the consequences of being the only human being on Mars. Would your race matter? How about the language you speak? Or your sexual orientation? It is around other human beings that our social identities become meaningful.

All human societies have structured systems of rules that determine the relationships between individuals, between individuals and the community, and between individuals and the society as a whole. Within these systems of relationship, certain identity characteristics are determined to be significant; however, the significance of each component of an individual's identity differs in the different relationship systems. Consider the example of Louise, a 73-year-old African American woman who lives with her daughter and grandchildren in an ethnically mixed neighborhood of New York City. Louise minds the children and manages the household while her daughter works long hours as a registered nurse. As head of her family, a deacon in her church, and a vocal member of her block association, Louise enjoys a high socioeconomic status in her community. However, on this day, Louise must travel to midtown Manhattan to visit her cardiologist. Returning the greeting of a local storekeeper as she enters the subway, Louise savors this last taste of her local status before she heads downtown, to the place where she feels like "an old, Black nobody." As the train travels farther downtown and the mix of the passengers changes from mostly poor and mostly Black and Latino to

REFLECTION EXERCISE **4.1**

Generic human

Take a moment to visualize a human being who is "generic."

What does this person look like?

Notice that it is impossible to imagine a human being who does not have skin color, sex, a certain age, and so on. Also notice, that what skin color, sex, age, and other visible markers the person has will change the way that person is responded to and treated.

Now, visualize a person who is "heroic."

What does this person look like?

What personal or physical characteristics do you tend to associate with this person?

How similar or different are the generic person that you visualized and the heroic one? What does this exercise tell you about yourself, your culture, your worldview, and any inherent biases you may have learned?

From where did these images of the generic person originate? What about the heroic person?

mostly middle class and mostly White, Louise feels herself steadily transforming from a respected pillar of the community to a woman primarily characterized by her race, her age, and her relative poverty. Walking to her doctor's office in a sea of young, fashionably dressed office workers on their way to work, she forces herself to "hold her chin up high." But in her heart she knows that it doesn't matter what she does—no one is going to look at her.

It is not simply the "culturally different" or "special" populations that have complex identities. What all these groups so labeled have in common is that a characteristic of theirs has been deemed significant and therefore served as a focus of discrimination for a society. These characteristics tend to separate and define a group through one facet of identity, whether it be an easily perceivable characteristic, such as sex, skin color, and age, or a less visible one of sexual orientation, socioeconomic class identity, or religion. It is significant that even with the less immediately perceivable characteristics, there is a tendency to assign visible attendant signifiers to those characteristics, no matter how valid or invalid they may be. For instance, there is a whole system of folklore that assigns certain visible differences by which to identify gays and lesbians, making the invisible difference comfortably visible to the dominant social group of heterosexuals.

Social dominance theory (Sidanius, Levin, Federico, & Pratt, 2001) suggests three basic types of hierarchical systems: (a) *age systems*, in which persons identified as adults have disproportionate power over those perceived as children; (b) *patriarchal systems*, in which men have greater power relative to women; and (c) *arbitrary-set systems*, where characteristics such as race, caste, social class, clan, ethnicity, estate, religion, region of origin, sexual orientation, or disability are salient in demarcating power among groups of people. Different societies vary in the degree to which they are hierarchically organized and in the relative emphasis of each of the three systems, so that in some societies the social hierarchy may be more patriarchal than in others, whereas in other societies the hierarchy is more age based. However, they share commonalities in the processes used to establish and maintain such systems, and all societies have some combination of these systems. The third category, of arbitrary-set hierarchies, varies most across societies and is the most sensitive to social context. Take, for instance, racial identity. Former U.S. Secretary of State Colin Powell would be classified as *Black* in the United States but *non-Black* in Brazil, based on the respective classification system used in each country.

REFLECTION QUESTIONS 4.1

Consider the following questions:

- What does oppression mean to you, and how has it affected your life?
- Do you remember the first time you began to understand that prejudice existed?
- What is the source of most of your views toward members of cultural groups different from your own?
- How do your beliefs affect the way you interact with people from these groups?
- How has oppression affected the lives of people close to you?
- Do you consider yourself privileged or nonprivileged, and if so, in what ways?
- How has your privilege or lack thereof affected your view of the world?
- How have privilege and oppression strengthened your ability to empathize with the lives of other people who may be either similar to or different from you?
- What are your potential blind spots when it comes to understanding the experiences of others who are similar to or different from you?

MANIFESTATIONS OF OPPRESSION

The arbitrary set of group-based characteristics that is used in developing hierarchies of oppression varies across societies. In U.S. society, certain salient characteristics have been determined to be significant, and each manifests as a particular kind of oppression, resulting in what are commonly referred to in the multicultural literature as the *isms*.

Racism, for instance, is defined as the belief that one race is superior to others and therefore has the right to dominate, as well as the institutional power to do so. It is a pattern of attitudes and behavior that systematically tends to deny access to opportunities to certain social groups while affording privileges to members of another group (Ridley, 1995). **Sexism** is the belief that one sex is inherently superior to the other, and therefore has the right to dominate the other, as well as the institutional power to enforce that belief

(Frye, 1995). Similarly, **ableism** is the belief of temporarily able people that the ways in which they perceive, do, think, and feel are the only correct and normal ways of perceiving, doing, thinking, and feeling, and that those who are disabled are inferior to them and abnormal. **Heterosexism** is the belief that intimate relationships between men and women are superior to intimate relationships between the same gender, and are therefore more acceptable. **Homophobia** is the fear and rejection of gays, lesbians, and bisexuals (McHenry & Johnson, 1993). Similarly, **classism** is the oppression, based on socioeconomic differences, of the working class and poor; **ageism** is oppression, based on age, of the very young and the very old; and **anti-Semitism** is the oppression of Jewish people, based on a complex of culture and religion. You can see that even though each of these oppressions is based on a different aspect of identity, the common characteristics of all these manifestations of oppression are that they are based on the concept that different can never be equal. Only one way is the right way, which justifies the use of power to systematically enforce and institutionalize that oppressive belief system.

DEFINING OPPRESSION

Systemic classification and its effects on institutional frameworks, social structures, as well as community and family and interpersonal interactions, go beyond discrimination. They become oppression. There are a number of interrelated components to conceptualizing oppression. The main ones are prejudice, discrimination, institutional power, and systematic inequality. We will discuss each of these concepts in turn, building toward a definition of oppression that is based on these aspects.

Prejudice

Prejudice means, most simply, to prejudge. Prejudice is an attitude: a combination of feelings, inclinations to act, and beliefs (Myers, 2002). The beliefs out of which prejudice grows are stereotypes, generalizations that seek to categorize and separate information into distinct groups. Stereotypes arise from the need to simplify the world. For instance, stereotyping the British as reserved, professors as absentminded, and women who assume the title of *Ms.* as more assertive are all attempts to summarize and categorize the world. They tend to be representations of categories of persons. In and of themselves, stereotypes may be helpful, but they are often inaccurate, overgeneralized, and resistant to change (Lee, Jussim, & McCauley, 1995).

Prejudice defines the way in which members of social groups are stereotyped to have certain characteristics simply because they are members of those groups. The judgment may be benign or detrimental depending on the positive or negative value assigned to members of that group. An example of prejudice would be to believe that women are emotional. Perhaps such a belief may be considered benign in that women are believed to have more access to their emotions in contexts that demand emotion. However, in this judgment, then, men would be oppositionally considered as lacking such openness. When a belief about women's emotionality is negative, it means they can be considered irrational and hysterical. What makes this belief a prejudice is when it is applied to all women simply because they are female rather than applied specifically to an individual in response to her behavior. Although a perspective of oppression concerns itself mainly with negative prejudice toward some groups, it is important to not lose sight of the inclusion of all social groups into the oppressive system.

REFLECTION QUESTIONS 4.2

- With what personal characteristics or categories do you tend to pre-judge people in a positive way? In a negative way? In what ways does that affect those people if you are aware of it?
- With what personal characteristics or categories have you been pre-judged by others in a positive way? In negative way? What was the context of that experience? How did it affect or change you, if at all?

Discrimination

The second major component of oppression is the behavior toward a group and its individual members because they are members of that group. Again, discrimination without context can be either positive or negative in effect. For instance, enlisting an African American student to be on the basketball team regardless of his actual performance in the sport based on a belief that all African Americans youth are innately talented at basketball is discrimination based on prejudice. Note, however, that such discriminatory actions may end up having positive effects for that student in that he is given an opportunity that he otherwise might not have received, though more often it simply sets him up for failure to meet unrealistic expectations. An example of negative discrimination is the phenomenon known as *driving while Black*, where police routinely stop African Americans drivers on the suspicion that they are far more likely to engage in criminal activity occurring than drivers of other ethnic groups.

According to social psychology studies, although discrimination and prejudice are linked, the link is not always causal. Our behavior as humans is influenced by both our internal beliefs and external situational variables (Myers, 2002). For instance, a White male business manager may not feel he has prejudices, but if business deals are discussed at the local country club that does not allow women or People of Color, he discriminates against these groups because they do not have access to the sites where deals are made. "Business as usual" becomes discriminatory business.

Often, a ready counterargument to perceived discrimination is that the person who complains is hypersensitive or trying to explain away his or her own incompetence. In other words, "those people" must just be whining too much. Do those who experience discrimination exaggerate the discrimination they receive? Are they indeed hypersensitive? Major and Ruggiero (1998) conducted an interesting study on perceived discrimination, where they gave groups of men and women and White men and Black men a test regarding their future success. Each group was told that a judge from the opposite gender would evaluate their test results and that this judge had a tendency to discriminate against their gender group. The level of discrimination the judge was supposed to use varied among 100%, 75%, 50%, and 0%. The subjects were all told they didn't do well and were asked to explain their poor performance with the options of discrimination, quality of the test, quality of their answers, or lack of personal effort. At every level of discrimination, the researchers found that the women and the Black men were less likely to use an explanation of discrimination in low-performance evaluations, whereas White men were the most likely to use discrimination as an explanation for their poor performance. Thus, even though African American men and women may experience frequent discrimination, when offered the option, it is the White men who infrequently experience it who are readiest to use such explanations.

REFLECTION QUESTIONS 4.3

- Can you think of a time when you discriminated against someone else? What were your thoughts and feelings around this experience at the time? What are your thoughts and feelings around this experience reflecting back on it at this point?
- Can you think of a time when you were discriminated against by someone else? What were your thoughts and feelings around this experience at the time? What are your thoughts and feelings around this experience reflecting back on it at this point?
- How can these experiences help you become a better counselor?

Institutional Power

The degree of access to opportunities in society is institutional power. In simple terms, it's the question of whose voice is heard. Being heard can be as simple as having the most money so that you can bombard television with advertisements that get your point across and drown out others. It can also be as complicated as being a member of a group that is perceived by society to be normal and noteworthy and worth listening to (Sue, 2003). Institutional power is held by those networks that control powerful systems such as finance, media, religious institutions, and government. The degree to which you have access to such networks is the degree of privilege you have. We will speak more about the concept of privilege a little later.

Discrimination becomes oppression when behavior is linked with a structured way of dealing with members of society that has the given effect of subordinating people of a certain group and uplifting people of an opposing group. There may be no negative prejudicial intent among individual members of a given society, but the practice of "the way things are done" has discriminatory effects. For instance, a police force might set a certain height requirement of over 5 feet 10 inches for all its officers. The institutional reasoning might be that in some way, height causes greater on-the-job-effectiveness. It may also systematically exclude most women, as well as people of certain ethnic groups who are typically of a smaller height.

Finally, we come to developing a comprehensive definition of oppression that uses all of the previous constructs:

$$\text{Oppression} = \text{Prejudice} + \text{Discrimination} + \text{Institutional Power}$$

Oppression is the culmination of prejudice and discrimination together with an institutional power to create structures that passively as well as actively discriminate against certain groups and their members. Oppression of a group is always relative to another social group that has been given privilege and power. The system of domination and subordination requires a relationship between a target group and an agent group (Hardiman & Jackson, 1997). All oppressed groups have a link with a group that in turn receives privileges; thus men and women, European Americans and People of Color, and heterosexuals and gays, lesbians, and bisexuals all dance together in complex patterns of interdependence. It is crucial to recognize the connections so that one not only turns the focus of understanding oppression on those who suffer from it but also notices those who benefit from it.

Hanna, Talley, and Guindon (2000) describe two ways in which oppression comes about: by force and by deprivation. Oppression by force or duress imposes on others an object, role, label, or experience that is detrimental to physical and/or psychological well-being. These can range from actual physical intimidation and violence (such as searing images of police restraining marchers during the civil rights struggles of the 20th century) to abusive messages that are designed to cause pain, and may foster negative and distorted beliefs. Beyond simply imposing unpleasantness, oppression by deprivation works to confiscate those objects, experiences, and living conditions that are conducive and necessary to physical and psychological health. An example of this sort of oppression might be the federal government banning of the use of peyote by the Native American church during their worship rituals. Demeaning roles can be imposed, and desirable roles can be removed. One type of oppression does not preclude the other, and in many cases, both types are present in varying degrees.

REFLECTION QUESTIONS 4.4

- In what ways do you benefit from existing institutional systems of power?
- In what ways do you suffer based on existing institutional systems of power?
- If there was one thing about existing institutional systems of power that you could change, what would it be and why?

Systemic Inequality

One of the core issues of oppression is its systemic nature. The systemic structuring of inequality between groups of people—between European Americans and People of Color, between men and women, and between heterosexuals and gays, lesbians, and bisexuals—leads to enduring inequality and thus to oppression. There are instances of temporary inequality that are different from oppression. For instance, the relationships between parents and children, teachers and students, and, possibly, counselors and clients are examples of temporarily unequal relationships. In instances of temporary inequality, the rationale is that the subordinate member of the dyad has some ability, knowledge, or quality to gain from the superordinate member of the dyad, which justifies the inequality. This temporary nature is part of the unwritten contract in that when the subordinate person is brought up to full parity through the efforts of the superordinate person, the relationship will be one of equals. The paramount goal of the relationship is to end the inequality (Miller, 1986).

However, these relationships of temporary inequality are by no means free of trouble. The balance often tips toward the superordinate person's needs being served, rather than those of the subordinate. Or, the subordinate learns through the relationship how to be a good subordinate rather than ever achieving equality. There is really no solid central theory or concept that defines how the movement from lesser to equal may be achieved. Perhaps some of the confusion may come from the second type of inequality that permeates the society, molding the ways in which we perceive and conceptualize ourselves and our relationships to others.

In the situation of permanent inequality, the situation of oppression, there is little belief that the relationship will one day be equal. The superordinate member is superior due to reasons of inherent superiority, which means that the inequality will always continue. In effect, unequal status breeds prejudice, which in turn legitimizes discrimination. Enslaved or conquered people are likely to be assigned attributes that justify their unequal position. Once these attributes are assigned, treatment that ensures the superiority of the dominant group is justifiable (Johnson, 2001). Nineteenth-century Europeans justified colonization by describing the peoples they colonized as "inferior" and "requiring protection," and by claiming it was the "white man's burden" to protect them (Giddings, 1990).

The circular nature of oppression implies that due to institutional structures, many people may participate in oppressive acts while holding no consciously negative attitudes. Yet, oppressive acts breed negative attitudes, ensuring the continuation of the cycle. In an early study, Worchel and Andreoli (1978) found that subjects who were required to shock others for giving "wrong" answers on a learning task were more likely to dehumanize them. After the shocks were given, the subjects were less able to remember unique characteristics of the person they hurt, and better able to recall attributes such as race and gender, depersonalizing the victim by identifying him or her solely as a member of a group. The self-justification of one's own hurtful acts may lie in explaining away the individuality of the victim, or else in shifting the blame to the victim.

 REFLECTION QUESTIONS 4.5

- In what ways do you benefit from existing systems of inequality?
- In what ways do you suffer from existing systems of inequality?
- If there was one thing about current systems of inequality in your community that you could change, what would it be and why?
- How might you address systems of inequality as a part of effective counseling services?

CYCLES OF OPPRESSION

One way of thinking about oppression is to look at the cycle of oppression (see Figure 4.1). As you can see, we begin by being born into social groups that already have a relative social status within the dominant culture. We are taught ways of thinking about and justifying our status. So, if we are born female, we may learn from our parents about appropriate gender roles of who should work and who should stay home, go to school and have our teachers treat us differently from boys, be told that our greatest happiness will come when we get married and lose our maiden name and take on an identity based on our husband's, and go to work and have our ambition taken less seriously because we are going to put family first. We may be treated as hysterical or hypochondriacal by the medical system, inept by the financial system, inferior by the religious system, and unimportant by the political system. Given these profound experiences, it is no surprise that women are good students and act out the roles that have been assigned. Women may, in turn, pass on to their daughters and sons what has been taught, continuing the cycle to the next generation. The only way to interrupt the cycle is to take responsibility to unlearn misinformation, learn correct information, challenge messages, and work toward change.

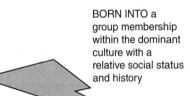

BORN INTO a group membership within the dominant culture with a relative social status and history

TAUGHT interpretations of history, explanations for injustice, norms (misinformation)

SIGNIFICANT TEACHERS: Parents, teachers, community, role models, religious authorities, political, leaders, media

MAINTAIN THE STATUS QUO by protecting and justifying privileges, inequities & unjust treatment, being thankful and not questioning structures, norms, messages, ideologies, etc.

TAKING RESPONSIBILITY FOR OURSELVES AND CHANGE by becoming aware of our roles in the perpetuation of oppression, taking personal, interpersonal, and organizational stands in our lives, unlearning misinformation and learning correct information, consciously and working towards change

REINFORCED & SANCTIONED BY culture, traditions, family, social institutions such as media, legal system, banks, government, education, health care, economy, language, religious institutions

PEOPLE "ACT OUT" PRESCRIBED ROLES of internalized oppression and externalized oppression

FIGURE **4.1** Cycle of Oppression

Source: Excerpted from Bobbie Harro, "The Cycle of Socialization," in M. Adams et al., *Readings for Diversity and Social Justice* (New York, Routledge Press). Copyright © 2000 Bobbie Harro. Reprinted with permission.

CASE STUDY **4.1**

The Case of Kara

Kara McGuire is a 32-year-old university librarian. She lives in San Jose, California, where she was born and raised. Kara's mother is first-generation Japanese American, and her father is Irish American. Kara is the oldest child in a family with three children. She has a younger sister and, in her words, a "baby brother." Kara has always wondered where she inherited her looks. She reports that her sister is tall and thin, and "looks white." Kara has always struggled with her weight, has dark eyes with a pronounced epicanthic fold, and has dark skin. Her family attended the local Catholic Church, which was located in a primarily Irish American community, but as she grew up, she reports that her family's church attendance fell away, and although they still are nominally Catholic, she thinks of herself as "lapsed." She feels she would have more in common with the Shintoism that was a part of her mother's upbringing, but knows little about it.

Kara has been under a lot of stress at work given the budget shortfalls that have left her understaffed. She says she has a hard time getting out of bed in the morning. She has gained 35 pounds in 3 months, and says that she seems to eat a lot in the evening, just sitting on the couch watching TV. "Its not that I'm hungry, either," she says, "but it's like I keep putting food in my mouth." She has been crying a lot; is socially withdrawn from her friends and family; finds it difficult to concentrate at work, where she has been making many mistakes; and has been drinking more alcohol to the point of becoming intoxicated most evenings.

Recently Kara and her colleagues were talking about the wife of a coworker. One of her White colleagues said, "She may have married White and rich, but she will always be a slanty-eyed Chink." Her colleague then said, "Don't take offense, Kara—I don't see you as Asian." Kara felt awkward but smiled and said, "Don't worry about it."

Kara has been married 6 years to an African American man, Tyler, but is currently separated from her husband, who moved out 2 months ago. For nearly 2 years, Kara had been feeling suspicious about Tyler. He was often out late or away from his job as a chiropractor for reasons of business or professional development. Kara had also found some receipts for gift purchases that were for a woman. When she asked Tyler if anything was wrong, he told her there wasn't.

She reports that she now knows he had been involved with various women throughout their marriage.

At a recent physical examination, Kara's physician noticed that in addition to her significant weight gain, her blood pressure was elevated. Kara has also been complaining of frequent headaches. Kara tearfully confided in her doctor about the challenges both at work and at home. Dr. Clemson diagnosed Kara's clinical depression and gave her a prescription for Wellbutrin. She also wrote down the name of a counselor and strongly recommended that Kara call her. Kara feels ashamed about her need for professional help, but she presents for counseling on the recommendation of her doctor. Her therapist is Ms. Carson, an African American woman with a master's degree in counseling.

Case Discussion
Thinking About This Case:
1. What are some aspects of Kara's presentation that could result from internalized oppression?
2. What are some aspects of Kara's presenting problems that could be due to the effects of oppression?
3. Might there be aspects of the relationship between the counselor and Kara that may be challenging for one or both?

In this case, it is important to notice how cultural heritage interacts with society's perceived valuing of that heritage to impact the individual experience. Although Kara and her sister are both Japanese American, Kara is impacted more by a sense of inferiority because of what she perceives as negative markers of darkness. Her experience as a woman also intersects with these markers. One example is an analysis of the ways that weight and size are constructed for women, particularly as markers of attractiveness and femininity. She may well blame herself for her husband's adultery, framing it in terms of her lack of attractiveness. With an African American female counselor, Kara may be able to address her feelings about being darker and how she was received. On the other hand, if the counselor does not reassure her adequately that such areas of discussion are a significant and valued part of the therapy, she may well work from a perspective that if she just fixes herself to be a better fit, everything will be fine. This would be very much an iatrogenic result, whereby her therapeutic work would suffer from the counselor's lack of receptivity.

Similar to the cycle of sexism, one can apply most forms of oppression within this model. The key component is to notice that the messages and structures of oppression are systematically taught and facilitated, and they have as much impact on those who benefit from that oppression as they do on those targeted by that oppression. Based on learned experiences, we may act out these messages targeting ourselves by acquiescing to the limitations placed on us, as well as act out against others. When we benefit from oppression, we tend not to notice the privileges that we get from being such beneficiaries.

CONTEXTS OF OPPRESSION

Just as oppression consists of prejudicial attitudes and beliefs, discriminatory behaviors, and social systems of dominance, it is maintained and perpetuated on different levels. The three levels of individual, institutional, and cultural and social oppression exist in the conscious and unconscious domains.

Individual Level

At this level, the focus is on the beliefs and behaviors of persons rather than social practices. This is the easily recognizable aspect of oppression as we look at acts of harassment, hate language, or exclusive behavior. What is more difficult to notice are the ways in which individuals who are agents or targets of oppression are influenced by social controls. Conscious individual acts include using racial slurs or a parent asking that his child's gay teacher be fired. The teacher who prides herself on being fair but ends up calling on boys far more often than on girls may well be acting unconsciously. In Example 4.1, the death of Vincent Chin was clearly an individual act. Yet, one can also see the social context of such individual acts, in the events that lead up to the attack as well as the consequences that followed.

EXAMPLE **4.1**
Murder of Vincent Chin

In 1982, a Chinese American man in Detroit, Michigan, was beaten to death by two European American men, Ronald Ebens and his stepson, Michael Nitz. Witnesses saw the two auto workers assail Chin with racial epithets, blaming people "like him" for the unemployment of auto workers resulting from the slump in the U.S. auto industry, as they beat him with a baseball bat. In 1983, they were convicted of manslaughter, and the judge sentenced them to fines and probation. The Asian Pacific American community sought the prosecution of the two on federal charges of violating Chin's civil rights. The U.S. Department of Justice filed the charges against Ebens and Nitz. In 1984, Ebens was convicted on one account and sentenced to 25 years in prison; Nitz was acquitted. But the conviction was overturned, and a retrial ordered. In 1987, a jury in Cincinnati cleared Ebens, saying that Chin's killing was not racially motivated.

Institutional Level

Oppression is shaped and maintained on this level through governmental, educational, corporate, religious, and familial institutions in the form of policies and procedures. At this level, we look at examples of housing discrimination against People of Color, denial of access to quality education for the poor and working class, and exclusions from country clubs, golf clubs, and civic groups of Jews, women, African Americans, and the poor.

A study (Center for Community Change, 2002) found that Latino and Black home owners with the same income as White counterparts paid much higher mortgage rates than did the White home owners. Often, such policies and procedures are not explicitly framed as exclusionary, but end up being so in practice. For instance, when colleges give preference to the children of alumni, such policies are not considered exclusive even though first-generation college applicants have a harder time getting in. A more lethal example of this kind of oppression was the Nazi Sterilization Program, based on the 1933 German law for the Prevention of Genetically Diseased Offspring. In this program, churches and doctors cooperated to register anyone known to have a "genetic illness" such as schizophrenia, epilepsy, blindness or deafness, "insanity," or "feeblemindedness" to the extent that 400,000 people were forcibly sterilized. After World War II, sterilization was never considered a war crime, and no one was held accountable for it, primarily because so many other countries (including the United States) had similar laws. As you can see from the examples above, institutional oppression can be both conscious and unconscious.

Cultural and Social Level

Norms and beliefs perpetuate values both explicitly and implicitly that shape the behavior of individuals and institutions. Philosophies about life, goodness, normality, health, deviance, and sickness often serve as justifications for the everyday acts that perpetuate oppression. A case in point is beliefs about men and women. If we believe that men get sex and women give sex, then it becomes easy to think about the difference between women's consensual sexual activity and forced sexual activity as simply a difference in degree rather than in kind. The step from belief to behavior leads to an ambivalent social attitude toward rape. So, whereas a victim of a mugging would never be told, "Well, you've given money to charity before, so how do we know you didn't want to give money in this case?" a victim of sexual assault might well be asked, "Well, you had sex before and wanted to, so how do we know you didn't want to in this case?"

In conscious cultural oppression, one might have movements such as the "English-only" movement that strives to place English as the official and only language of the United States, often with statements that it is the foundation of the country and that all immigrants should be expected to come in and learn this language. Such a position, of course, takes no account of the fact that English, too, is an immigrant import and that we might as well demand that everyone learn the local indigenous American Indian language. On unconscious levels, we might base standards of beauty among women on specific ethnic norms, privileging blond hair and blue eyes as universally beautiful norms to be aspired to.

Vertical and Horizontal Oppression

Oppression can be both vertical and horizontal. Vertical oppression is when members of the dominant group enforce subordinate status on members of an oppressed group. For instance, middle- and upper-class European American men often pass laws that directly impact poor women and People of Color. One of the fundamental tenets of the Revolutionary War was "no taxation without representation," where peoples in the United States refused to be subject to laws in which they had no voice. However, when there is no sufficient representation in Congress of People of Color and women, the process of government becomes vertical rather than participatory. Citizens who have been convicted of felonies, or who are below the age of 18, have no voice in any of the laws that directly affect their well-being and freedoms.

Horizontal oppression occurs in two ways. In one, members of the dominant group enforce status with other members of their group. Boys who don't conform to traditional "masculine" behaviors are often harassed by other boys. Similarly, when a European American girl is discouraged by her parents from dating a Chinese American boy, her dominant status is being enforced despite her own wishes. In the other form of horizontal oppression, members of marginalized groups enforce subordinate status amongst themselves. When African American adolescents make fun of their peers who strive to succeed in school, or gays oppose the participation of other gays in Pride marches who act too "stereotypical," subordinate status is being imposed.

PRIVILEGE

As mentioned earlier, privilege accrues from the access one has, based on one's membership in a socially dominant group. However, what makes that particular passport to being heard privilege is the degree to which that access is denied to others. Privilege creates a yawning divide in levels of income, wealth, dignity, safety, health, and general quality of life. In Example 4.2, see an excerpt from a famous article by Peggy McIntosh (1998), where she began to detail the ways in which she had invisible privilege as a White, heterosexual, middle-class woman. One of the key aspects of the privileges listed below and many others you may uncover for yourself is that they require no intentional activity. In essence, they are invisible because they do not have to be counted and, as McIntosh argues, are designed to engender obliviousness.

Johnson (2001) suggested that privilege isn't just a problem for those who don't have it, because privilege is always in relation to others. Because one person's access and opportunity are at someone else's expense, everything that is done to maintain it, however passive, results in deprivation for another. To be in a society where privilege is attached in various contexts to being White, male, heterosexual, middle class, Christian, or able-bodied means that persons who fall into those categories are part of the problem as long as they are not part of the solution.

Cullinan (1999) described three major presumptions of having privilege, namely, the presumption of innocence, the presumption of worthiness, and the presumption of competence. As an example of the first given of "innocent

EXAMPLE **4.2**
Invisible Knapsack

1. I can, if I wish, arrange to be in the company of people of my race most of the time.
2. I can avoid spending time with people whom I was trained to mistrust and who have learned to mistrust my kind or me.
3. If I should need to move, I can be pretty sure of renting or purchasing housing in an area which I can afford and in which I would want to live.
4. I can be reasonably sure that my neighbors in such a location will be neutral or pleasant to me.
5. I can go shopping alone most of the time, fairly well assured that I will not be followed or harassed by store detectives.
6. I can turn on the television or open to the front page of the paper and see people of my race widely and positively represented.
7. When I am told about our national heritage or about "civilization," I am shown that people of my color made it what it is.
8. I can be sure that my children will be given curricular materials that testify to the existence of their race.
9. I can be fairly sure of having my voice heard in a group in which I am the only member of my race.
10. I can go into a book shop and count on finding the writing of my race represented, into a supermarket and find the staple foods that fit with my cultural traditions, [and] into a hairdresser's shop and find some-one who can deal with my hair.
11. Whether I use checks, credit cards, or cash, I can count on my skin color not to work against the appearance that I am financially reliable.
12. I did not have to educate our children to be aware of systemic racism for their own daily physical protection.
13. I can be pretty sure that my children's teachers and employers will tolerate them if they fit school and workplace norms; my chief worries about them do not concern others' attitudes toward their race.
14. I can talk with my mouth full and not have people put this down to my color.
15. I can swear, or dress in secondhand clothes, or not answer letters, without having people attribute these choices to the bad morals, the poverty, or the illiteracy of my race.
16. I can be late to a meeting without having the lateness reflect on my race.
17. I can speak in public to a powerful male group without putting my race on trial.
18. I can do well in a challenging situation without being called a credit to my race.
19. I am never asked to speak for all the people of my racial group.

(continues)

Example **4.2** *(continued)*

20. I can choose blemish cover or bandages in "flesh" color and have them more or less match my skin.
21. I can remain oblivious to the language and customs of persons of color who constitute the world's majority without feeling in my culture any penalty for such oblivion.
22. I can criticize our government and talk about how much I fear its policies and behavior without being seen as a cultural outsider.
23. If a traffic cop pulls me over or if the IRS audits my tax return, I can be sure I haven't been singled out because of my race.
24. I can easily buy posters, postcards, picture books, greeting cards, dolls, toys, and children's magazines featuring people of my race.
25. I can be sure that if I need legal or medical help, my race will not work against me.
26. I can easily find academic courses and institutions that give attention only to people of my race.
27. If I have low credibility as a leader, I can be sure that my race is not the problem.
28. I can go home from most meetings of organizations I belong to feeling somewhat tied in, rather than isolated, out of place, outnumbered, unheard, held at a distance, or feared.
29. I can think over many options, social, political, imaginative, or professional, without asking whether a person of my race would be accepted or allowed to do what I want to do.
30. I can be pretty sure of finding people who would be willing to talk with me and advise me about my next steps, professionally.
31. If I declare there is a racial issue at hand, or there isn't a racial issue at hand, my race will lend me more credibility for either position than a person of color will have.
32. I am not made acutely aware that my shape, bearing, or body odor will be taken as a reflection on my race.
33. I can take a job with an affirmative action employer without having my coworkers on the job suspect that I got it because of my race.
34. If my day, week, or year is going badly, I need not ask of each negative episode or situation whether it has racial overtones.

Source: Excerpted from P. McIntosh, "White Privilege and Male Privilege: A Personal Account of Coming to see Correspondences Through Work in Women's Studies," Working Paper 189 from the Wellesley College Center for Research on Women, Wellesley MA 02181. Copyright © 1988 by Peggy McIntosh. Reprinted with permission.

until proven guilty," if you are privileged and are leaving a store when the alarm goes off, many times you will be asked kindly to return as the sales clerk checks the bags to see where she made a mistake in not demagnifying an item. On the other hand, those not so privileged are often assumed to have been stealing before their accusers look for explanations of mistakes.

The experience of those without privilege is "guilt by association." If other members of your group are suspected of being guilty, you are more likely to be. So, if a crime is committed by a Latino man, all Latino men in that community are treated with suspicion.

The second presumption of worthiness is that those with privilege believe that they are generally deserving of the attention, success, services, and respect that they receive. The opposite of this presumption, of course, is that others are immoral, bad, and undeserving. This leads to what has been called the "just world belief" (Lerner, 1998), where people get what they deserve and deserve what they get. In other words, when bad things happen to people, they must have deserved them. This may lead to blaming the victim for what has occurred to them.

The final presumption of competence, the belief that certain persons can do the work and meet expectations, is withheld from those without such privilege. For instance, because of misunderstanding about the ways that affirmative action works, People of Color are often judged incompetent until they can prove differently. The powerful nature of such beliefs about our competence or incompetence was strikingly demonstrated by what is known as the *Pygmalion effect* (Rosenthal & Jacobson, 1968), based on a study where young children whose new teachers were told about the children's fictitious levels of competence had began to display the level of competence expected of them by their teachers, regardless of their previous performance.

CASE STUDY **4.2**

The Case of Johnny

Mrs. J, an African American woman in her early 30s, brought in her 14-year-old son Johnny to see you in November. She is a single parent. She reported that she was concerned because in the last couple of months, Johnny was having problems at home and in school. Johnny had three younger siblings living at home. Mrs. J is a full-time waitress and works from 5 a.m. until late in the evening. Mrs. J's mother often assists with the children, and a neighbor looks after them occasionally. Johnny took care of them in the morning, giving them breakfast that Mrs. J had laid out, and got them on the bus. After he returned from school, he made sure they ate and did their homework. Mrs. J's sister, Mary, with her two children, a boy and a girl of 13 and 10, recently moved into the house while their own apartment was being repaired. Because Mary is not working currently, she has taken over the morning and afternoon rituals with the children. She complains that Johnny does not

seem to listen to her, and Mrs. J too has found Johnny very silent and "different" at home lately.

Mrs. J reported that Johnny's problems of acting out, being disrespectful and talking back to teachers at school, and fighting seemed to be escalating, and she worries that he will join a gang. His teachers at a primarily European American high school where he is a freshman told Mrs. J that Johnny is very threatening and uncooperative. She says he did not have those problems in his middle school, which was more diverse. When he moved to the high school, he had to take the bus and early on complained to his mother that he was being harassed. Lately he does not say much. One of the few teachers he does not seem to have a problem with is Ms. Williams, who is an African American social studies teacher. He also enjoys working with Mr. Simmons, who teaches shop and is an older European American man. Johnny himself is unresponsive, and does not seem

(continues)

to say much. He is almost six feet tall, and his mother says that this last growth spurt happened almost overnight, and it is hard to keep him in clothes that fit.

Case Discussion

Thinking About This Case

1. How might you conceptualize the problems Johnny is having?
2. In working with Johnny, what sorts of interventions might be helpful and effective?
3. How might your identities and understanding of oppressions influence the therapeutic relationship you can build with Johnny?

Although this is a common problem in schools, where African American youth are often characterized as troublemakers, it is important to notice issues such as timing. A cue to the contextual nature of the situation is that Johnny's new reputation as a troublemaker has only developed in the last couple of months after entering a new, largely White school. Although it might be easier to see this as Johnny's problem to adapt to the situation and that his conflicts arise from his inability to deal with his new environment, an effective helper must acknowledge that he has complained of harassment. Realistically, he is probably experiencing micro-insults and aggressions on a daily basis. His recent silence may well be a result of his deciding that no one can help him rather than a sign that the harassment has ended. Given that he is comfortable with the African American teacher and the male teacher, he is not universally perceived as threatening. Because his mother says he has recently shot up to his new height, another aspect is how African American males are perceived through an oppressive lens. When he was smaller, behavior that would have been seen as impulsive but unexceptional might suddenly be perceived as threatening when acted out by a 6-foot-tall Black male. Johnny himself may be getting accustomed to his new body. African American youth may well react to being continually misperceived as threatening by deciding to assert themselves in the only way allowed to them and evoke fear to get power if no other means is provided. Another cue is that Johnny is used to being a caretaker with his siblings, being the man of the house. He has now been displaced at home in that role with the arrival of his aunt and feels his identity assaulted everywhere. Like every other adolescent, he is striving to find a place for himself in the world, while being beset by oppressive and racist forces.

White Privilege and White Supremacy

Given the nature of the Unites States as a nation founded on ideals of liberty and justice, yet also paradoxically built with slavery, racism is an underlying factor in much of society. Smith (2007) developed a historical treatise tracing the development of racial groupings as a social construct that developed into a systemic and pervasive caste system. In this text, we use the term *European American* to distinguish actual peoples who carry a European ethnic heritage from the oppressive structure of *Whiteness*, a way of separating people into dominant and subordinate groups. **White privilege** is based on advantages that accrue from being designated White. Because it is based on being born into a racial categorization, many people who are not intentionally racist will still benefit without wishing to or knowing it. White privilege works because it seems normative such that those who do have it may not even notice it, whereas those without it carry an extra layer of burden. Reflection Exercise 4.2 highlights some examples of these subtle and pervasive privileges. **White supremacy** is a term that may seem intimidating to many people who associate it as a descriptor of hate groups such as the Ku Klux Klan, and associate it with overt aggressive violence. Actually, it is used to refer to an entire system designed to maintain White economic, legal, political, and social privilege. It is a historically based system of exploitation and domination that was originally used to justify slavery and

REFLECTION EXERCISE **4.2**

The Privilege Chart

Fill in the following chart by listing as many privileges as you can think of that you either have or do not have based on each of the dimensions of your own personal and cultural identity.

Dimensions of Personal and Cultural Identity	Privilege	Nonprivilege
Ability and attractiveness		
Age		
Ethnicity and race		
Gender		
Generational status and history		
Language and nationality		
Religion and spirituality		
Sexual orientation		
Socioeconomic class		

Questions for Reflection:

- What feelings and insights occur to you as you create your list of privileges or nonprivileges?
- What important life memories and critical incidents does this stir up for you?
- How might you use what you've learned from this exercise to better assist your clients?

colonization, but has become entrenched as a means of justifying and consistently advantaging White people (Smith, 2007). It consists of layers, so that one level might be the overt discrimination of public segregation, and another level is an absence of protection for People of Color, police and other public servants who enforce discriminatory laws, and individual citizens who obey those laws.

INTERNALIZED OPPRESSION

If dominant groups require certain attitudes and beliefs to justify their privileges, this must have some effect on the subordinate groups. Oppression resides not only in external social institutions and structures but also within the human beings who make up such systems (Fanon, 1967; Freire, 1970; Miller, 1986). Identity formation is an interactive process between the individual and society that is highly influenced by the norms and values of the family and society at large (Erikson, 1968). Members of subordinate groups get the same messages that dominant group members do. However, in this case the content of the message has negative implications about their capacity to succeed, their power, and, even more simply, their presence, giving rise to significant influences on identity and worldview.

It is hard to miss the impact of the different social values given to different groups. For instance, research shows that children of color can differentiate between their own color and the color they would like to be. In a famous early study asking young Black children to color a figure the color they were and to color another figure the color they like, 90% of the children colored the first figure dark, and over 50% colored the second figure with a light crayon (Clark and Clark, 1950). Most children of color have experienced hearing derogatory ethnic slurs in the schoolyard, which are often reinforced more covertly by authority figures (Aboud, 1988). If one is consistently rejected, one would understandably begin to question and doubt whether one and one's group really deserve any more respect from society than what they are given [See Example 4.3]. Oppression is introjected, such that the oppressed member perceives himself or herself as the despised and self-despising other. No stigmatized groups can escape the intrapsychic effects of oppression; thus, they may define themselves in terms of the stigmatized characteristics, with some degree of ambivalence, guilt, alienation, and self-hatred. Studies of different types of stigma show that no matter what the stigma, individuals from those stigmatized groups go through a process in which they have the task of integrating the stigmatized aspect into their identities. Feelings of shame, guilt, confusion, and alienation result when the person discovers or admits to belonging to the stigmatized group, and strives to fit the negative stereotypes into his or her self-image and make meaning of them (Fein & Nuehring, 1981; Hanley-Hackenbruck, 1989; Masterson, 1988; Sanders & Kroll, 2000).

EXAMPLE **4.3**
Sexist Messages to Women

When a woman believes she is inferior to men, could it be that she has internalized a long history of subordinate-status messages demonstrated across history, culture, and religion such as the following?

- "One hundred women are not worth a single testicle."—Confucius (551–479 BCE)
- "A proper wife should be as obedient as a slave" and "The female is a female by virtue of a certain lack of qualities—a natural defectiveness."—Aristotle (384–322 BCE)
- "In childhood a woman must be subject to her father; in youth to her husband; when her husband is dead, to her sons. A woman must never be free of subjugation."—The Hindu Code of Manu (c. 100 CE)
- "Men are superior to women."—The Koran (c. 650)

(continues)

Example 4.3 *(continued)*

- "Woman in her greatest perfection was made to serve and obey man, not rule and command him."—John Knox (1505–1572)
- "The souls of women are so small that some believe they've none at all."—Samuel Butler (1612–1680)
- "What a misfortune to be a woman! And yet, the worst misfortune is not to understand what a misfortune it is."—Kierkegaard (1813–1855)
- "Blessed art thou, O Lord our God and King of the Universe, that thou didst not create me a woman."—Daily prayer, still in use, of the Orthodox Jewish male
- "It seems to me that nearly every woman I know wants a man who knows how to love with authority. Women are simple souls who like simple things, and one of the simplest is one of the simplest to give.... Our family Airedale will come clear across the yard for one pat on the head. The average wife is like that. She will come across town, across the house, across to your point of view, and across almost anything to give you her love if you offer her yours with some honest approval."—Episcopal Bishop James Pike in a letter to his son (1968)

It is necessary to simultaneously see the similarities in the experience of oppressed groups as part of an overall experience of oppression, while perceiving the differences in that experience. Groups oppressed by racism have a set of within-group constructs, such as a shared experience of racism within the family and community (if the person of color has not been adopted by a European American family). One is born into an oppressed situation in racism by virtue of birth as a person of color.

Women, on the other hand, although being born into oppression by virtue of sex transformed to a social construction of gender, have oppression within their families and communities in the presence of intimate oppressor models of fathers and brothers. With these male relatives, there are often ties of affection as well as oppression, such that a daughter might get both tenderness from her father and messages from him regarding her fragility and a refusal to allow her to obtain higher education on the grounds that it is wasted on girls.

Gays, lesbians, and bisexuals, when they come to a realization of their sexual orientation, give up the privileges of a heterosexual identity and take on a stigmatized identity. In the process, they may have to sacrifice affectional ties with those kin who reject them for their sexual orientation. Persons who are not born with disabilities have to similarly give up the ideal of an able-bodied identity, and perceive themselves as the focus of the stigma of disability that they have learned about others.

These different experiences of oppression and resulting differences in identity have profound effects on internalized oppression and the process of accepting or reclaiming the stigmatized identity. Thus, although a gay man may have to come to terms with his fears about society's reactions to his sexual orientation, he may also have to work through his own internalized self-loathing based on messages he has heard from his own family about homosexuality. On the other hand, an Asian girl may receive messages at school about being too passive, but she also has her family and community's contradictions of those messages.

One of the significant results of such differential experiences is that members of an oppressed group may not wish to count themselves as oppressed. For instance, a woman may say that she doesn't like other women and prefers men. Such a statement echoes the messages she has received about women, which she has managed to apply to all women other than herself. By allying herself with men, she can distance herself from the negative messages. Such a statement is often received benignly by those around her. Now imagine a man saying as publicly that he doesn't like men and prefers to be with women. Such a statement will be less well received and may carry connotations that the man isn't properly masculine.

An oppressed group has to concentrate on survival. In a society dominated by an outlook and belief system that characterize members of the group negatively, honest, direct response to oppressive treatment must be restricted. Open, self-initiated actions have resulted—and still can result, in some cases—in death. After all, both Malcolm X and Martin Luther King Jr. were assassinated.

In less overt ways, individuals who do not conform to the belief system and who challenge it may find economic hardship, social ostracism, and psychological isolation as their rewards (Frye, 1995). It is hardly surprising, then, that members of a subordinate group may resort to disguised and indirect ways of acting and reacting, with actions designed to accommodate the dominant beliefs while often containing hidden defiance.

To be able to play this dangerous game, oppressed peoples have to know their oppressors very well. They have to be attuned to and extremely sensitive to dominant group members' reactions and their implications (Hanna et al., 2000). Examples of this sensitivity and knowledge can be seen in the behavior of African Americans during the segregation era. Knowing the needs of European Americans, they shuffled their feet, always used an honorific such as "sir" or 'ma'am," and spoke in dialectical English when addressing European Americans. All of this confirmed for European Americans their inherent superiority and made them safe, because, as African Americans knew, if that sense of superiority was threatened, the lives and well-being of African Americans would be threatened in retaliation (Giddings, 1990).

If the survival of oppressed groups depends on knowing their oppressors very well, there may be little possibility or purpose in knowing oneself. Self-knowledge comes from action and interaction; to the extent that the range of action or interaction of oppressed groups is limited, so will a realistic sense of self be limited. A paradoxical effect may occur. On the one hand, members of oppressed groups have internalized negative beliefs, while at the same time they have experiences and perceptions that reflect different truths about themselves and the injustice that they experience. These within-group, self-generated concepts may collide with the internalized mythology of the oppressors, creating a continuing and internal sense of dissonance (Sue, 2003).

OPENING THE DIALOGUE ON OPPRESSION, POWER, AND PRIVILEGE

With all of the topics discussed in this chapter, you are now challenged to think through how you would utilize this information in session with any number of clients from a variety of cultural backgrounds and worldviews. Questions for reflection offered to you throughout this chapter also serve as excellent process questions for opening the dialogue with clients on oppression, power, and privilege. Some of these questions are listed here to assist you in terms of opening the dialogue with your clients:

- What does oppression mean to you, and how has it affected your life as well as your presenting issue?
- Do you remember the first time you began to understand that prejudice existed?
- What is the source of most of your views toward members of cultural groups different from your own?
- How do your beliefs affect the way you interact with people from these groups?
- How has oppression affected the lives of people close to you?
- Do you consider yourself privileged or nonprivileged, and if so, in what ways?
- How has your privilege or lack thereof affected your view of the world as well as your presenting issue?

Prejudice

- With what personal characteristics or categories do you tend to prejudge people in a positive way? In a negative way? In what ways does that affect those people if you are aware of it?
- With what personal characteristics or categories have you been prejudged by others in a positive way? In a negative way? What was the context of that experience? How did it affect or change you, if at all? How does it affect your presenting issue in counseling?

Discrimination

- Can you think of a time when you discriminated against someone else? What were your thoughts and feelings around this experience at the time? What are your thoughts and feelings around this experience reflecting back on it at this point?
- Can you think of a time when you were discriminated against by someone else? What were your thoughts and feelings around this experience at the time? What are your thoughts and feelings around this experience reflecting back on it at this point?

- How have these experiences affected what it is you are bringing to counseling, and what it is that you are struggling with? How have the ways that you dealt with these experiences empowered you to be able to deal better with any variety of struggles?

Institutional Power

- In what ways do you benefit from existing institutional systems of power?
- In what ways do you suffer based on existing institutional systems of power?
- If there was one thing about existing institutional systems of power that you could change, what would it be and why? How could you go about making this change, and how can I help?

Systemic inequality

- In what ways do you benefit from existing systems of inequality?
- In what ways do you suffer from existing systems of inequality?
- If there was one thing about current systems of inequality in your community that you could change, what would it be and why? How could you go about making this change, and how can I help?
- How might we address systems of inequality as a part of effective counseling services for you?

Privilege

- What feelings and insights occur to you as you create your list of privileges or nonprivileges?
- What important life memories and critical incidents does this activity stir up for you?
- What insights does this offer to you based on what you are struggling with right now in your life?
- How might you use what you've learned from this exercise to help you better deal with your issue(s) or make some constructive life choices for yourself?

CONCLUSION AND IMPLICATIONS

Incorporating a framework of oppression into the structures of counseling has a number of implications on a variety of levels, including diagnosis, intervention, and process in terms of the therapeutic relationship itself. On another level, there are implications for what counseling sees as part of its purpose, and the need to develop new ways to meet that purpose. Counseling can be more destructive than any distress when the chaotic context of our lives is invalidated by the expert to whom we have come to get help.

In devising interventions and treatment plans to work with the presenting issues of the client, counselors need to keep in mind the contexts in which people live. There can be a huge problem of denial if one ignores the power of systems of oppression that begin operating as soon as children come in contact with the world outside of themselves, and that continue to exercise power throughout their adult lives. Counselors who devise interventions that do not take into account the support systems and resources that need to be in place before systemic thinking can be challenged should not be surprised at the failure of their interventions.

Similarly, in the process of counseling, awareness of the client's experience or struggle with oppressions enables the therapist to be more effective. The process can be affected by both the client's and the counselor's unexamined privilege. Client resistance or anger toward a counselor during critical pieces of work can be fueled by oppressive assumptions that the client holds about the counselor's group membership. Hardy (1993) reported a case of working with a 9-year-old White boy who confronted him with the words "I want a White doctor" (p. 50). Hardy went on to say that as the boy continued to use racist stereotypes and argue with him, he did not know what to do. Nothing in his training had addressed the issue of being perceived as less than competent because of his African American identity.

An unspoken assumption that may permeate counselor training is that dealing with oppression is marginal to the task of counseling. Somehow, when clients present their problems, oppressive attitudes, beliefs, and behaviors, whether acted out by the client or acted upon the client, are considered peripheral to their *real* issues. Hardy (1993) found that the social forces that control the ways in which we relate to each other do not respect the sanctity of the counseling room, and will not be left at the door. They are as present in counseling as they are anywhere else. Yet Hardy's training team, who were all European American, told him to ignore the content of the boy's speech, advising him instead to focus on the "underlying process and deeper therapeutic dynamics" (Hardy, 1993, p. 52). If training programs for counselors do not acknowledge and address these realities effectively, they will churn out counselors who consciously or unconsciously deny oppression in the lives of their clients and themselves, and paralyze either the client or themselves in the process.

At present, counselors work with the visible *symptoms* of oppression, seeing client after client who has an endless stream of issues such as low self-esteem, a lack of self-confidence, loneliness and fears, self- and other-destructive anger, substance abuse problems, eating disorders, and depression. Training programs continue to focus on ways to treat these manifest symptoms while downplaying the systemic causal factors that cluster the effects among socially oppressed groups of people. Simultaneously, counselors work with remanded or mandatory clients who have abused others and committed other crimes against others who are members of oppressed groups. Yet, the counseling profession has been muted traditionally about acknowledging and addressing oppression in counseling.

At the deepest level, the most critical implication of acknowledging the presence and impact of oppression is the imperative to challenge it. Being systemic, oppression becomes part of the way things are. If counselors accept the task of challenging and confronting oppression in counseling, the invisible walls that are structured to divide us become apparent. Only in recognizing the interconnecting bars of the cage can we take seriously the immobilization of the prisoner. Recognition of imprisonment leaves an ethical obligation on the part of all well-intentioned helpers to act in ways that release prisoners from imprisonment rather than further restricting them.

To complete the circle, we end with a metaphor of another imprisoned bird. There is a story told in rural parts of north India (and probably other places too, because it seems apocryphal) of a man who went to a sage revered for his knowledge, determined to ask an unanswerable question. He caught a bird and held it in his hands behind his back, resolving to ask the sage if the bird was alive or dead. If the sage answered, "Alive," the man would crush the bird to death, and if the sage answered, "Dead," the man would open his hands to reveal a live bird. Either way, the supposedly wise sage would be wrong. The man then came to the sage and triumphantly asked, "Oh master, tell me if this bird I hold in my hands is alive or dead?" The sage replied quietly, "It is in your hands."

In forthcoming chapters, we will be examining in detail the constructs such as race, gender, socioeconomic class, sexuality, disability, age, and religion, as well as the ways in which holding a particular aspect of identity shapes individual experience. As we continue to explore these concepts, there are some important points to keep in mind.

No one is born wanting to oppress or be oppressed. As the musical *South Pacific* articulates, "We have to be carefully taught to hate and fear." The identities into which we are born are not chosen. Therefore, none of us can be blamed for the identities we hold on an innate level. However, although we cannot be blamed for being White or male or straight or Christian or able-bodied, we can be held accountable for the privileges we have based on status. Although we cannot change the past, we are responsible for the present and the collective future. No one is completely responsible, and no one is let off the hook. Due to the number of identities, alternative sets of characteristics used to justify oppressive hierarchies in society, the majority of persons simultaneously hold both oppressive and oppressed positions. It is this interplay of experiences that shapes our perspectives (Croteau, Talbot, Lance, & Evans, 2002). Ultimately, because life is a one-way journey, all of us, no matter how many privileges of identity status we hold, will get old and face a society that does not care for us. Acknowledging these dimensions of oppression allows us to move past guilt and paralysis into action and emancipation. After all, although the structures of the systems of oppression may be beyond us, the action we can take is in our hands.

GLOSSARY

Ageism: Individual, interpersonal, and institutional discrimination toward and subordination of people based on their age, such that the very old and very young have little power or status.

Ableism: Individual, interpersonal, and institutional discrimination toward and subordination of people based on their physical or mental abilities. Those people designated as able-bodied have status and privilege compared to those designated as disabled.

Anti-Semitism: A system of prejudice and discrimination against Jewish people.

Classism: Individual, interpersonal, and institutional discrimination toward and subordination of people based on their socioeconomic status. Those peoples designated as ruling class, upper class, or rich have status and privilege compared to those designated as poor or working class.

Heterosexism: Individual, interpersonal, and institutional discrimination toward and subordination of people based on their sexual orientation. Those people designated as heterosexual are considered normative, and have status and privilege compared to those designated as gay, lesbian, bisexual, or transgender.

Homophobia: Fear of and hatred toward people identified as gay, lesbian, bisexual, or transgender, expressed in prejudice and discriminatory acts, including emotional and physical violence.

Oppression: The domination of subordinate groups in society through prejudice, discrimination, and access to political, economic, social, and cultural power.

Oppression is exemplified by specific manifestations of racism, sexism, classism, ableism, ageism, heterosexism, anti-Semitism, and religious discrimination.

Privilege: Advantages, favors, or immunities specially accrued through membership in a dominant group that are withheld from members of subordinate groups.

Racism: Individual, interpersonal, and institutional discrimination toward and subordination of peoples based on their racial classification. Those people designated as White have status and privilege compared to those designated as People of Color.

Religious discrimination: Individual, interpersonal, and institutional discrimination toward and subordination of people based on their religious affiliation. In the United States, those people designated as Christian have status and privilege compared to those who are affiliated with Judaism, Islam, Hinduism, Buddhism, Zoroastrianism, Wicca, and other indigenous or nature-based spiritual belief systems.

Sexism: Individual, interpersonal, and institutional discrimination toward and subordination of people based on their gender classification. Those peoples designated as male have status and privilege compared to those designated as women.

White privilege: Advantages that are assigned based on being designated as White.

White supremacy: An entire system designed to maintain White economic, legal, political, and social privilege.

REFERENCES

Aboud, F. (1988). *Children and prejudice*. New York: Basil Blackwell.

Center for Community Change. (2002, May 1). Study of racial disparities found in costs of mortgages. *New York Times*, Retrieved from http://www. nytimes.com/2002/05/01/us/wide-racial-disparities-found-in-costs-of-mortgages.html.

Clark, K. B., & Clark, M. P. (1950). Emotional factors in racial identification and preference among Negro children. *Journal of Negro Education. 19*, 341–350.

Croteau, J. M., Talbot, D. M., Lance, T. S., & Evans, N. J. (2002). A qualitative study of the interplay between privilege and oppression. *Journal of Multicultural Counseling and Development*, 30(4), 239–258.

Cullinan, C. (1999). Vision, privilege, and the limits of tolerance. *Electronic Magazine of Multicultural Education.* Retrieved from http://www.eastern.edu/publications/emme/1999spring/cullinan.html

Erikson, E. H. (1968). *Identity, youth, and crisis.* New York: Norton.

Fanon, F. (1967). *Black skin, white masks.* New York: Grove Press.

Fein, S., & Nuehring, E. (1981). Intrapsychic effects of stigma: A process of breakdown and reconstruction of social reality. *Journal of Homosexuality*, 7, 3–13.

Freire, P. (1970). *Pedagogy of the oppressed.* New York: Seabury.

Frye, M. (1995). Oppression. In P. S. Rothenberg (Ed.), *Race, class, and gender in the United States: An integrated study* (3rd ed., pp. 81–84). New York: St. Martin's Press.

Giddings, P. (1990). *When and where I enter: The impact of Black women on race and sex in America.* New York: Bantam.

Hanley-Hackenbruck, P. (1989). Psychotherapy and the "coming out" process. *Journal of Gay & Lesbian Psychotherapy*, 1(1), 21–39.

Hanna, F. J., Talley, W. B., & Guindon, M. H. (2000). The power of perception: Towards a model of cultural oppression and liberation. *Journal of Counseling and Development*, 78(4), 430–441.

Hardiman, R., & Jackson, B. (1997). Conceptual foundations for social justice courses. In M. Adams, L. A. Bell, & P. Griffin (Eds.), *Teaching for diversity and social justice: A sourcebook.* New York: Routledge.

Hardy, K. (1993). No refuge from racism: War of the worlds. *Family Therapy Networker*, 17(4), 50–57.

Harro, B. (2000). The cycle of socialization. In M. Adams, W. J. Blumenfeld, R. Castañeda, H. Hackman, M. Peter, & X. Zúñiga (Eds.), *Readings for diversity and social justice: An anthology on racism, anti-Semitism, sexism, heterosexism, ableism, and classism.* New York: Routledge.

Johnson, A. G. (2001). *Privilege, power, and difference.* New York: McGraw-Hill.

Lee, Y. T., Jussim, L. J., & McCauley, C. R. (1995). *Stereotype accuracy: Towards appreciating group differences.* Washington, DC: American Psychological Association.

Lerner, M. J. (1998). The two forms of belief in a just world: Some thoughts on why and how people care about justice. In L. Montada & M. J. Lerner (Eds.), *Responses to victimizations and belief in a just world* (pp. 247–270). New York: Plenum.

Major, B. N., & Ruggiero, K. M. (1998). Group status and attributions to discrimination: Are low or high status group members more likely to blame their failure on discrimination? *Personality and Social Psychology Bulletin*, 24(8). Retrieved from http://www.hrzone.com/articles/see_discrimination.html

Masterson, J. (1988). *The search for the real self.* New York: Free Press.

McHenry, S., & Johnson, J. (1993). Homophobia in the therapist and gay or lesbian client: Conscious and unconscious collusions in self-hate. *Psychotherapy*, 30(1), 141–151.

McIntosh, P. (1988). White privilege and male privilege: A personal account of coming to see correspondences through work in women's studies (Working Paper 189). Wellesley, MA: Wellesley College Center for Research on Women.

Miller, J. B. (1986). *Towards a new psychology of women.* Boston: Beacon Press.

Myers, D. G. (2002). *Social psychology* (7th ed.). New York: McGraw-Hill.

Ridley, C. R. (1995). *Overcoming unintentional racism in counseling and therapy: A practitioner's guide to intentional intervention.* Thousand Oaks, CA: Sage.

Rosenthal, R., & Jacobson, L. (1968). *Pygmalion in the classroom.* New York: Holt, Rinehart & Winston.

Sanders, G. L., & Kroll, I. T. (2000). Generating stories of resilience: Helping gay and lesbian youth and their families. *Journal of Marital and Family Therapy*, 26(4), 433–442.

Sidanius, J., Levin, S., Federico, C. M., & Pratt, F. (2001). Legitimizing ideologies: The social dominance approach. In J. T. Jost & B. Major (Eds.), *The psychology of legitimacy: Emerging perspectives on ideology, justice, and intergroup relations* (pp. 307–331). New York: Cambridge University Press.

Smith, C. (2007). *The cost of privilege: Taking on the system of White supremacy and racism.* Fayetteville, NC: Camino Press.

Sue, D. W. (2003). *Overcoming our racism: Journey to liberation.* San Francisco: Jossey-Bass.

Worchel, S., & Andreoli, V. M. (1978). Facilitation of social interaction through deindividuation of the target. *Journal of Personality and Social Psychology*, 36, 549–556.

CHAPTER 5

Race and Ethnicity

Those who cannot feel the littleness of great things in themselves are apt to overlook the greatness of little things in others.

—Okakura Kakuzo (cited in Robinson-Wood, 2009, p. 107)

One of the cornerstones of multicultural counseling competence in this country is a clear understanding of the constructs of race and ethnicity. The earliest movements in advocating for such competence were race-based, though they have since broadened in scope. However, the concepts of race and ethnicity have been defined in a variety of ways often leading to confusion in terms of meaning, significance, scope, and application. Regardless, there is no denying their impact on the experiences of people from all walks of life.

In this chapter, we provide a review of the origins of these concepts in a historical context to reflect the changing ways in which they have been conceptualized and defined. Following this, a multidisciplinary overview of theoretical approaches to race and racial classifications is offered along with an overview of ethnicity as a social construct. The chapter then offers brief overviews of various racial/ethnic groups that include African Americans, Asian Americans, Latinos/Hispanic Americans, Native Americans, Jewish Americans, and European Americans. Finally, we conclude with a discussion of the impact of racism on various members of racial and ethnic groups with implications for counseling.

REFLECTION QUESTIONS 5.1

Questions for Reflection:

- How do you define race? How do you assess/recognize a person's race? What elements make up that construct for you?
- How have your racial ideas about different groups been formed? How much of your knowledge is based on first-hand contact and information?
- How do you define your own race and ethnicity? Where, when, and how did you learn this?
- How do you define the race and ethnicity of others who are different from you? Where, when, and how did you learn this?
- As you learn more about the impact of racism on various groups, you may well find that you have prejudicial attitudes and biases against a particular group. How might the information here shape a new understanding of the experience of members of this group?
- How can you take a deeper understanding of the impact of racism and move through emotions of guilt, anxiety, or pity, to be able to act rather than react?
- How will better understanding the race, ethnicity, and the experience that members of various racial and ethnic groups have with racism make you a better counselor?
- How might you work toward positive social change with regard to the racism that exists in your own life at the individual, group, and societal levels?
- To what extent do you value a person's race or ethnicity as a sign of his or her worth?
- Have you ever stood up for someone being harassed or oppressed on the basis of race or ethnicity? If not, why not? Has anyone ever stood up for you in this way?
- What does it mean to you to be multiculturally-competent in the areas of race and ethnicity?

HISTORICAL OVERVIEW

Race as a Biological Construct

It has been suggested that, "race is neither biological nor scientific." According to Dr. Silvia Spangler of the Human Genome Project, "race is something we do to one another". If this is true, does the notion of racism make sense? There have been discussions regarding race and racism for decades and in multiple settings. For instance, scholars have explored and discussed race and racism in scholarly arenas, everyday citizens have held town hall meetings, and even former President Clinton commissioned a task force to encourage dialogue around race and racism. For a concept that is neither biological nor scientific, it has certainly received a great deal of attention and its impact on the daily lives of people has been tremendous.

Race originated as a biological construct grouping populations by their difference on biological measures. Diverse categories of peoples were classified into races based on skin pigmentation and morphology (features and build). From this perspective, race was a fundamental organizing principle of human affairs. Everyone had a race, and only one. The races were biologically separate and potentially in conflict with one another. The most important aspect of racial classifications was in the boundaries that basically separated them.

These boundaries were framed differently in different societies. In the United States, they were framed by descent rather than by phenotype (Omi, 1999). For instance, in the early part of this century, across nine southern states, a person with 15 White ancestors four generations back and a single African American ancestor was reckoned a 'Negro' in the eyes of the law (Spickard, 1989). The "one drop rule," as it has been referred to, came out of America's early experience with slavery and afterward in the Jim Crow south. The commonly understood story of race in the United States has largely taken place in terms of race relations between Blacks and Whites, with other groups occasionally making an appearance, usually in opposition to Whites. What is important to realize is that such categorization of human beings is not accidental and has historical roots that need to be explored.

From the 14th century onwards, with the increasing durability, skill, and sophistication of ships being built in Europe, the rush for colonization was started by Portugal and Spain, later joined and dominated by the Northern European nations such as Britain, France, and Germany. In their discovery of new lands, colonizers also discovered peoples hitherto unknown to the Europeans. Africans and indigenous peoples of Australia, Americas, and the Caribbean were seen as part of the discovered resources to be used (Takaki, 1989). To justify this use, they needed to be placed in a different category from the Europeans. In the 16th century, the concept of race was used by Europeans to rationalize the enslavement of peoples who were considered racially "inferior" (Feagin & Feagin, 2003). For instance, in explaining the Spanish conquest of Indians, Juan Gines de Sepelveda, a Spanish lawyer, used Aristotle's doctrine that some groups were by their nature of being barbarous and subhuman, naturally slaves (Takaki, 1993). Similarly, in a famous 1838 "Memoir on Slavery," Chancellor Harper of the South Carolina College defended slavery by arguing, "If there are sordid, servile, and laborious offices to be performed, is it not better that there should be sordid, servile, and laborious beings to perform them?" and then went on to conclude that since Africans were "nearer to the brute creation than perhaps any other people on the face of the globe ... [they represented] the very material out of which slaves ought to be made." (pp. 51–59, Harper, 1838, quoted in Frederickson, 1988).

The typological view of races developed by Europeans arranged the peoples of the world hierarchically, largely based on physical abilities and moral qualities with Caucasians at the top, Asians next, then Native Americans, and Africans at the bottom. The racial categorizations and the accompanying descriptions of each racial grouping demonstrate such perspectives. Linneaus (1806, in Gould, 1994) was the first scientist to classify humanity into different types. In the mid 1700s, he sorted *Homo sapiens* into four finite categories of white, red, yellow, and black, which were stereotyped phenotypically and behaviorally. For example, while he described the European type as fair and brawny, blue eyed, inventive, and governed by laws, he epitomized the Asian type as sooty, black eyed, melancholic, haughty, and governed by opinion. In the 18th century, Blumen-bach (1795, in Marks, 1995) coined the term Caucasian, after a skull from the Caucasus Mountains of central Eurasia. He described the skull as perfectly formed and Europeans came to be called Caucasians because they were thought to be descendents of the "perfect" people from the Caucasus area. On the other hand, Negroid came about in derivation from the Greek word *nekros* meaning the dead. As the unknown world was explored and different indigenous people encountered, naturalists, the scientists of the time, described their physical characteristics and classified different populations as to their relatedness. Until late into the 20th century, this approach was used to classify humanity. The numbers of categories shifted, with some recognizing five major categories of Caucasoid, Negroid, Mongoloid, Semitic, and Amerindian, while others put the number at considerably more. For instance, in 1976, the *Brazilian Institute of Geography and Statistics* developed a classification system determined by skin color and came up with 135 categories. Table 5.1 demonstrates the shifting number of categories that emerged and changed based on the needs of the times.

TABLE **5.1**
Census Racial Categories over the Years (Population Reference Bureau, 2003)*

	1790	1860	1890	1900	1970	2000
Race	White	White	White	White	White	White
	Other	Black	Black	Black	Negro or Black	Black, African American, Negro
	Slave	Mulatto	Mulatto a person who was 3/8 to 5/8 Black	Indian	Indian (Amer.)	American Indian or Alaska Native
			Chinese	Chinese	Chinese	Chinese
			Indian	Japanese	Japanese, Filipino, Korean, Chinese	Japanese, Filipino, Asian Indian, Korean, Vietnamese, Other Asian
			Quadroon 1/4 Black		Hawaiian	Native Hawaiian, Guamanian, Chamorro, Samoan, Other Pacific Islander
			Octoroon 1/8 Black		Mexican, Puerto Rican, Central/ So. Amer., Cuban, Other Spanish	Mexican, Mexican American, Chicano, Puerto Rican, Cuban, Spanish/ Latino/ Hispanic
					Other	Some Other race

*Note: Prior to the 1970 census, respondents wrote in the race of individuals using the designated categories. In subsequent censuses, respondents filled in circles next to the categories. Also beginning with the 1970 census, persons choosing American Indian, other Asian, other race, or (for the Hispanic question) other Hispanic categories, were asked to write in a specific tribe or group. Hispanic ethnicity was asked of a sample of Americans in 1970 and of all Americans beginning with the 1980 census.
Source: Population Reference Bureau. (2003). *200 Years of Census Taking: Population and Housing Questions 1790-1990*. U.S. Bureau of the Census. Retrieved December 12, 2003 from http://www.prb.org

The categorization of race was used to systematically appropriate privilege and exclude persons from participation. In 1790, the Naturalization Act was approved by Congress to grant citizenship only to 'free white persons', excluding all others from citizenship. This exclusion applied to Native Americans, considered 'domestic foreigners' and ineligible. By the same token, up until the 1860's, Chinese persons were considered to be Indian because of the theory that Native Americans were Asians who had crossed the Bering Straits into North America (Spring, 2004).

While early definitions of 'white' applied only to those of British Protestant descent, by the early twentieth century, it was being applied to any who were of European descent. Although it was a struggle for Southern and Eastern Europeans, and the Irish to gain acceptance primarily due to different religious beliefs, their compatible complexions allowed them to assimilate by blending in, a method that was not possible for Native Americans, Asians, Mexicans and enslaved African Americans (Ignatiev, 1995).

Montagu (1942) was among the first to question the scientific validity of race in his classic work, *Man's Most Dangerous Myth: The Fallacy of Race*. He argued that over the course of the 19th century, both social and physical sciences such as anthropology, biology, psychology, medicine, and sociology became instruments for the "proof" of the inferiority of various races as compared with the white race. According to Winston (2004), research endeavors in psychology supported the 19th century ideology about racial typology and the biological basis for hierarchical ranking up until the 1930s. A shift did occur in which psychologists began to study prejudice, and by the 1950s it was clearly evident that a small but growing number of psychologists took a stance against racial injustices. However, this discourse also promoted racism. For example, Winston comments that during the 1940s and 1950s when societal issues centered on the segregation of African Americans, the research on race in psychology also shifted to focus on racial differences between Blacks and Whites in intelligence, a highly controversial and much debated topic. A classic example is The *Bell Curve*, a much publicized work, by Herrnstein and Murray (1994) in which they argued that the reason that African Americans were disadvantaged was due to a one-dimensional construct of intelligence based in genetics rather than slavery, segregation, or historical and continuing discrimination.

Claims that race mixing known as "hybridity" would produce people of inferior mental and physical abilities that posed a major threat to the well-being of society was a central theme in psychology's history. This discourse was alive and well during the early part of the 20th century, in which research supported and promoted this perspective (e.g., studies by T.R. Garth (1923) compared the intelligence of Mexicans, and mixed and full blood Native Americans). However, several landmark publications emerged that challenged the debates on race. One such publication was Guthrie's (1976, 1998) *Even the Rat Was White: A Historical View of Psychology*, whose writings about the inherent racism in all aspects of the discipline, profoundly influenced the shift from so-called "race psychology" to the study of prejudice (Winston, 2004). Today as Winston cogently articulates "... race and racial differences have been persistent and troublesome issues for the discipline. Even after a century of severe criticism, discussions of the size of Black versus White brains still appear in psychology journals, race is still treated as a set of distinct biological categories, and racial comparisons of intelligence test scores are still presented as meaningful scientific questions" (p. 3).

Livingstone (1964) suggested that a more legitimate and fruitful approach to understanding contemporary human biological variation was to focus on patterns of biological differences across space, rather than on differences between and among populations. Such an approach would yield greater insight into their adaptive significance since environmental parameters that drive natural selection vary systematically across geographic areas.

With the increasing sophistication in the science of genetics, it became clear that people are biologically quite varied. Typically, the external biological characteristics are hereditarily influenced and the hundreds of internal biochemical characteristics are genetically determined. The external features such as skin color, facial features of nose type, epicanthic eye folds, height of cheekbones, texture and color of hair are the ones that people tend to associate with racial variation and use to categorize individuals into one or another race. In reality, the internal qualities are many-fold more varied than those observable with the eye.

Relative to classification, molecular genetics has revolutionized our understanding of groups because of science's ability to compare individual's DNA; consequently, genotypes, or the genetic makeup of an organism, now take precedent as a viable means of comparison. According to the data derived from the Human Genome Project (2003), any two humans on this planet are more than 99.99 percent identical at the molecular level, indicating that racial differences are indeed only skin deep. Ironically, two Caucasians of different heights represent more of a genetic difference than a Caucasian and a person of color (Ponterotto & Pedersen, 1993; Helms & Cook, 1999).

Race as a Social Construct

By the late twentieth century, race had been redefined as a social construct rather than solely biological in nature (Omi & Winant, 1986). Such a definition subsumed ethnic identity and allowed for recognition of the historical identification of persons in various groupings. The social construction of race also sheds light on the political context of racial categorization.

Interestingly, the movement of race from a biological to sociological concept did not result in less emphasis being placed on the hierarchy of group rankings. However, explanations for the differential experience and success of groups of persons shifted from being based in biology to culture. From being biologically inferior beings, low-ranking racial groups became culturally inferior. Much of this cultural inferiority or disadvantage was blamed on conditions of past racism, but still ended up blaming the victim. For instance, Elkin (1959) reworked the stereotype of the grinning, shuffling, primitive African American, presenting it as being a result of slavery rather than biology, leading to a childlike dependency on the part of its victims. Even though such a thesis was refuted by scholars such as Blassingame (1972, in Frederickson, 1988) who argued that far from being dependent on their masters, slaves had to marshal substantial resources of discipline, will, intelligence, and endurance to resist

EXAMPLE **5.1**
Susie Gregory Phipps

In 1977, Susie Gregory Phipps who had considered herself white all her 43 years was shocked to find that she had been designated by the State of Louisiana as colored. According to the State's genealogical investigation, Ms. Phipps' great-great-great-great grandmother was a Black woman slave named Margarita. By 1970 Louisiana state law, since Ms. Phipps was at least 1/32nd Black, she was considered Black. When Ms. Phipps sued the State of Louisiana to change her racial designation, she lost. In 1983, the state Supreme Court upheld the state's right to classify and quantify racial identity (Omi and Winant, 1994).

Source: From Omi, M., & Winant, H. (1994). Racial formation in the United States from the 1960s to the 1990s. New York: Routledge.

oppression and maintain a sense of their dignity and worthiness, others echoed similar themes. Some like Fogel and Engerman (1974, in Frederickson, 1988) argued that plantations were models of efficiency and that slaves were willing collaborators in such capitalist endeavors. Thus while being unable to defend a biological construct of race, many still believed that racial minorities were intellectually and morally inferior and that they should not mix with Whites.

The 1965 Moynihan Report was a case in point. Entitled, *The Negro Family: The case for national action*, it essentially argued that through the legacy of slavery and discrimination, a matriarchal family structure had developed in the African American community. The heart of the problems facing inner city life was this matriarchal family structure that did not allow African Americans to assimilate into the middle class. The role of extended family ties, the readiness to offer sustenance to neighbors and friends, and the frequent presence of women as heads of household, were all presented as pathological features. One of the striking contentions was that "the present tangle of pathology is capable of perpetuating itself without assistance from the white world"(p.47), reframing the problems of African Americans as based in their own family dysfunction rather than on unrelenting and historical segregation and discrimination.

Laws stemming from the 1896 Plessy vs. Ferguson decision that upheld the separate yet equal doctrine had continued to be used to segregate Whites from African Americans and other minorities. This peaked in the 1960's, and today African Americans are more segregated than any other group, have experienced segregation longer than any other group and are segregated at every income level (Bonilla-Silva, 1999). In another view of the notion of segregation, some might argue that Whites are the most self-segregated group in the United States, with the most choices of being able to live in neighborhoods and communities that are largely White. In the new millennium, race is obviously still a thorny issue, continuing to be a social construction that sets apart and privileges European immigrant groups from all others.

Without a biological foundation, race now only exists as a societal mechanism of classification, and although genetic research continues to destroy the reality of race as a valid biological construct, our society's perception of race continues to divide us and cripple us as a nation (Axelson, 1999; Brown, 2002; Helms & Cook, 1999; Kivel, 1996). Our society is so entrenched in racial boundaries that the lines of division entangle every aspect of our existence from economics to education to even our religious practices. We try to erase the racial lines that are so prevalent in our society with bumper stickers that claim we are all part of the "human race" and yet we are quick to react to the phenotype, or physical appearance, of an individual. Even textbooks dedicated to examining the damaging effects of racism and how to combat them as educators and counselors struggle with a definition of race; they deny its reality and yet, still depend on the term as a frame of reference (Axelson, 1999; Ponterotto & Pedersen, 1993). The term persists because of its link to racism, which in reality would be better termed "colorism"; this term adequately describes our society's insistence on maintaining an "us" and "them" mentality necessary for the dominance of one group economically, politically, and socially over others.

With the concept of race so questionable, other terms have surfaced in an attempt to describe the differences that exist between different groups of people; two of the terms include *ethnicity* and *culture*. Rose (1964) described *ethnicity* as a group of individuals "who share a unique social and cultural heritage (e.g., language, custom, religion) passed on between generations" (Ponterotto & Pederson, 1993, p. 6). This definition relies on characteristics that seem to be inherent in a way of life rather than biological considerations. This term seems acceptable until one reviews the definition of **culture** as referring to the values, beliefs, language, rituals, traditions, and other behaviors that are passed from one generation to another within any social group. Confusion between the two terms is compounded by the fact that many texts use the terms interchangeably or expand on these definitions using the term "racial" or "socioracial" as part of their explanation (Helms & Cook, 1999).

Ethnicity as a Social Construct

According to Guzzetta (1995), the term *ethnic* that comprises the word *ethnicity* was "originally derived from a Greek word for 'nation' and was used to distinguish particular national groups from other national groups not identified by nation, such as Jews or Gypsies" (p. 2508). However, over time, many factors have influenced the overall interpretation of the term including experiences with time, place, and context, among other things. Robinson (2005) points out that the construct of ethnicity first entered into professional/academic discourse in the U.S. in 1910 at the University of Chicago where researchers were interested in examining how (with the more than 1 million immigrants that were entering the country each year) more than 20 nationalities were managing conflicts associated with the process of assimilation. At that time, most immigrants coming into the U.S. were quick to adapt in any way possible, to the existing mainstream American culture that they found here at that time. An excellent example of this was the tendency to change last names to "sound more American," and therefore, avoid identification with home country/culture if possible for political, social, economic, or psychological reasons. According to Robinson (2005), "the process of assimilation among White ethnic microcultures differs greatly from that among people of color. Historical differences between race and ethnicity originated from U.S. policies such as the 1790 Naturalization Law, which essentially stated that only "White" immigrants would be eligible for naturalized citizenship in the U.S. Remaining in effect for over 162 years, Native people, for example were denied citizenship until 1924, and Asian people were not allowed citizenship until 1952. By contrast, people of color found themselves barred from many of the privileges and liberties enjoyed by their White counterparts. Policies such as these were not only created out of racist attitudes, beliefs, and practices, but have served to perpetuate those attitudes, beliefs, and practices to this day on the social, political, economic, and psychological levels.

Ethnicity, by general definition, refers to one's sociocultural heritage based on commonalities represented in such dimensions as collective history, religion, nationality, regional origin, language, and others. It is the collective experience of one's socially-constructed identity that can be (1) chosen or (2) ascribed. Chosen aspects of ethnic identity can include any number of dimensions on which people can self-define; religion is a good example of this. Ascribed aspects of one's ethnic identity include any number of dimensions that are assigned by external forces; racial classifications designated by the U.S. Bureau of the Census are examples of this. Overall, characteristics associated with ethnicity include loyalty to and identification with group membership based on:

- Shared group image and sense of identity derived from values, behaviors, beliefs, or language
- Shared political, social, and economic interests
- Shared history of family immigration
- Shared history of group segregation, separation, or assimilation
- Shared group visibility, cohesiveness, and density in localized regions of the country

To be clear, Robinson (2005) points out that people can be of the same ethnicity (e.g., Latino, for example) but not be of the same racial group (e.g., White, Black, Asian, bi- or multiracial). At the same time, people can be of the same racial group (Asian), but not of the same ethnicity (e.g., Chinese, Vietnamese, Cuban, Japanese, Korean, Filipino, Asian Indian, and so forth).

In general, issues around race, ethnicity, and culture are never simple, and historical context out of which these concepts arise is quite extensive. However, having grounding ourselves in the historical development and current impact of the constructs of race and ethnicity, it now becomes important to explore the impact of racial categorizations and racism on various groups that have established a presence in U.S. society, including African Americans, Asian Americans, Latinos/Hispanic Americans, Native Americans, Jewish Americans, and European Americans.

RACE-ING AND E-RACING

African Americans

For **African Americans**, race is something one lives with everyday because of being constantly reminded that one is different, in other words, that you are not White. Racism takes many forms including individual and institutional; within these two groupings, racism is expressed covertly, overtly, and even unintentionally (Axelson, 1999; Brown, 2002; Cole, & Omari, 2003; Koch, Gross, & Kolts, 2001; Wade, & Bielitz, 2005; Kivel, 1996; Ponterotto & Pedersen; Ridley, 1995). Even at a young age, African American children internalize the negative messages associated with being a African American as part of their racial identity development; such negativity could have a direct impact on the direction of their life and has been linked to alienation in school, high failure rates, increasing number of dropouts as well as increased involvement with the juvenile justice system. Later in life, the compounded effects of racism or colorism could be expressed as mental illness, physical illness, or a combination of both (Axelson, 1999; Ball, Armistead, & Austin, 2003; Chadiha, Rafferty, & Pickard, 2003; Jang, 2004; Lee, 1999).

When we think of racism, we tend to think of individual or isolated incidents. This allows some [Whites] to avoid seeing the true impact of racist experiences on the psychological well-being of African Americans. It could also be argued that focusing on individual and/or isolated incidents of racism allows African Americans to endure the cumulative impact of racism. Unfortunately, this cumulative effect of racism and prejudice takes its toll affecting the individual's capacity to cope effectively with life's injustices. Even the effects of "small stuff" can accumulate over time and eventually break a person's spirit. Sue (2003) refers to the "small stuff" as micro-insults. These micro-insults may be viewed as unimportant events or incidents in the lives of some African Americans; however, these incidents tend to collect in the unconscious psyche of African Americans until their collective weight creeps into the African American conscious and, for some, interfere with the healthy development of the individual's identity. Researchers suggest that these experiences result in the activation and, in some cases, development of a cultural mistrust (Hunter, 2002; Phelps, Taylor, & Gerard, 2001) or healthy cultural paranoia, also referred to as paranorm (Sue & Sue, 2003). These defense or survival mechanisms allow African Americans to minimize the impact of such negative experiences. Researchers (Vontress and Epps, 1997) even suggest that these experiences also contribute to historical hostility. Vontress and Epps define (1997) historical hostility as a reaction to current and past experiences of prejudice and racism. These experiences can even be past down from generation to generation in the form of stories relating the experiences of family members.

In an effort to avoiding the full impact of prejudice and racism, some African Americans have made attempts to assimilate into the lifestyle or ways of being identified with White America. This assimilation, while seeming necessary for survival on the one-hand it is problematic on the other. For example, African American boys who apply themselves academically may be considered "sell-outs" by trying to be White or being a "sissy." African American men who wear neckties and suits on a regular basis as well as speak Standard English are oftentimes looked upon as "acting White or not being real". To believe that only White men can and should dress professionally indicates how images of self are internalized early and shape cultural perceptions. The flip side of this issue is when White Americans significantly notice and are surprised by the attire of an African American male who is dressed professionally in a suit and tie as opposed to "thug gear." Both examples show how racism and prejudice have impacted African Americans. Other areas affected by racism and prejudice, on a more institutional level, include the disparities in housing, education, employment, and health care, including mental health services, with a final prominent area being the justice system.

REFLECTION QUESTIONS 5.2

- What are some of the beliefs, images, or stereotypes you have held about African Americans?
- Where did these beliefs, images, or stereotypes come from?
- How have they changed over time and if so, what caused them to change for you?
- How do these beliefs, images, or stereotypes affect your work with members of this population?
- What have been some of your experiences with members of this population, both positive and negative?

Asian Americans

The identification of *Asian* or **Asian American** as a racial category emerges from the shadow of Linnaeus and Blumenbach's first designation of yellow people. In the 19th century, the term "yellow peril" signified this notion of geopolitical conflict, as White colonizers in the American West feared that the Chinese laborers they had imported would become a horde that threatened Anglo-Saxon civilization. The 1882 Chinese Exclusion Act was the attempt by the state to control the immigration of Chinese to this country. Along with the 1917 barred zone act and the supplementary 1924 act that excluded any Asians from being classified as white, there were systematic attempts to keep out Asians. The only exception were Filipinos who, being denizens of the only U.S. Colony in Asia, were labeled American nationals and served as surrogates and replacements for Chinese and Japanese labor.

In a sense, given the vast sweep of persons with diverse geographic origins who fall under the term, Asian is a racial category rather than an ethnic description. For instance, Hmong and Malaysians are no more alike than Ukrainian and Irish, but are grouped together by a racial categorization.

Most descriptions of Asian communities in the United States follow the myth of immigration whereby the United States operates as a land of promise and freedom to teeming masses. In this version, Asians, sometimes referred to as the "Model Minority," are proto-whites, not really white but designated as a minority success story to be held up in rebuke to other minority groups. In the 1980's, President Ronald Reagan thanked them for their example, saying, "we need *your* values, *your* hard work ... [within] *our* political system." (italics added, in Takaki, 1989, p. 475). In 1986, several major television news shows aired special segments on Asian Americans reporting them to be very successful in the level of income they had, outperforming most other ethnic groups other than Whites. What the media downplayed was that there were often more people in an Asian household that were working, which contributed to this higher income. The face of this racialized model Asian was also usually Japanese or Chinese, suppressing the struggle of many Cambodian and Vietnamese Americans to survive in abject poverty.

Historically the movie industry has portrayed the Asian as evil, plotting in the shadows, from Dr. Fu-Manchu in the early black-and-white films, to the more recent James Bond film that demonstrate that even when an Asian changes his face to look white, underneath he is still the same villain. Many of the major wars that the U.S. has fought have had enemies with Asian faces, from Japan in World War II through Korea and Vietnam.

Seen as essentially alien along with the familiar statement that "they all look the same," Asian American participation in the construction of the United States has been marginalized. Politically, this has lead to large-scale invisibility of Asians in active participation in the society. For instance, when the Transcontinental Railroad was completed in 1869, the photographs managed to render invisible the thousands of Chinese workers who had worked the railroad. As Takaki (1989) reported, when the great histories of immigrants who made America are presented, Asians are rarely included. It has also meant that Asians are vulnerable to being targeted as not really American. One reason often given is that Asians do not assimilate into the population as Europeans do. In denying naturalized citizenship to Asian Indians in 1923 because they were not White, the Supreme Court remarked that, "the children of English, French, German, Italian, Scandinavian and other European parentage, quickly merge in to the mass of our population and lose the distinctive hallmarks of their European origin." (*U.S. v. Bhagat Singh Thind*, 261 U.S. 215, 1923, in Takaki, 1989).

Perhaps the most significant aspect of the racial construction of Asians as foreign is that while there are Chinese and Japanese Americans who are fourth and fifth generation American, they can still expect to be asked casually, "Where are you from?" In national crises, the Anti-Asian rhetoric often emerges, from the barrage of diatribes against Japan in the mid-1980's for "buying up America," to the current panic of jobs being relocated to India. Over and over again, the foreignness of Asians is seen as threatening in a country that is comprised of immigrants from all over, but quintessentially determines its national identity as European American (Constantine, Okazaki, & Utsey, 2004; Goto, Gee, & Takeuchi, 2002).

 REFLECTION QUESTIONS 5.3

- What are some of the beliefs, images, or stereotypes you have held about Asian Americans?
- Where did these beliefs, images, or stereotypes come from?
- How have they changed over time and if so, what caused them to change for you?
- How do these beliefs, images, or stereotypes affect your work with members of this population?
- What have been some of your experiences with members of this population, both positive and negative?

Latinos/Hispanic Americans

Historically, categories used to classify and describe people have largely been based on genealogical and biological characteristics. As noted earlier, the rigid and mutually exclusive racial categorization of people (e.g., Black or White) with skin color as the dominating criteria has been the source of much confusion when applied to the Latino population. Part of this confusion stems from the incredible variability in the population's physical characteristics, and because of the way that race has been conceptualized in this country. The issue of race and Latinos can be examined in two ways: 1) how the U.S. government views (historical and present day) the population, and 2) how the population see themselves.

It is important to note that the term **Hispanic** was created in 1978 by Directive 15 of the Office of Budget and Management defined as a "person of Mexican, Puerto Rican, Cuban, Central or South American, or other Spanish culture of origin" (Marín & Marín, 1991, p.20). This label was created to categorize a group of people who come from Spanish-speaking countries. One of the main problems with this designation is that it promotes the view that Hispanics are a homogeneous group when in reality they come from 21 Spanish-speaking countries, each with a unique history and indigenous roots, as well as distinct foods and customs (Santiago-Rivera, Arredondo, & Gallardo-Cooper, 2002). Although the term was not intended to be a racial category, there is an erroneous perception held by many that it is. The confusion lies in the variations in labeling and categorizing Hispanics on the U.S. decennial census, sometimes using race, and on other occasions using ethnicity as the main identifier. For example, Mexicans were categorized as "nonwhite" in 1930, as "persons of Spanish mother tongue" in 1940, as "white persons of Spanish surname" in the 1950 and 1960 censuses, but by only five Southwest states. It changed, once again, in 1970 to "persons of both Spanish surname and Spanish mother tongue", and finally in 1980, 1990, and 2000 the census reflected the increasing diversity in the population by listing specific groups, namely, Mexican, Puerto Rican, Cubans, and other Spanish/Hispanics. Moreover, the 1980 census was the first time in the history of decennial data collection that Latinos were asked to identify their race as well as their country of origin (Spanish roots) (Moore & Pachon, 1985; Rodriguez, 2000).

Accordingly, a number of interesting patterns have emerged in terms of how they self-identify with respect to race. For example, census data show that there is a steady increase of Latinos who self-identify as "other race," meaning that they are not choosing the traditional categories of Black, White, Asian or Native American, but rather using the "Hispanic" label. In fact, Logan (2003) describes this group as the "Hispanic Hispanic" (p.2). In addition, a small but significant segment of the Latino population self-identify as Black whereas the majority report being White.

When comparing across groups within the Latino population, there are also interesting trends. For instance, there is a tendency for Puerto Ricans and Dominicans to self-report as being Black, whereas Cubans tend to identify as White. In essence, **Latinos** can be of any race and are often referred to as the "rainbow" people because of the varied phenotypes, particularly skin color (Comas-Díaz, 2001; McConnell, & Delgado-Romero, 2004). The point to be made here is that although Latinos may choose a standard racial category, perhaps because of the insistence of government census data-collection methods, they also self-identify with their country of origin. Further complicating the issue is Clara Rodriguez's (2000) claims that socio-economic class, generation (e.g., first or second generation born in the U.S.), and the size and extent to which the referent group is accessible contribute to self- identification.

It has been argued that the recent Latino immigrant has a different view of race compared to the view held by American society. Many scholars allege that Latinos, undergo a "racialization process" in which they are confronted with the dominant society's perception of who they are that often times does not match their self-perception (e.g., Obler, 1999; Rodriguez, 2000; Spanakis, 2004; Torres, 2003; Torres, 2004). The use of discrete racial categories is so widespread in this country that it is hard to resist accepting them. Nonetheless, leading scholars argue that Latinos still perceive the notion of race as associated with culture, the socialization process and country of origin rather than a pure biological and genealogical phenomenon (Rodriguez, 2000). This is clearly evident in the Spanish term **la raza**, which means "race" in English but has a significantly different connotation in that it encompasses culture and heritage, and equally important, a political consciousness.

Related to race and Latinos is the notion of **mestizaje** defined as the mixing of races, particularly, White, African, and indigenous populations in the various Spanish speaking countries. As Acosta-Belén and Sjostrom (1988) pointed out this race mixing occurred during the Spanish conquest and colonization period of the Americas that resulted in a diverse group of people not only in cultural traditions, but also in physical characteristics, and how they see themselves. In essence, the construction of race and how Latinos experience it remains a complex issue.

REFLECTION QUESTIONS 5.4

- What are some of the beliefs, images, or stereotypes you have held about Latinos/Hispanic Americans?
- Where did these beliefs, images, or stereotypes come from?
- How have they changed over time and if so, what caused them to change for you?
- How do these beliefs, images, or stereotypes affect your work with members of this population?
- What have been some of your experiences with members of this population, both positive and negative?

Native Americans

In the earliest accounts of race, explorers, colonizers and settlers described the indigenous peoples they encountered as savage (Garrett, & Garrett, 2003). The label of *los indios* was placed upon the first peoples of the Arawak nation encountered by Christopher Columbus on the mistaken belief that he had reached India (Trimble & Jumper-Thurman, 2002). According to Trimble (1996), this term has been used to classify almost all indigenous peoples of the Western hemisphere. In the Curtis Act of 1898, the term American Indian was defined by blood heritage. While this has been revised several times, currently the Bureau of Indian Affairs (BIA) continues to designate as American Indian a person whose Native blood quantum is at least one-fourth and/or is an official member of one of more than 500 federally recognized tribes (Thomason, 1995). Members of those tribes who did not sign formal treaties with the US government, or were part of scattered groups are eliminated by this definition. Numerous tribes have also changed the blood inheritance criteria used by the BIA, in some cases lowering it to as low as 1/28th while in others increasing it to 1/2. This is the only ethnic group that still has to prove their identity through blood inheritance and carry a card to prove they are who they say they are.

Currently, some of the preferred terms for designating these groups are **Native Americans**, American Indians, First Nations Peoples, and Indigenous Peoples. In Canada, the preferred term has become First Nations Peoples. In many cases, the term used is based on political affiliation. Those who wish to claim affiliation with all indigenous peoples, use terms reflective of that, while others may use their own nation, tribe, or region's designation. Thus, Athabascan people may use a collective designation of Alaskan Native, while the original inhabitants of Hawaii may use the term Native Hawaiian.

One of the ways in which this racialized construct of Indians has impacted Native Americans is through reducing a diverse set of peoples to a single category. The blanket label reduces the cultures of many nations, such as Hopi, Osage, Navajo, Sioux, Seneca, Mohawk, to a single dimension. Neither does this label acknowledge the indigenous heritage of Mexican Americans in the Southwest, Puerto Ricans, or Chamorro of Guam, or native Hawaiians for whom the labels of Hispanic or Pacific Islander must fit. It also conflates and diminishes and separates the multiple identities of many who are biracial and multiracial. For instance, the Cherokee Nation was widely distributed and many African Americans may also have Cherokee ancestry. However, the insistence on having a singular racial identity led many to claim African American as their primary identity. The physiognomic characteristics of race, where people of one race are supposed to look similar has resulted in a stereotypical definition of what a Native American should look like, that does not fit the appearance of many African Americans. In the latest Census, where respondents had the opportunity to mark multiple racial categories, there was a huge increase in the number of respondents identifying with sharing American Indian or Alaskan Native heritage.

On the other hand, the emergence of a pan-ethnic identity of American Indian has also created a political force by bringing together diverse peoples who share a common history of broken treaties with the U.S. government. An example is the modern Powwow, a term that came from the Algonkian-speaking Narragansett Indians of the Northeast. The word used to refer to a shaman or a teacher, a dream or a vision, or a council or a gathering, but now it signifies a collection of dances and celebration that knows no tribal boundaries. Songs and dances that once were sung or danced only by a specific tribe or group are now performed by Native people from other parts of the country. The contemporary powwow provides an opportunity for people to celebrate their identification with Native cultures and have become pan-Indian and inter-tribal expressions of pride (Portman & Garrett, 2006).

Sociopolitically, the historical discriminatory racial policies and practices devastated the lives of Native Americans. The massacre of Wounded Knee in 1890 where hundreds of Native American men, women, and children were killed when they were penned in a relocation camp signaled the end of the Frontier age. Francis Amasa Walker was the commissioner of Indian Affairs in the 1870's and pursued a policy of social engineering, where civilization would be brought to the savage Indian (Takaki, 1993). Beyond the massacres, broken treaties, loss of traditional lands, forced relocation, unemployment, disease and epidemic, government agencies began a deliberate policy of enculturation to coercively assimilate Native Americans into mainstream society (Garrett & Carroll, 2000; Garrett & Pichette, 2000). One method was to foster children away from their indigenous cultures and families, and in pursuit of this goal, Native children were moved to boarding schools where they were not allowed to speak their language, wear traditional clothes, or see their families. In the 1950's, there were specific policies encouraging the placement of Native children away from their families and tribes into White families and environments. The BIA, which was charged to facilitate the government-to-government relationship between the Federal government and Native tribes often behaved more like an enforcer of the repressive policies.

An example of the continuing racial objectification of Native Americans is the issue of mascots. Many sports teams use Native American peoples as mascots (Garrett & Garrett, 2003). The Atlanta Braves, Washington Redskins, and Cleveland Indians are some examples of these stereotyped depictions that include red skin, big nose, and a full headdress. There are "Cherokee" Jeeps and "Cheyenne" trucks, "Thunderbird" and "Pontiac" automobiles, "Mohawk"-carpets, "Pequot" sheets, "Oneida" tableware, "Big Chief" writing tablets, "Red Man" chewing tobacco, "Land O' Lakes" Butter (with its Indian princess on the label), "Eskimo" Pies, Piper "Cherokee" and "Navaho" airplanes, "Winnebago" motor homes, and of course the ironically named "Apache" and "Comanche" helicopters used by the U.S. military. There is no equivalent example for other peoples whose names are so objectified that they can be used as designations to sell products.

 REFLECTION QUESTIONS 5.5

- What are some of the beliefs, images, or stereotypes you have held about Native Americans?
- Where did these beliefs, images, or stereotypes come from?
- How have they changed over time and if so, what caused them to change for you?
- How do these beliefs, images, or stereotypes affect your work with members of this population?
- What have been some of your experiences with members of this population, both positive and negative?

Jewish Americans

The U.S. Census does not have a racial category of Semitic or Jewish, and places being Jewish in a religious category. The racial categorization of Whiteness has been applied to **Jewish Americans**, since the majority of Jewish Americans are Ashkenazi, having a common origin of Central and Eastern Europe, and fit the physiognomy of Whiteness in terms of skin pigmentation and morphology. They also have a common language of Yiddish (combining mostly Hebrew and German elements). Sephardic Jews, darker of skin tone and hair color, who trace roots back to Spain and Portuguese often migrated to South and Central America as well as the Caribbean and are not highlighted as normatively Jewish American. Yet being Jewish has historically been perceived not only as a religious identity but as part of the Semitic racial identity, even though Jewish Americans can trace their roots back to many parts of the world other than the Middle-east. The mythos of a Jewish race has been used historically to commit acts of oppression, such as the ghettoization of Jews in much of Europe, the pogroms of Eastern Europe, as well as the horrific genocide during World War II. The term ghetto was first used to describe the Jewish quarter of all European cities. Often not allowed to own land, and capriciously persecuted, Jewish peoples had to remain mobile in their occupations and often could only be part of a narrow range of trades and professions.

Since the Christian dominant societies were enjoined against usury, but needed the function of loans, money lending was seen as a Jewish function that was simultaneously highly stigmatized. The distinct constellation of stereotypes that have applied to Jews had consistently focused on the manipulation of money. The figure of Shylock in Shakespeare's play, the Merchant of Venice, is the exemplar of these stereotypes. One can see the racial construction of Jews in the ascription of both psychological and biological traits to people of Jewish descent. Jews are imagined to be intrinsically concerned with money, and the actual wealth and power of members of this group is vastly overestimated. The first organized Jewish community established in 1677 in the United States was Sephardic (Hertzberg, 1989). It was during the late 1800; however, that the sizable immigration waves from Germany and Eastern Europe made the Jewish American presence a significant one. Demographically, the population is little more than 2% of the total U.S. population. In 1990, the U.S. Census reported 3,137,000 Jews.

The question of who is a Jew is tricky. Membership is counted either through descent from a Jewish mother, or by conversion. The kind of conversion required shifts and changes from the Orthodox, Conservative and Reform denominations of Judaism. However, when someone is born of a Jewish mother, he or she is considered Jewish without having to practice the religion. So, it is possible to be secular or non-religious and Jewish, which is a membership that is more ethnically and culturally consistent.

In the colonial period, anti-Semitism was muted as there were minimal Jewish settlements. The entrance of the Eastern European Jews brought about more intense hostility in the 1880's, when Jews began to be barred from resorts, clubs, and college fraternities. During the 1920's, the Ku Klux Klan targeted Jews as widely as its anti-Black campaigns and Henry Ford's newspaper, the *Dearborn Independent* made virulent attacks citing a "world Jewish conspiracy" (Dinnerstein, 1994). This notion was based on an Anti-Semitic tract called the *Protocols of the Elders of Zion* circulated originally by the Russians to justify oppressive policies against the Jews. This was also used by Hitler as an ideological base for Nazi policies. The oppression in the United States at this time appeared to be mainly policies of exclusion and restriction as opposed to the systematic violence and the genocidal conditions in Europe (Dinnerstein, 1994). Anti-Semitism expressions largely died down in the post World War II period and began to take place on a sporadic basis, increasing in the 1990's with acts of vandalism by young men parroting Nazi propaganda. Even the anti-Semitism expressed by African Americans, most notoriously by members of the Nation of Islam, represented situational antagonism rather than traditional hostility. However, that which persists is a racialized construction that continues to ascribe certain stereotypes, subscribe to discriminatory practices, and keep Jewish Americans as tentatively accepted members of the dominant society, who could forfeit their privilege capriciously.

REFLECTION QUESTIONS 5.6

- What are some of the beliefs, images, or stereotypes you have held about Jewish Americans?
- Where did these beliefs, images, or stereotypes come from?
- How have they changed over time and if so, what caused them to change for you?
- How do these beliefs, images, or stereotypes affect your work with members of this population?
- What have been some of your experiences with members of this population, both positive and negative?

European Americans

It may be surprising to examine the racialized construction of European Americans, but in many ways, the systems of race focus on this group. Rather than use the racial term of Caucasian, since most **European Americans** do not come from the Caucasus Mountains, we will use the term White to distinguish the impact of racial notions from ethnicity. The construction of Whiteness has not only marginalized people of African, Asian, native, and Hispanic descent, but has also created a peculiarly narrow identity for people of European descent. The colonization of the land that would become known as the United States was carried out first by the English, though the Spanish, French, and Dutch also established early settlements.

The national identity of citizens of the fledgling state was rooted in being racially Anglo-Saxon. Those who came from Southern and Eastern Europe, such as the Italians and the Polish, experienced discrimination and marginalization until they could assimilate into an ostensibly ethnically neutral construction of Whiteness. Joining in a racially defined identity of Whiteness allowed entry into society and access to White privilege. It also often meant giving up a specific ethnic identity. In the 1800, many immigrants from Eastern and Southern Europe changed their names for a more anglicized version, so that they could blend in. They were often characterized by what Gans (1985) called a symbolic ethnicity, of a nostalgic allegiance to the culture of origin in the forms of traditions that were nevertheless separated from daily behavior. Roediger (1999) describes the Irish immigrants who came to the United States in droves during the Great Famine of the late 1800 as imagined in racial terms to be savages, despised as close kin to the African, Mexican, and Native peoples. In their own land, they had been identified as enslaved and felt pushed out of Ireland by British colonialism, but upon immigration, the complexity of racial stereotypes lead them to strive to transform their despised identity to an acceptable Whiteness by attacking African Americans. Historically, the hostility between the Irish and African Americans began because the two groups were too close in status. The notion of a racial divide helped the Irish to become White and climb out of the marginal status of a despised people.

Essentially, a racial construction of Whiteness offers access to opportunities and privileges, but the cost is assimilation, diving into the melting pot (Hanna, Talley, & Guindon, 2000). Such racial notions also allow for the sense of a majority that can withstand the minorities. After all, if one counted peoples by ethnic identity rather than race, there would be no dominant White majority of 75% in this country (U.S. Census, 2000). Instead, every group would have to negotiate power and access in multiple contexts. Whiteness in the United States allowed for 500 years of Affirmative action that favored White identity over other groups. This very fact necessitates further discussion and understanding of the impact that racism has on the lives of people who may be our potential clients.

 REFLECTION QUESTIONS 5.7

- What are some of the beliefs, images, or stereotypes you have held about European Americans?
- Where did these beliefs, images, or stereotypes come from?
- How have they changed over time and if so, what caused them to change for you?
- How do these beliefs, images, or stereotypes affect your work with members of this population?
- What have been some of your experiences with members of this population, both positive and negative?

THE IMPACT OF RACISM

It is well documented that racism affects the lives of people. Being targeted by racism is hurtful and humiliating. The experience of racism can occur in many contexts and forms, during hate crimes, political activities that are against a particular group, backlashes against racial equity efforts, or expressions of racial intolerance, hostility and violence through the Internet, print media, or in person. People can experience racism in multiple contexts: 1) interpersonally through direct and vicarious experiences of bias; 2) collectively through group disparities in achievement, literacy, education, employment, salary, and inequitable treatment in the medical, financial, and justice systems; 3) culturally and symbolically through portrayals in the media, arts, scholarship, and sciences that reflect the values and beliefs of society; as well as 4) sociopolitically in the public discourse about race and its impact on governance and political process (Harrell, 2000).

Along this line of reasoning, Harrell (2000) defined racism-related stress as "the race-related transactions between individuals or groups and their environment that emerge from the dynamics of racism and that are perceived to tax or exceed existing individual and collective resources or threaten well-being" (Harrell, 2000, p. 44). She further elaborated that the stress of racism includes both the incidence and the subjective experience of the person, including the resistance of others to validate the experience. In this context, Harrell details six types of racism-related stress:

1. *Racism-related life events,* such as being racially profiled by police, which while significant, are infrequent and time-limited;
2. *Vicarious racism experiences,* which include experiences through observation and report that invoke heightened psychological and emotional states, such as following the high-profile media report of a hate crime;
3. *Daily racism microstressors,* which are typified by subtle or covert forms of degrading and marginalizing incidents that occur as everyday reminders of one's position and status and has been colorfully expressed by Margaret Cho as "the death of a thousand paper cuts";
4. *Chronic-contextual stress* reflects social, political, and institutional inequities that lead to unfair distribution of resources and opportunities that have to be survived such as crumbling infrastructures of schools, high-priced grocery stores, or poor public transportation;
5. *Collective experiences* impact the individual in their observation of how their group is collectively impacted through stereotypic portrayals, lack of political representation, or economic conditions; and
6. *Transgenerational transmission* refers to historical contexts of group experiences that are passed from generation to generation such as the experience of slavery for African Americans, the removal of tribal lands for Native Americans, the Holocaust for Jewish Americans, the Vietnam

War for Vietnamese Americans, or the genocidal experience of Bosnian Muslims.

Accordingly, racism-related stress affects us physically such as causing hypertension, as well as psychologically leading to trauma, general distress, substance abuse, disordered eating, psychosomatization, and violence. One's ability to trust, develop and maintain close relationships, achieve in school, perform at work, and function as a parent can all be impacted by racism-related stressors. Similarly, *racial* micro-agressions defined as "brief and commonplace daily verbal, behavioral, and environmental indignities, whether intentional or unintentional, that communicate hostile, derogatory, or negative racial slights and insults to the target person or group" (p. 273, Sue, Capodillupo, Torino, Bucceri, Holder, Nada & Esquilin, 2007) can operate in ways that may be harmful. Sue, et al. (2007) offer a number of examples that call attention to their impact on the individual such as 1) deliberate actions, such as serving Whites first at a restaurant, or calling someone "colored" (*micro-assult*), 2) statements that are more subtle but clearly convey the message that underrepresented groups are inferior such as "I believe in affirmative action, but we must admit qualified students of color into our program" (*micro-insult*), and 3) invalidation of the experiences of persons of color that can be manifested in actions, such as "I don't see racial differences and treat everyone the same" or "You are being overly sensitive about the situation, it wasn't racist"(*micro-invalidation*). Sue et al. (2007) also note that micro-aggressions extend beyond racial groups to include gender, disability, and sexual orientation.

The dehumanizing and degrading nature of racism can also threaten one's spiritual well-being and faith. Although there is very limited research on the impact of micro-aggressions as of this writing, Sue, Capodilupo and Holder's (2008) qualitative study offer tentative results showing that there are profound effects. In an African American sample of 10 participants, several themes emerged that support the effects of exposure to micro-aggressions, such as feeling powerless, invisible and less valued than Whites and pressure to represent his/her racial group in such a way as to not promote stereotyping. In order to better understand some of the possible issues and challenges associated with counseling people who are dealing with issues of racism, let us consider the following case.

OPENING THE DIALOGUE ON RACE, ETHNICITY, AND THE IMPACT OF RACISM

With all of the topics discussed in this chapter, you are now challenged to think through how you would utilize this information in sessions with any number of clients from a variety of cultural backgrounds and worldviews. Questions for reflection offered to you throughout this chapter also serve as

CASE STUDY **5.1**

The Case of Steve

Steve is a 43-year-old African American male. He is the CEO of a non-profit organization that he founded 15 years ago. He is currently separated from his wife for one year with no children. Steve lives in a middle-class suburb of a large metropolitan city in the Northeastern part of the U.S. Steve grew up in a public housing development in a small Southwestern city. His mother and father were divorced when he was 10 years of age. His father died when he was 15 years old, and he reports that he had no other male role model in his life with the exception of his high school counselor who was also an African American male. It is important to note that his mother worked as a domestic and, before his death, his father was employed as a janitor in a local hospital. Even though his parents were divorced, they instilled in Steve and his two siblings a strong work ethic and often relayed the message that if they worked hard enough they would earn the respect of others and experience happiness and success. Steve was taught by his parents that education was a "Black man's freedom" and to be truly free "a man had to be educated." As a teenager, Steve was an average student, but, according to Steve, his parents and his counselor saw him as more than "average." Growing up, his only role model besides his parents, was his high school counselor who he recalled telling once "… Mr. X you are just like Dr. Martin Luther King."

After several months of severe depression, Steve stated to a close friend that "I feel like I'm losing my mind … it seems that all my life, no matter how hard I work, some White person blocks my chance at happiness." Concerned about Steve, his friend encouraged him to seek professional help. Steve was adamant about not seeing a therapist and told his friend that "only crazy people and White people go to shrinks, and I am a long ways from being crazy or White." However, after much encouragement from his friend, he agreed to see a therapist. Steve's friend, an Asian American, suggested that Steve make an appointment with a therapist that he went to several years ago. Even though the therapist was a White male, Steve agreed to go. After several sessions, Steve reveals to the therapist that he has been experiencing severe depression and his only relief came from drinking himself to sleep. When asked by the therapist what he thought was the source of his depression, Steve stated "I don't know. It's not just one

thing. It seems like all my life, no matter how hard I work, someone has blocked my road to happiness." To which the therapist asked "who do you think has blocked you road to happiness?" Steve's responded with "White people! Every since I can remember some White person has done something to keep me from being happy or experiencing success." The therapist became very uncomfortable, and Steve noticed right away. Steve continued with his response …"I remember incidents as far back as elementary school … for example, I can remember when I had a crush on my best friends sister … they were White, and when his father found out that I had a thing for his daughter, they were told that they could no longer be friends with me because I was the wrong color. I can still remember being a confused and hurt. In high school, I worked at a Chinese restaurant, and right before graduation, I had to go graduation rehearsal and when I arrived late to work the owner of the restaurant pointed her finger in my face and shouted 'nigger too late, nigger too late.' During undergraduate at a predominately White institution, I remember being accused of cheating on an Algebra/Trig test because I scored a perfect score on the test. The professor, a White woman, stated that 'there's no way you could have made an A without cheating because you people aren't that smart in Math.' At the same institution during my master's program, I was the youngest, and the first African American to be enrolled in that particular master's program, the professor informed me in front of the entire class 'that you don't belong in this program.' It didn't stop there, one Christmas, I was shopping in a large department store and a White lady's shopping bag broke and when I attempted to assist her, she responded by clutching her purse and calling security … these are only a few of the experiences I have had as a Black man who has worked hard all of my life. I don't get it … I just don't understand why I'm so feared and despised. I'm a good person … a hard worker. My parents always told me all I had to do was work hard and I'd be respected and successful. Unfortunately, this has not been my experience."

Steve reluctantly confides to the therapist that in order to deal with the stress, his fears, anger, frustration, and depression, he has begun to drink heavily. He states, "it is the only way I can get through the day."

(continues)

Case Discussion

Thinking About this Case:

1. How might you respond to Steve, and what should your focus be?
2. What do you conceptualize Steve's issues to be, and what might be the best approach to take?

This case study represents the complexity and magnitude of issues faced by some African Americans. While many of the presenting issues are not exclusive to African Americans, many are intensified by the overwhelming external or environmental influences (i.e., historical, societal and political influences) in the life experiences of African Americans. Crawley and Freeman (1993) suggest that racism and prejudice are omnipresent in the life of African Americans as they try to negotiate life. Crawley and Freeman (1993) also suggest that young African Americans are faced with challenges during early adolescence, which require them to learn how to negotiate situations where race and/or culture are an issue. Failure to master this task could prove to be problematic later in life. Steve reports a series of negative experiences that may or may not have resulted from his being African American and male. However, if he believes that his ethnicity and gender are the causes of these experiences, it will be important for the counselor to explore these possibilities with him. Using Harrell's (2000) framework may be helpful in charting his life along the various dimensions and modalities to identify the racism-related stressors with which he is coping.

Being that this is Steve's' first counseling experience as an African American, it will be important to explain to Steve what counseling is and is not. Furthermore, allowing Steve to ask questions regarding the counseling process could be important in helping to alleviate any fears or misconceptions he may have. Using basic counseling or helping skills first is recommended. For example, it will be extremely important to develop rapport with Steve by allowing him to tell his story, listening carefully to his experience, and summarizing his experiences as you have heard them. This will allow him to hear his own experiences as someone else does. This will also provide him with an opportunity to clarify for the counselor and himself how he has made sense of these experiences and their impact on his life experience.

As this chapter suggests, counselors must be sensitive to the effects of racism and be willing to explore openly with their clients. For White counselors, it will be extremely important to be aware of your reactions to the clients' experiences. It is imperative that the counselor be careful not to discount the client's experiences or assume that they never happened. For White counselors, exploring your own biases and attitudes regarding men and African Americans in particular, before entering a therapeutic relationship with them becomes critical. Failure to do so could result in appearing less than genuine and create a sense of mistrust or exacerbate the clients' current level of mistrust. In this case, a counselor of color may well be faced with challenges as you may need to manage your reactions and responses to Steve's experiences and the ways they may resonate with your own. It would be important to maintain boundaries between your own understandings of race and racism and allow Steve to express and make sense of his experience.

Steve has presented several incidents in which he felt he was treated unjustly. Given his upbringing and his belief that "if you work hard you will earn the respect of others," these incidents do not describe his experience. It will be important to have Steve recount his experiences where he has experienced "respect." This should not be done to discount the negative experiences, but to bring to the forefront his experience as an African American.

It is important to acknowledge that there is no single approach to working with African American clients. However, patience on the part of the therapist will be critical to working with African Americans. Once a working alliance has been established, it will be critical for both parties to become clear as to which issue they will address first. Once this decision is made, a discussion regarding Steve's coping strategies will assist in identifying what has worked for him in the past and what has not with a major focus on what has worked. While no one can guarantee Steve that he will not experience similar experiences in the future, empowering him to gain control over how he responds could prove to be helpful. It will also be helpful to assist Steve with understanding how the use of alcohol only masks his depression and possibly exacerbates his feelings of victimization. If the counselor has limited knowledge of substance use and abuse, he or she may want to arrange consultation with a colleague who is more knowledgeable in that area.

If at the onset of the counseling intervention you realize that you are not prepared to directly address the issues of racism (as it relates to Steve's experience) or substance abuse, it may be important to refer Steve to someone who is more equipped to do so. Since this is his first experience with counseling, a good first experience will be critical if he is to continue with the counseling experience. A bad first experience could lead to irreversible actions. It is most important that counselors from all backgrounds understand the power of both racism (overt and covert) and prejudice. Coupled with depression and substance use/abuse, these collective experiences can lead to serious bouts of depression and other physical and psychological consequences.

excellent process questions for opening the dialogue with clients on issues of race, ethnicity, and experiences with racism. Some of these questions are listed here to assist you in terms of opening the dialogue with your clients:

- Who are you racially and ethnically? How important is this in your personal/cultural identity, and what impact do these dimensions have on how you view the world and live your life?
- How did your racial and ethnic definition of yourself develop, and who were some significant people in your life that helped to shape this definition?
- How has your view of race and ethnicity been reinforced or challenged during your life?
- What does your culture say about race and ethnicity?
- What does your family and community say about race and ethnicity both in terms of beliefs and practice?
- How do issues of power and privilege influence your view of race and ethnicity and concept of racism?
- How has your view of race and ethnicity affected the way you define yourself now and at previous points in your life?
- How will your view of race and ethnicity continue to affect the way you define yourself and the way others see you or treat you?
- How has your view of race and ethnicity affected the way you interact with others who are similar to you versus different in age to you at different points in your life?
- Who are some people of your own race and ethnicity that you look up to and why?
- How might the difference or similarity in race and ethnicity between you (client) and I (counselor) affect your experience in the process of counseling as well as the relationship between us?
- When and how did you first become aware of racism? What was your initial reaction, and how did that reaction change over time?
- What have your experiences with racism been and in what ways have those experiences shaped who you are as a person, as well as the issues you are dealing with now?
- What efforts have you made to work toward positive social change with regard to the racism that exists in your own life at the individual, group, and societal levels, and what other kinds of efforts would you like to make?
- To what extent do you value a person's race or ethnicity as a sign of his or her worth?
- Have you ever stood up for someone being harassed or oppressed on the basis of race or ethnicity? If not, why not? Has anyone ever stood up for you in this way?
- How do race and ethnicity play into the issues you are bringing to counseling, and how can we address this in a way that is most helpful to you?

CONCLUSION AND IMPLICATIONS

In today's diverse society, counselors will inevitably encounters clients of differing racial and ethnic backgrounds. As such, we must be knowledgeable about race and ethnicity, as well as their historical contexts. Likewise a clear understanding of the saliency of race, ethnicity, or both in a client will undoubtedly help establish a stronger therapeutic alliance and facilitate the counseling process. In your role as a counselor, it is particularly important for you to understand and be sensitive to the profound impact racism has on the physical and psychological well-being of individuals. Counselors need to be especially aware of life events and situations, whether it be micro-aggressions or race-relate stressful encounters, that may contribute to client problems or life-circumstances. As illustrated in the case study the magnitude of issues faced by some clients may be compounded by external or environmental influences (i.e., historical, societal and political). It is essential for counselors to validate a client's lived experiences.

We began this chapter with the notion that multicultural counseling competence requires an effective understanding of the constructs of race and ethnicity. The concepts of race and ethnicity have been problematic both by their existence in our consciousness and the way they have been used in a way that has placed very real limitations and abuses on the rights and privileges of specific people in this country throughout its history. The concepts of race and ethnicity have been defined in a variety of ways often leading to confusion in terms of meaning, significance, scope, and application. Overall, a review of the origins of the constructs of race and ethnicity were provided in a historical context to reflect the changing ways in which race and ethnicity have been conceptualized and defined. Following this, a multidisciplinary overview of theoretical approaches to race and racial classifications were offered. The chapter then offered brief overviews of various racial/ethnic groups that included African Americans, Asian Americans, Latinos/Hispanic Americans, Native Americans, Jewish Americans, and European Americans. Finally, we concluded with a discussion of the impact of racism on various members of racial and ethnic groups with implications for counseling. It is important to understand the impact that race and ethnicity continue to have on the experiences of people from all walks of life, and therefore, the critical importance they play in achieving multicultural counseling competence in order to facilitate optimal delivery of effective therapeutic services in a variety of settings.

GLOSSARY

African American: All persons having origins in any of the Black racial groups of Africa.

Asian American: All persons having origins in any of the original peoples of the Far East, Southeast Asia, or the Indian subcontinent including, for example, Cambodia, China, India, Japan, Korea, Malaysia, Pakistan, the Philippine Islands, Thailand, and Vietnam. Also, sometimes considered within this category is Native Hawaiian or Other Pacific Islander–All persons having origins in any of the original peoples of Hawaii, Guam, Samoa, or other Pacific Islands.

Culture: Values, beliefs, customs, traditions, language, and other behaviors that are passed on from one generation to another within a particular group.

Ethnicity: A group of people who share a particular social and cultural heritage, which includes language, customs and traditions, clothing, and history.

European American (sometimes referred to as White, Not of Hispanic Origin): All persons having origins in any of the original peoples of Europe, North Africa, or the Middle East.

Hispanic: A U.S. government term created to classify a group of people who come from Spanish-speaking countries.

Jewish American: The majority of Jewish Americans are Ashkenazi, having a common origin of Central and Eastern Europe, and fit the physiognomy of Whiteness in terms of skin pigmentation and morphology; they also have a common language of Yiddish (combining mostly Hebrew and German elements).

La Raza: Means "race" in English; however, the term encompasses culture, heritage and political consciousness.

Latino/Hispanic American: All persons of Mexican, Puerto Rican, Cuban, Central or South American, or other Spanish culture or origin, regardless of race. The term, "Spanish origin," can be used in addition to "Hispanic or Latino."

Mestizaje: The mixing of races (e.g., Spaniards from Spain and indigenous peoples, Blacks and Spaniards from Spain, Europeans and indigenous peoples from Spanish-speaking countries).

Micro-aggressions: Persistent verbal, behavioral and environmental assaults, insults and invalidations that can occur in such subtle ways that they are hard to identify. Micro-aggressions can be unintentional or intentional and convey hostility and intolerance.

Native American: (sometimes referred to as American Indian or Alaska Native): All persons having origins in any of the original peoples of North and South America (including Central America), and who maintain tribal affiliation or community recognition attachment.

Race: Originally based on biological characteristics based on skin pigmentation, physical features, hair and body type. Race was used to classify people into groups based on these characteristics. A contemporary view defines race as a "social construction," which encompasses the sociopolitical and historical contexts of racial classification.

REFERENCES

Acosta-Belén, E., & Sjostrom, B. R. (Eds.). (1988). *The Hispanic experience in the United States.* New York: Praeger.

Adams, M. (2001). Cross processes of racial identity development. In C. Wijeyesinghe & B. W. Jackson III (Eds.), *New perspectives on racial identity development: A theoretical and practical anthology* (pp. 209–242). New York: New York University Press.

Aldarondo, F. (2001). Racial and ethnic models and their application: Counseling biracial individuals. *Journal of Mental Health Counseling*, 23, 238–255.

American Anthropological Association. (1998). *Statement on "Race".* Retrieved December 8, 2003, from http://www.aaanet.org/stmts/racepp.htm

Arredondo, P. (2002). Mujeres Latinas-santas y marquesas. *Cultural Diversity and Ethnic Minority Psychology*, 8(4), 308–319.

Atkinson, D. R., Morten, G., & Sue, D. W. (1989). A minority identity development model. In D. R. Atkinson, G. Morten, & D. W. Sue (Eds.), *Counseling American minorities* (pp. 35–52). Dubuque, IA: William C. Brown.

Axelson, J. A. (1999). *Counseling and development in a multicultural society.* Pacific Grove, CA: Brooks/Cole.

Ball, J. Armistead, L., & Austin, B. (2003). The relationship between religiosity and adjustment among African American, female, urban adolescents, *Journal of Adolescence*, 26, 431–446.

Beale Spenser, M., Noll, E., Stoltzfus, J., & Harpalani, V. (2001). Identity and school adjustment: Revising the "acting white" assumption. *Educational Psychologists*, 36, 21–30.

Bernal, M. E., & Knight, G. P. (1993). *Ethnic identity: Formation and transmission among Hispanics and other minorities.* Albany, NY: State University of New York Press.

Bonilla-Silva, E. (1999). The new racism. In P. Wong (Ed.), *Race, ethnicity, and nationality in the United States: Towards the twenty-first century* (pp. 55–101). Boulder, CO: Westview Press.

Brown, C.S. (2002). *Refusing racism: White allies and the struggle for civil rights.* New York: Teachers College Press.

Castillo, L. G., & Hill, R. D. (2004). Predictors of distress in Chicana college students. *Journal of Multicultural Counseling and Development*, 32, 235–249.

Chadiha, L. A., Rafferty, J., & Pickard, J. (2003). The influence of caregiving stressors, social support, and caregiving appraisal on marital functioning among African American wife caregivers. *Journal of Marital and Family Therapy*, 29, 479–490.

Choney, S. K., Berryhill-Paake, E., & Robbins, R. R. (1995). The acculturation of American Indians. In J. G. Ponterotto, J. M. Casas, L. A. Suzuki, L. A., & C. M. Alexander (Eds.), *Handbook of multicultural counseling* (pp. 73–92). Thousand Oaks, CA: Sage.

Cole, E. R. & Omari, S. R. (2003). Race, class and the dilemmas of upward mobility for African Americans. *Journal of Social Issues*, 59, 785–802.

Comas-Díaz, L. (2001). Hispanics, Latinos, or Americanos: The evolution of identity. *Cultural Diversity and Ethnic Minority Psychology*, 7, 115–120.

Constantine, M. G., Okazaki, S., & Utsey, S. O. (2004). Self-concealment, social self-efficacy, acculturative stress, and depression in African, Asian, and Latin

American international college students. *American Journal of Orthopsychiatry*, 74, 230–241.

Cross, W. (1971). The Negro- to- Black conversion experience. *Black World*, 20, 13–27.

Cross, W. (1995). The psychology of Nigrescence: Revising the Cross Model. In J. G. Ponterotto, J. M. Casas, L. A. Suzuki, L. A., & C. M. Alexander (Eds.), *Handbook of multicultural counseling* (pp. 93–122). Thousand Oaks, CA: Sage.

Cross, W., & Vandiver, B. J. (2001). Nigrescence theory and measurement: Introducing the Cross Racial Identity Scale (CRIS). In J. G. Ponterotto, J. M. Casas, L. A. Suzuki, L. A., & C. M. Alexander (Eds.), *Handbook of multicultural counseling* (pp. 371–393). Thousand Oaks, CA: Sage.

Davey, M., Stone Fish, L., Askew, J., & Robila, M. (2003). Parenting practices and the transmission of ethnic identity. *Journal of Marital and Family Therapy*, 29, 195–208.

Elkins, S. (1976). *Slavery: A problem in American institutional and intellectual life.* Chicago: University of Chicago Press.

Erikson, E. H. (1968). *Identity: Youth and crisis.* New York: Norton.

Feagin, J. R., & Feagin, C. B. (2003). *Racial and ethnic relations* (7th ed.). Upper Saddle River, NJ: Prentice-Hall.

Ferdman, B. M., & Gallegos, P. I. (2001). Racial identity development and Latinos in the United States. In C. L. Wijeyesinghe & B. W. Jackson III. (Eds.), *New perspectives on racial identity development: A theoretical and practical anthology.* (pp. 32–66). New York: New York University Press.

Fischer, A. R., & Moradi, B. (2001). Racial and ethnic identity: Recent developments and needed directions. In J. G. Ponterotto, J. M. Casas, L. A. Suzuki, L. A., & C. M. Alexander (Eds.), *Handbook of multicultural counseling* (pp. 342–370). Thousand Oaks, CA: Sage.

Frederickson, G. M. (1988). *The arrogance of race: Historical perspectives on slavery, racism, and social inequality.* Hanover, NH: Wesleyan Press.

Garrett, M. T., & Barret, R. L. (2003). Two-spirit: Counseling Native American sexual minority persons. *Journal of Multicultural Counseling and Development*, 31, 131–142.

Garrett, M. T., Brubaker, M. D., & Torres-Rivera, E, & West-Olaunji, C., Conwill, W. (2008). The medicine of coming to center: Use of the Native American centering technique—Ayeli—to promote wellness and healing in group work. *Journal for Specialists in Group Work*, 33, 179–198.

Garrett, M. T., & Carroll, J. (2000). Mending the broken circle: Treatment and prevention of substance abuse among Native Americans. *Journal of Counseling and Development*, 78, 379–388.

Garrett, M. T., & Garrett, J. T. (2002). Ayeli: Centering technique based on Cherokee spiritual traditions. *Counseling and Values*, 46, 149–158.

Garrett, M. T., & Garrett, J. T. (2003). *Native American faith in America.* New York: Facts on File.

Garrett, M. T., Garrett, J. T., Wilbur, M., Roberts-Wilbur, J., & Torres-Rivera, E. (2005). Native American humor as spiritual tradition: Implications for counseling. *Journal of Multicultural Counseling and Development*, 33, 194–204.

Garrett, M. T., & Pichette, E. F. (2000). Red as an apple: Native American acculturation and counseling with or without reservation. *Journal of Counseling and Development*, 78, 3–13.

Portman, T. A. A., & Garrett, M. T. (2005). Beloved women: Nurturing leadership from an American Indian perspective. Invited publication for the *Journal of Counseling and Development: Special Issue on Women and Counseling*, 83, 284–291.

Portman, T. A. A., & Garrett, M. T. (2006). Native American healing traditions. *International Journal for Disability, Development, and Education*, 53, 453–469.

Garrett, M. T. (2004). Profile of Native Americans. In D. Atkinson (Ed.), *Counseling American minorities* (6th ed., pp. 147–170). NY: McGraw-Hill.

Goto, S. G., Gee G. C., & Takeuchi, D. T. (2002). Strangers still? The experiences of discrimination among Chinese Americans. *Journal of Community Psychology*, 30, 211–224.

Guthrie, R.V. (1976). *Even the rat was White: A historical view of psychology.* New York: Harper & Row.

Guthrie, R.V. (1997). *Even the rat was White: A historical view of psychology.* New York: Harper & Row.

Guzzetta, C. (1995). White ethnic groups. In R. L. Edwards (Ed.), *Encyclopedia of social work* (19th ed., pp. 2508–2517). Washington, DC: NASW Press.

Haley, A., & X, M. (1987). *Autobiography of Malcolm X* (reissued). NY: Ballantine Books.

Hanna, F. J., Talley, W. B., & Guindon, M. H. (2000). The Power of perception: Toward a model of cultural oppression and liberation. *Journal of Counseling & Development*, 78, 430–441.

Harrell, S. P. (2000). A multidimensional conceptualization of racism-related stress: Implications for the well-being of people of color. *American Journal of Orthopsychiatry*, 70(1), 42–57.

Helms, J. E. (1990). *Black and White racial identity: Theory, research and practice*. Westport, CT: Greenwood.

Helms, J. E. (1995). An update of Helms's White and People of Color Racial Identity Models. In J. G. Ponterotto, J. M. Casas, L. A. Suzuki, L. A., & C. M. Alexander (Eds.), *Handbook of multicultural counseling* (pp. 181–198). Thousand Oaks, CA: Sage.

Helms, J. E. (1996). Toward a methodology for measuring and assessing racial as distinguishing from ethnic identity. In G. R. Sodowsky, & J. C. Impara (Eds.), *Multicultural assessment in counseling and clinical psychology* (pp. 143–192). Lincoln, NE: Buros Institute of Mental Measurement.

Herrnstein, R., & Murray, C. (1994). *The bell curve: Intelligence and class structure in American life*. New York: Free Press.

Herring, R. D. (1999). *Counseling with Native American Indians and Alaska Natives: Strategies for helping professionals*. Thousand Oaks, CA: Sage.

Horse, P. G. (2001). Reflections on American Indian identity. In C. L. Wijeyesinghe & B. W. Jackson III. (Eds.), *New perspectives on racial identity development: A theoretical and practical anthology* (pp. 91–107). New York: New York University Press.

Hunter, M. L. (2002). "If you're light you're alright:" Light skin color as social capital for women of color. *Gender & Society*, 16, 175–193.

Ignatiev, N. (1995). *How the Irish became White*. New York: Routledge.

Jang, S. J. (2004). Explaining religious effects on distress among African Americans, *Journal for the Scientific Study of Religion*, 43, 239–260.

Kerwin, C., & Ponterotto, J. G. (1995). Biracial identity development: Theory and research. In J. G. Ponterotto, J. M. Casas, L. A. Suzuki, L. A., & C. M. Alexander (Eds.), *Handbook of multicultural counseling* (pp. 199–217). Thousand Oaks, CA: Sage.

Kim, J. (2001). Asian American identity development theory. In C. L. Wijeyesinghe, & B. W. Jackson III. (Eds.), *New perspectives on racial identity development: A theoretical and practical anthology* (pp. 67–90). New York: New York University Press.

Kivel, P. (1996). *Uprooting racism: How White people can work for racial justice*. Gabriola Island, British Columbia: New Society.

Kivisto, P., & Nefzger, B. (1993). Symbolic ethnicity and American Jews: The relationship of ethnic identity to behavior and group affiliation. *Social Science Journal*, 30, 1–12.

Koch, L. M., Gross, A. M., & Kolts, R. (2001). Attitudes toward Black English and code switching. *Journal of Black Psychology*, 27, 29–42.

Lee, W. M. L. (1999). *An introduction to multicultural counseling*. Philadelphia, PA: Taylor & Francis.

Lieberman, L. (1968). The debate over race: A study in the sociology of knowledge. *Phylon*, 39, 127–141.

Lieberman, L., & Byrne W. G. (1993). Race and how to teach it in the 21st Century. *Teaching Anthropology*, 2–3.

Lieberman, L., & Jackson, F. L. (1995). Race and the three models of human origin. *American Anthropologist*, 97(2), 231–241.

Linneaus, C. (1806). *Systema Natura* [Natural System]. London: Lackington, Allen, and Co.

Livingstone, F. B. (1964). On the non-existence of human races. In F.A. Montagu (Ed.), *The concept of race* (p. 46–60). New York: Free Press.

Logan, J. R. (2003, July). How race counts for Hispanic Americans. Mumford Center for Comparative Urban and Regional Research. Retrieved on February 9, 2004 from http://mumford1.dyndns.org/cen2000/report.html

McConnell, E. D., & Delgado-Romero, E. A. (2004). Pan-ethnic options and Latinos: Reality or methodological construction? *Sociological Focus*, 4, 297–312.

Marín, G. (1992). Issues in the measurement of acculturation among Hispanics. In K. F. Geisinger (Ed.), *Psychological testing of Hispanics* (pp. 235–251). Washington, DC: American Psychological Association.

Marín, G., & Marín, B. V. (1991). *Research with Hispanic populations*. Newbury Park, CA: Sage.

Marks, J. M. (1995). *Human biodiversity: Genes, race, and history*. New York: Aldine deGruyter.

McConnell, E. D., & Delgado-Romero, E. A. (2004). Pan-ethnic options and Latinos: Reality or methodological construction? *Sociological Focus*, 4, 297–312.

McLaughlin, D. (1994). Critical Literacy for Navajo and other American Indian learners. *Journal of American Indian Education*, 33, 47–59.

Montagu, M. F. A. (1942). *Man's most dangerous myth: The fallacy of race.* New York: Coumbia University Press.

Moore, J., & Pachon, H. (1985). *Hispanics in the United States.* Englewood Cliffs, NJ: Prentice-Hall.

Munford, M. B. (1994). Relationship of gender, self-esteem, social class, and racial identity to depression in blacks. *Journal of Black Psychology*, 20, 157–174.

Nobles, M. (2000). *Shades of citizenship: race and the census in modern politics.* Stanford, CA: Stanford University Press.

Obler, S. (1999). Racializing Latinos in the United States: Toward a new research paradigm. In L. R. Goldin (Ed.), *Identities on the move: Transnational processes in North America and the Caribbean Basin* (pp. 45–68). Albany, NY: Institute for Mesoamerican Studies.

Office of Policy Planning and Research. (1965). *The Negro Family: The Case for National Action.* Washington, DC: Department of Labor.

Omi, M. (1999). Racial identity and the state: Contesting the Federal standards for classification. In P. Wong (Ed.), *Race, ethnicity, and nationality in the United States: Towards the twenty-first century* (pp. 25–33). Boulder, CO: Westview Press.

Omi, M., & Winant, H. (1986). *Racial formation in the United States from the 1960s to the 1980s.* New York: Routledge.

Omi, M., & Winant, H. (1994). *Racial formation in the United States from the 1960s to the 1990s.* New York: Routledge.

Parham, T.A. (2002). *Counseling persons of African descent: raising the bar of practitioner competence.* Thousand Oaks, CA: Sage.

Phelps, R. E., Taylor, J. D., & Gerard, P. A. (2001). Cultural mistrust, ethnic identity, racial identity, and self-esteem among ethnically diverse Black university students. *Journal of Counseling and Development*, 79, 209–216.

Phillips Smith, E., Walker, K., Fields, L., Brookins, C. C., & Seay, R. C. (1999). Ethnic identity and its relationship to self-esteem, perceived efficacy and prosocial attitudes in early adolescence. *Journal of Adolescence*, 22, 867–880.

Phinney, J. S. (1989). Stages of ethnic identity in minority adolescents. *Journal of Early Adolescence*, 9, 34–49.

Phinney, J. S. (1990). Ethnic identity in adolescents and adults: Review of research. *Psychological Bulletin*, 108, 499–514.

Phinney, J. S. (1992). The Multigroup Ethnic Identity Measure: A new scale for use with diverse groups. *Journal of Adolescent Research*, 13, 156–176.

Phinney, J. S. (1993). A three-stage model of ethnic identity development in adolescence. In M. E. Bernal, & G. P. Knight (Eds.), *Ethnic identity: Formation and transmission among Hispanics and other minorities* (pp. 61–79). Albany, NY: State University of New York Press.

Phinney, J. S. (1996). When we talk about American ethnic groups, what do we mean? *American Psychologist*, 51, 918–927.

Phinney, J. S., & Chavira, V. (1992). Ethnic identity and self-esteem: An exploration longitudinal study. *Journal of Adolescence*, 15, 271–281.

Ponterotto, J. G, & Pedersen, P. B. (1993). *Preventing prejudice: A guide for counselors and educators.* Newbury Park, CA: Sage.

Population Reference Bureau. (2003). *200 years of census taking: Population and housing questions 1790-1990.* U.S. Bureau of the Census. Retrieved December 12, 2003 from http://www.prb.org

Portman, T. A. A., & Garrett, M. T. (2006). Native American healing traditions. *International Journal for Disability, Development, and Education*, 53, 453–469.

Poston, C. W. (1990). The Biracial Identity Model: A needed addition. *Journal of Counseling and Development*, 69, 152–155.

Pyant, C. T., & Yanico, B. J. (1991). Relationship of racial identity and gender-role attitudes to Black women's psychological well-being. *Journal of Counseling Psychology*, 38, 315–322.

Robinson, T. R. (2005). *The convergence of race, ethnicity, and gender: Multiple identities in counseling* (2nd ed.). Upper Saddle River, NJ: Pearson.

Robinson-Wood, T. (2009). *The convergence of race, ethnicity, and gender: Multiple identities in counseling* (3rd ed.). Upper Saddle River, NJ: Prentice-Hall.

Ridley, C.R. (1995). *Overcoming unintentional racism in counseling and therapy: A practitioners guide to intentional intervention.* Thousand Oaks, CA: Sage.

Rodriguez, C. E. (2000). *Changing race: Latinos, the census, and the history of ethnicity in the United States.* New York: New York University Press.

Santiago-Rivera, A. L., Arredondo, P., & Gallardo-Cooper, M. (2002). *Counseling Latinos and la familia.* Thousand Oaks, CA: Sage.

Sellers, R. M., Smith, M. A., Shelton, J. N., Rowley, S. A. J., & Chavous, T. M. (1998).

Multidimensional Model of Racial Identity: A re-conceptualization of African American Racial identity. *Personality and Social Psychology Review*, 2(1), 18–39.

Shanklin, E. (1994). *Anthropology and race*. Belmont, CA: Wadsworth.

Sodowsky, R. G., Kwan, K. L. K., Pannu, R. (1995). Ethnic identity of Asians in the United States. In J. G. Ponterotto, J. M. Casas, L. A. Suzuki, L. A., & C. M. Alexander (Eds.), *Handbook of multicultural counseling* (pp. 123–154). Thousand Oaks, CA: Sage.

Soto-Carlo, A., Delgado-Romero, E. A., & Galván, N. (2005). Challenges of Puerto Rican Islander students in the US. *Latino Studies Journal*, 3, 288–294.

Spanakis, N. C. (2004). Difficult dialogues: Interviewer, White inner voice, and Latina Interviewee. *Journal of Multicultural Counseling and Development*, 32, 249–254.

Spanakis, N. C. (2004). Difficult dialogues: Interviewer, White inner voice, and Latina Interviewee. *Journal of Multicultural Counseling and Development*, 32, 249–254.

Spickard, P. (1989). *Mixed Blood: Intermarriage and ethnic identity in twentieth-century America*. Madison, WI: University of Wisconsin Press.

Spring, J. (2004). *Deculturalization and the struggle for equality* (4th ed.). New York: McGraw-Hill.

Sue, D. W., Capodilupo, C. M., & Holder, A. M. B. (2008). Racial micro-aggressions in the life experience of Black Americans. *Professional Psychology: Rsearch and Practice*, 39, 329-336.

Sue, D. W., Capodilupo, C. M., Torino, G. C., Bucceri, J. M., Holder, A. M. B., Nadal, K. L., & Esquilin, M. (2007). Racial micro-aggressions in everyday life. *American Psychologist*, 62, 271–286.

Sue, D. W., & Sue, D. (1999). *Counseling the culturally different: Theory and practice* (3rd. ed.). New York: John Wiley.

Sue, D. W., & Sue, D. (2003). *Counseling the culturally diverse: Theory and practice* (4th ed.). New York: NY: John Wiley & Sons.

Tajfel, H. (1981). *Human groups and social categories: Studies in social psychology*. London: Cambridge University Press.

Takaki, R. (1989). *Strangers from a different shore: A history of Asian Americans*. New York: Penguin Books.

Takaki, R. (1993). *A different mirror: A history of multicultural America*. Boston: Little, Brown & Co.

Thomason, T. C. (1995). Counseling Native American students. In C. Lee (Ed.), *Counseling for diversity: A guide for school counselors and related professionals* (pp. 109–126). Needham Heights, MA: Allyn & Bacon.

Thompson, C. E., & Carter, R. T. (1997). An overview and elaboration of Helms' Racial Identity Development Theory. In C. E. Thompson, & R.T. Carter (Eds.), *Racial identity theory: Applications to individuals, group, and organizational interventions* (pp. 15–32). Mahwah, NJ: Erlbaum.

Torres, J. B., Solberg, S. H., & Carlstrom, A. H. (2002). The myth of sameness among Latino men and their machismo. *American Journal of Orthopsychiatry*, 72(2), 163–181.

Torres, V. (2003). Influences on Ethnic Identity Development of Latino College Students in the First Two Years of College. *Journal of College Student Development*, 44, 532–547.

Torres, V. (2004). Familial influences on the identity development of Latino first year students. *Journal of College Student Development*, 45, 457–469.

Trimble, J. E. (1996). Towards an understanding of ethnicity and ethnic identification and their relationship with drug use research. In G. J. Botvin, S. Schinke, & M. A. Orlandi (Eds.), *Drug abuse prevention with multiethnic youth* (pp. 3–27). Thousand Oaks, CA: Sage.

Trimble, J. E., & Jumper-Thurman, P. (2002). Ethnocultural considerations and strategies for providing counseling services to Native American Indians. In P. B. Pedersen, J. G. Draguns, W. J. Lonner, & J. E. Trimble (Eds.), *Counseling across cultures* (5th ed., pp. 53–92). Thousand Oaks, CA: Sage.

U.S. Department of Energy. (2003). Human Genome Project. Retrieved on December 12, 2003, from http://www.ornl.gov/sci/techresources/Human_Genome

Vontress, C. E., & Epps, L. R. (1997). Historical hostility in the African American client: Implications for counseling. *Journal of Multicultural Counseling and Development*, 25, 170–184.

Wachtel, P. (1999). *Race in the mind of America: breaking the vicious cycle between Blacks and Whites*. New York: Routledge.

Wade, T. J., & Bielitz, S. (2005). The differential effect of skin color on attractiveness, personality evaluations, and perceived life success of African Americans. *Journal of Black Psychology*, 31, 215–236.

Wijeyesinghe, C. L. (Ed.). (2001). Racial identity in multiracial people: An alternative paradigm. In C. L. Wijeyesinghe & B. W. Jackson III (Eds.), *New perspectives on racial identity development: A theoretical and practical anthology.* (pp. 129–152). New York: New York University Press.

Winant, H. (2000). Race and race theory. *Annual Review of Sociology, 26,* 169–185.

Winston, A. S. (Ed.). (2004). *Defining differences: Race and racism in the history of psychology.* Washington, DC: American Psychological Association.

Zak, I. (1973). Dimensions of Jewish American identity. *Psychological Reports, 33,* 891–900.

CHAPTER 6

Age

Dr. Thomas Baskin, University of Wisconsin-Milwaukee

The Road Not Taken

Two roads diverged in a yellow wood,
And sorry I could not travel both
And be one traveler, long I stood
And looked down one as far as I could
To where it bent in the undergrowth;

Then took the other, as just as fair,
And having perhaps the better claim,
Because it was grassy and wanted wear;
Though as for that the passing there
Had worn them really about the same,

And both that morning equally lay
In leaves no step had trodden black.
Oh, I kept the first for another day!
Yet knowing how way leads on to way,
I doubted if I should ever come back.

I shall be telling this with a sigh
Somewhere ages and ages hence:
Two roads diverged in a wood, and I—
I took the one less traveled by,
And that has made all the difference.

Robert Frost (1946, p. 117)

The goal of this chapter is to discuss age in a way that leads to an understanding of its affirming role in people's lives and in counseling. This is a challenge, as there has been a history in modern Western society of having biases and stereotypes about people's age. The well-known poem by Robert Frost that opened this chapter reveals an important metaphor that shows the nature of age and why age is important in counseling, yet avoids many of the pitfalls of making assumptions about people based on their age. The metaphor is that of a path. The nature of paths is both with distance and with choice. Where people are on their life path reveals where they have been, what choices they have made, and what choices are ahead of them. The path metaphor reveals how people cannot do everything but must make choices, and that people who have traveled the same distance may still be in very different places, whereas people may be at similar places having traveled different distances. Thus, in this chapter, we will explore how this view leads to a contextual understanding of age.

To do this, we will begin by defining the concept of age, then exploring how age has been studied historically. Next, we will review critical stages of life from a counseling perspective, including how counseling is different in each of those respective stages (what will be called *counseling life stages*) that informs the counseling of people at different places in their life paths. Then, keeping in mind Duncan and Loretto's (2004) assertion that negative biases around age tend to be highest regarding our society's youngest and oldest persons, we will look at ageism. This is important because discrimination due to age has become rampant and accepted in our society and has long-lasting effects on clients from all walks of life. Subsequently, we will look at ways that counselors can be an influence for positive change. Last, we will discuss selected special topics related to age and counseling. All of these areas will be explored together to convey a contextual understanding of age in counseling.

AGE DEFINED

Webster's (1983) dictionary definition of **age** is as follows: "The whole duration of a person … since … beginning" (p. 35). This definition is helpful, as it points to the potential of looking at a person from a holistic viewpoint. It suggests that a person is not just a moment in time but also a collection of his or her life experiences. The problem is that, commonly, this definition is not maintained. People are not thought of in their entirety, but by merely a chronological amount of years—a number. Assumptions are then often made about what that number represents for the person. As counselors, we need to look beyond a number. We need to take seriously Thornton's (2002) warning about the too prevalent problem of "mythmaking" about what aging means. In mythmaking, much like stereotyping, to make sense of our world our mind tends to simplify people and situations into basic categories. As counselors we need to view people as unique individuals, and learn to understand people of different ages, without oversimplifying what it means to be a certain age.

REFLECTION QUESTIONS 6.1

- What is your definition of age and aging?
- Where did that definition originate, and how has it been reinforced or challenged during your life?
- How do issues of power and privilege influence your definition of age and concept of aging?
- How has your definition of age affected the way you define yourself now and at previous points in your life?
- How will your definition of age and aging continue to affect the way you define yourself and the way others see you or treat you?
- How has your definition of age and aging affected the way you interact with others who are similar in age to you versus different in age to you at different points in your life?
- How does your definition of age and aging affect your ability to work with clients from a range of ages?
- How will your definition of age change as you grow older?

CASE STUDY **6.1**

The Case of Joyce

Consider Joyce, an 80-year-old Chinese-American woman. She lives in San Francisco, California, where her family has lived for generations. Joyce has made choices to marry, have children, and live close to her immediate and extended family. She describes her life as fulfilling; valuing the time she can spend with her adult children and grandchildren. But in recent years her physical health has been declining. She recently fell while going down the stairs and broke her hip. She is showing symptoms of depression because she can't do some of the things that she used to do. She is beginning to feel "less useful." Her children reassure her that she will always be taken care of within the family, but Joyce is thinking more about how many years she has left to live, and whether her declining health will be a burden to her family.

Case Discussion
Thinking About This Case
1. What does this case tell you about your own understanding of age? About your beliefs or biases?

2. What are some of your reactions in general to this scenario, and what kinds of things would you want to attend to from a therapeutic standpoint?
3. What limitations are you aware of in terms of working with aspects of age?

This case is an example of an individual who is transitioning to another life-stage. Although Joyce believes that she has family support, she still wants to remain valued, especially since her physical health is declining. The counselor can work with Joyce to find new meaning in her relationships and help support self-esteem as she is feeling less valued. Because Joyce may be entering a stage where there is reduced functioning, the counselor can work with her to identify specific activities that she can and can't do. In addition, involving members of the family in counseling is highly recommended, especially since Joyce reports that they are supportive.

THE HISTORICAL STUDY OF AGE

One of the early proponents of the scientific study of aging was Francis Bacon (Woodruff-Pak, 1988). He was born in the 16th century and believed that through scientific observation, we could learn many things about people and the natural world, including the causes of the aging process. Although his theory of why people age has since been disproved, he did help open the way toward a logical examination of aging as a process.

A Belgian named Quetelet can be considered to be the first gerontologist (Birren, 1961). He received his doctorate in science with the study of mathematics from the University of Ghent in 1819. He created some major statistical tools, including important work on what we now call the *bell-shaped curve*, or *bell curve*. He noticed that natural measurements, such as the height of a woman, tend to distribute in a predictable way. He looked at data related to many things, including age. In particular, he analyzed the productivity of French and English playwrights in comparison to their ages. He also analyzed data on how long people lived. In these ways, Quetelet furthered the scientific study of age.

In the late 1800s, Sir Francis Galton collected information on 17 different characteristics regarding things such as grip strength, vision, and reaction time from over 9,000 people aged 5 to 80 (Woodruff-Pak, 1988). He was then able, statistically, to show the influence of age in relationship to many of these characteristics. This examination is helpful in terms of understanding age in a logical manner; however, it is wise to remember that people are not only a measure of their physical features.

A 19th-century psychologist named G. Stanley Hall helped shift the study of age from physical measurement toward an examination of psychological development. In 1922, Hall's book *Senescence, the Last Half of Life* was published. Although Hall had done major work with children, and actually coined the term *adolescence,* in this book he emphasized the psychological states of older persons to be important in terms of thoughts, feelings, and will. He also emphasized the importance of individual differences amongst older persons. In these ways, Hall opened the door for modern developmental psychology and counseling to understand the importance of psychological changes as people age.

About 100 years after Hall, stage theories became important within psychology. Piaget and Inhelder's (1969) theory of cognitive development suggests that children go through four distinct stages in terms of how they make sense of the world cognitively. Additionally, Erikson (1950, 1997) proposed that there are psychosocial stages of development that form important foundations for human development. Erikson first considered eight stages of psychosocial development, and then added a ninth stage for the most advanced years of life. These nine stages outline how different stages of life bring different psychological challenges. In regard to counseling there are similar, yet different, life stages that can be kept in mind when counseling people of different ages. They are not rigid stages but are flexible guidelines for counseling people at different places along their life paths.

REFLECTION QUESTIONS 6.2

- How has the historical context of defining and studying age affected the way you look at this concept today?
- To what extent is your view of aging influenced by society at large, including media influences?
- What does your culture say about age?
- What do your family and community say about age in terms of both beliefs and practice?

COUNSELING LIFE STAGES

In terms of counseling, one can divide the life span loosely into 10 stages that influence where a person is at along their path, and how they may have unique needs within a counseling relationship. These stages can be seen as (a) preschool age; (b) school age—primary school; (c) school age—middle school; (d) school age—high school; (e) young adulthood; (f) middle adulthood; (g) advanced adulthood; (h) senior adulthood; (i) senior adulthood—reduced functioning; and (j) senior adulthood—limited functioning. The descriptions that follow for each stage include a definition of what each stage is, how it relates to counseling, and what some of the key things are that tend to differentiate people at this stage. An understanding of the differences at these stages can be key to not stereotyping a person who is at any given stage (Erikson, 1997; Levinson, 1978, 1996).

Preschool Age (birth to 5 years old)

As the name implies, this stage is from birth until a child goes to school. It is typified by a heavy dependence on one's parents; most of the major choices of this stage are predetermined for the child by his or her parents. It is also typified by a sense of potential. Children are at the beginning of their path of life, and their life, for the most part, has yet to unfold.

Counseling in this stage will tend to focus on the family and on the child's behavior. Because the child is so dependent on the family at this stage, therapy often occurs within the family. At times, however, it will be individual and will usually involve play therapy, or other ways of attaching meaning to behavior, as behavior at this age will tend to hold more meaning than verbal communication (such as that expressed in insight-oriented verbal therapies).

Most of the choices that differentiate persons in this stage are choices that are made by the parents. This can involve whether the child has a parental caretaker or goes to day care, the socioeconomic level of the parents, and how many siblings the child has.

Consider counseling a 4-year-old girl whose parents feel that she is always "fussy" and challenges everything that they say. What more would you want to know about the child?

School Age—Primary School (5 to 10 years old)

This stage covers children from grades kindergarten through fifth grade. The main shift is that they now have many more social tasks at this stage than they did at the previous stage. They now spend a large amount of time dealing with the social environment of the classroom, rather than having as close an association with a caregiver. Children at this age, however, still are very associated with their parents in terms of identity and range of life choices.

Counseling at this stage will continue to value behavior, as with the first stage, although there is more of an opportunity to help the child verbally. Furthermore, especially within the school context, there is more of an opening to help children developmentally to learn healthy ways of navigating their environment as individuals.

Differentiation at this stage again involves family choices more than individual ones, which is critical for all children. This may include where the family lives, leading to who neighborhood friends will be, what the quality of the school is, and what after-school opportunities exist. The availability of an extended family at this age can also be significant.

Consider counseling a second-grade boy who is constantly anxious and doesn't want to go to school. What questions would you ask him and his parents to try to assess what he is struggling with?

School Age—Middle School (10 to 14 years old)

This stage covers approximately fifth through eighth grades, although development can vary from individual to individual and from environment to environment. In this stage, children are making new strides to be individuals and to see themselves within their social context. They are more aware of the social norms and pressures around them, and of how they are being viewed socially by others. Furthermore, this is often the start of wanting to be seen more individually, although family can still be very important. Peers generally start becoming more important at this stage.

Counseling at this stage can start focusing on the individual choices that the person is making. This can still be seen within the contexts of the child's family and his or her culture, but children are also starting to make more significant choices about how they want their path in life to unfold. Groups can also be especially effective at this age, as students now tend to have fairly well-developed verbal skills, and tend to value the norms and opinions of a group.

Differentiation can include cultural values of how individualized a person is expected to be, and what being an individual may represent. Some children at this age spend most of their time with their nuclear family, others with their extended families, and still others away from their families. Each of these three directions will guide people toward different paths. Additionally, academic, athletic, and social abilities tend to distinguish individual paths at this stage.

Consider counseling a seventh-grade girl who was born in Bolivia, is ethnically Japanese, and doesn't want to study her math as hard as her parents feel that she should. How might you guide this family?

School Age—High School (14 to 18 years old)

This stage covers approximately ninth through 12th grades. These are the adolescent years of development. Individuals at this stage continue along the themes of middle schoolers by being more independent and by having an expanded emphasis on their social environment. Furthermore, differentiation according to academic, athletic, and social abilities tends to become more pronounced. Students tend to form into different social groups or cliques largely based on these abilities, and based on family wealth and a family's cultural values. These groups can stereotypically take on names such as *jocks*, *brains*, and the like. Although these groups may not be rigid in their boundaries, there is often a sense for people at this age to try to find a group of other students to belong with.

Counseling at this stage often remains in the context of school counseling; however, as persons become more and more mature, there are renewed opportunities to have successful individual counseling sessions. Furthermore, counseling sessions can become more verbal and insight oriented at this age. As with all ages, cultural values play an important role at this stage. These adolescents will often be struggling with individual concerns that are in conflict with family and social norms. Each culture will have influence on how persons at this stage are expected to develop. For example, in some families there will be a family business, such as a restaurant; a person in this life stage may be expected by his or her family to work at this business for many hours per week. In contrast, in some families, both parents are often away on business trips, and their children are frequently left alone at this age. These two types of families have very different day-to-day ways in which one belongs to the family. This is important to keep in mind during counseling, as these students' needs may be very different.

As previously stated, differentiation at this stage is heavily influenced by the social groups mentioned above. As adolescents at this age form into social cliques (or fail to be a part of social groups), their development is affected. These patterns will continue to influence their future paths, based on the amount of time that they put into different activities. Another important factor at this stage is finding a partner. At this stage, many students are first experimenting with committed partnerships. Paths can change based on early marriage versus not having a partner. And pregnancy and parenthood at this age are for the first time possible, and clearly will influence one's life path. Furthermore, the issues of finding a partner and career trajectory may be interrelated, as Parkes, Wight, Henderson, and West (2009) found that those who were sexually active at a younger age tended to participate less in tertiary education. Consequently, in this and other stages, counselors need to keep in mind not only the main struggles of clients but also how these challenges may interact with each other.

Consider a Latino male who is in the 11th grade and wants to join the military when he graduates high school, whereas his parents want him to go to a local college. Furthermore, his girlfriend is going to a distant college, and wants him to join her. How might you address him individually in counseling?

Young Adulthood

This stage is marked by high school graduation, or turning 18 years old. It is the stage when, socially, people are starting to be considered adults. People at this stage can choose what level of involvement they would like to have with their parents, in a way that was often not a choice previously. People may choose to become fully independent at this stage by finding employment and disengaging from their families; however, this is not the social trend in today's society. The trend is actually for an extended adolescence at this stage, where people are largely dependent on their family of origin for financial support as they continue their education.

Counseling at this age can more clearly focus on the choices that a person is making, as she or he tends to have more freedom and responsibility at this age. These freedoms commonly give students dilemmas between independence and family responsibilities. For example, a student may be supported in college by her parents and wants to smoke marijuana. The parents may threaten to cut off support if the drug use continues. Here counseling can help the student to address this dilemma, in which she feels old enough to make an independent choice about smoking marijuana, yet financially is not ready to be independent.

Differentiation can take the forms of student status, economic opportunity, and parental status. People pursuing a full-time college education will be highly influenced by this endeavor. It will often define where someone lives, how he or she spends an average day, and what resources are available. Although being considered adults, college students retain many similarities to, and responsibilities of, high school students. This is contrasted with those who enter the workforce full-time, who will experience more of a change if they are no longer a student. Involvement as a college student versus a full-time employee can also be seen on a continuum, where many people will work part- or full-time and go to school part- or full-time based on available economic resources. In this way, the number of years one spends in college can vary greatly. Also a key issue at this stage is parental status. Those having children at this age find themselves with many more responsibilities than those who do not. Becoming a parent can be the catalyst for moving from adolescence to adulthood.

Consider a 21-year-old African American female who has graduated from an Ivy League college in engineering, but wonders if she is not more interested in a career in dance. How might you counsel her in this dilemma?

Middle Adulthood

A range of issues can be important in the transition to middle adulthood. These can include issues relating to one's job, partnership(s), relation to parents, and decision to have children. In the area of employment, someone at this stage would tend to be finished with school and would have a more stable job or career than they may have had in young adulthood. Partnership status at this stage is also very important, with the typical pattern being more of a sense of permanence with a partner, rather than the movement between partners that can be more typical in young adulthood. Furthermore, at this stage there is a tendency to be less financially dependent on parents, and to view parents more as peers. Finally, having children of one's own often solidifies the transition to middle adulthood. However, in all of these areas there are great individual differences that need to be considered in effective counseling.

Possibly more than at any other stage, there will be considerable variance in what issues people want to address in counseling. It may be that they have too demanding of a job, or not enough to do in their job. It may be that they are unhappy with their partner and are thinking of leaving the relationship, or that they are wishing they had a partner. Typically the contrast with young adulthood will be that job, partners, and family will more likely raise long-term issues where they foresee the situation being more of the same for years, and they are looking for ways to deal with it. In young adulthood, more often a sense of a new job or partner could be seen as a solution, whereas in middle adulthood there is often a sense of having tried different options and of wanting to make the best of the current situation.

Differences in careers can start to show more and more at this stage. Those in higher income areas such as business and the professions can often have very high salaries at this time. Also, jobs that have few options for advancement may become more frustrating. Partnership status can be very diverse at this stage, too: from having no partner, to having a partner for over a decade who one adores, to having a partner for a few years who one is tired of being with, and all other variations on the spectrum. Also critical at this stage is parenthood status. Having no children, or one older child, or many young children are all possible, and will all inform a person's life path at this stage.

Consider the previous African American client who graduated from an Ivy League college in engineering. She is now 35 years old, has two kids, and did not pursue dancing, but has worked as an engineer for 14 years. She now wonders if she shouldn't have pursued dancing instead of engineering. How might your counseling differ than it would have when she was 21 years old?

Advanced Adulthood

In advanced adulthood, a common theme is that there is a sense of wanting to have fulfillment in every domain, but each domain may look very different. One may be happy in work, but not in partnership, and vice versa. As with other stages, there may be great differences in people's life paths, and the challenge of counseling is to be sensitive to an individual's specific situation.

In counseling, the concern is to help clients manage their great variety of triumphs, tragedies, and challenges for the future at this point in life. People will now have a number of years of life experience, and, as suggested above, they will have a mixture of experiences. As a counselor, the goal will tend to be to help them mourn their failures and commit to current or new goals for the future.

The stage of advanced adulthood can be seen through the lenses of career, partnership, and family concerns. A person may be moving into the highest stages of a corporate ladder, or may have been laid off and need to find a new job or career. A person may be happily married for many years, or seeking a divorce. A person may be the caretaker for their limited-functioning parents and for their own children, or may have no one dependent on them. Because these domains can be so disparate, it can be important in counseling to help clients to be dedicated to reality. A successful CEO may have a hard time facing a marriage that he sees as a failure. It can be hard to face pain in one domain when another seems so positive, but this can also help a person to overcome any mental health concerns.

Financially, this stage has taken a different shape for many in light of the Great Recession starting in 2008. Some who thought they could retire at 55 years of age are now looking at working much longer. Others have much less money in their retirement accounts than they previously had. For many, what they thought would be a period of leisure has become a period of continued stress. Related to this, some have had a shift in mind-set where they are much more cautious in their spending, and see the world as a riskier place than they once did. For counselors, there can be value to understanding the economic mind-set and circumstances of clients, and to realize that these may be very different at different life stages.

Consider a 60-year-old European American male who has been downsized from his company. He needs to find a job, as his savings are not enough for him to retire. He is single. How might you counsel him differently than a 20 year old in a similar position?

Senior Adulthood

The transition from advanced adulthood to senior adulthood takes place around the age of 65 years old. This can look very different for different individuals, but it predominately focuses around retirement. This is a significant transition because in retirement, there is a great shift in social expectations for how persons are expected to contribute economically. The social norm is that at this stage, there are not the same expectations that most people will have full-time jobs. Also at this stage, the level of health or illness that a person struggles with can become more and more of a factor in his or her life.

Counseling at this stage can often focus on transitions and new roles. This transition can be seen as bimodal in that many people are delighted with retirement, and others are so immersed in their jobs that they can't imagine life without them. This latter group will have a tougher transition to retirement. In the book *Retire Smart, Retire Happy: Finding Your True Path in Life*, Schlossberg (2004) gives the perspective that assisting people in the transition to retirement can be seen as helping them in another transition in life. That they've already undergone many transitions, and this is merely another one for them to tackle. Furthermore, for those where work has been critical, there are identity issues around how they view themselves. Helping them to maintain their identity in a meaningful way can be vital at this age.

Besides how much people had felt attached to their careers, there are also key differences around whether they are financially well-off or have limited resources. Also, there can be a large difference between those who are involved with an extended family and those who are not. Similarly, those with active social networks will tend to do better in retirement than those who lack such networks. There may be a need to reestablish a social network apart from one's work world. Indeed, Siegler, Bastian, Steffens, Bosworth, and Costa (2002) highlight that a major misconception about old age is that there is little variance among older people, when quite the opposite is actually the case.

A 70-year-old retired schoolteacher is depressed because many of her friends have died, and she lives far from her three children. How might one counsel her about staying in the home where her husband and she have lived for 50 years, or moving to where one of their three children are?

Senior Adulthood—Reduced Functioning

Advancement to this stage is defined in terms of functioning rather than age, as functioning determines many other factors at this stage. An 80 year old who still drives may more closely resemble a newly retired 65 year old who drives than another 80 year old who does not drive due to health concerns. The start of this stage is when health or mental concerns lead to reduced functioning, but they still can take care of their basic needs, such as feeding and dressing themselves.

This can be a critical stage for counseling to help people prioritize their lives and invest their reduced physical resources. Finding meaning in relationships and activities can be a challenge, as options are reduced, yet there can also be a great rediscovery of interests, social groups, and the importance of family. Furthermore, counseling that supports self-esteem can help to buffer the impact of physical declines (Jonker, Comijs, Knipscheer, & Deeg, 2009).

Differentiation includes connection to family and social groups, and whether there are tasks and interests that a person enjoys being involved with. Also critical at this stage are whether a partner is still alive, whether they are able to be helpful to their partner, and whether they themselves need help from their partner or others.

A 75-year-old woman has been taking care of her 85-year-old bedridden husband for the past 10 years. She is now becoming unable to care for him, as she is becoming more limited in her functioning. She does not want to sell her house, but cannot afford in-home care. How might you work with this couple in counseling?

Senior Adulthood—Limited Functioning

This final stage of life again focuses on functioning. People of limited functioning cannot care for themselves in their basic functions and may be confined to a bed. Finding meaning and meaningful connection can be especially challenging at this stage.

Counseling may be unconventional at this stage, and may come from a social worker or other caregiver. Support can be given by helping people to find meaning within their circumstances and to reflect on the meaning that their lives have held. Another important support in this challenging stage of life can be a person's spirituality and/or religion.

Three critical differences for people at this stage include whether they have care at home or in an institution, whether they have family and friends to visit or not, and what their financial resources involve. These facets may interrelate: For example, family involvement in institutional care can be complicated (Whitaker, 2009). As with all stages, finding meaning in the midst of challenge is vital for persons at this stage.

Consider a 90-year-old woman who cannot walk. She is not in pain, but her husband and two children have died, and she has no visitors. She feels that she would rather die than sit in bed all day. How might you support this person?

REFLECTION QUESTIONS 6.3

- What counseling life stage are you in, and based on that, what would you most need from a counselor?
- What counseling life stage are you most comfortable with, and why?
- What counseling life stage are you least comfortable with, and why?
- What age group are you most likely to listen to or value, and why?
- What age group are you least likely to listen to or value, and why?
- With which counseling stage(s) are you most or least effective as a counselor?

AGEISM

Everyone will age, and yet popular culture seems to deny this fact. For example, the obsession with remaining youthful in appearance is clearly evident by the proliferation of anti-aging beauty products, such cosmetic procedures to diminish or remove wrinkles; the use of hair dyes to eliminate the gray in one's hair; and the preponderance of images of happy and successful people who are under the age of 50. Quite often, one receives messages about the aging "baby boomers" who may potentially become a burden to society and families (Thornton, 2002), or see images of the "old" as sick, unproductive, and dependent. Even marketing strategies targeting the "retirement age" group tend to promote a quality of life that may not be attainable by a significant percentage of the population because of limited resources (McHugh, 2003). These and countless other examples of ways in which we continue to perpetuate ageist stereotypes have become a critical issue in our society (Thornton, 2002). At varying points in our lives, we probably have had ageist thoughts and perceptions due, in part, to our socialization experiences, including the multitude of messages we have and continue to receive from many sources about aging.

Ageism can be defined as negative perceptions and/or behaviors toward an individual exclusively based on age, and it can be unintentional, operating at the unconscious level of awareness (e.g., Greenberg, Schimel, & Martens, 2002; Levy & Banaji, 2002). Although the term *ageist* was coined by Butler (1969) over 30 years ago to refer to negative attitudes and actions toward those individuals who are of advanced age, the term is now applied to any age group. From this perspective, the definition of ageism consists of (a) negative feelings about the age group, (b) preconceived stereotypes about a person in that age group, and (c) how one differentially treats the individual in that age group.

Interestingly, ageism has received very limited attention in psychology's empirical and theoretical literature compared to racism and sexism. Even more surprising is that the existing literature tends to focus primarily on the aging adult population. Scholars such as Nelson (2002) speculate that this may be due to the widespread acceptance of prejudice against older individuals in the United States and other countries. In many respects, ageism is a complicated phenomenon because it also involves prejudice and discrimination in favor of older people. An example is the exclusionary nature of the Medicare insurance

REFLECTION EXERCISE **6.1**

Ageism and Word Associations

People of all ages commonly hold negative attitudes about aging. When you think about children or teenagers, what words come to mind? What do you notice about attitudes toward young people? Now, answer the same questions for older adults. Just as young people may be influenced by negative stereotypes, how might older adults be affected?

Source: From National Academy for Teaching and Learning About Aging (n.d.).

program, for which the young and middle-aged populations are not eligible (Wilkinson & Ferraro, 2002). The fact that ageist attitudes, beliefs, and behaviors are so engrained in our society (i.e., institutionalized and therefore influencing policy decisions) makes the process of heightening sensitivity to this issue, as well as breaking down barriers, especially difficult.

As noted earlier, ageism plays out in ways that devalue the worth of individuals who are older. For example, although the Social Security Act of 1935 was established to provide support to individuals who retire at the age of 65, it also promoted the perception that people who reach this age and retire become financially dependent (Calasanti & Slevin, 2001). The current debate about dwindling Social Security benefits is particularly troublesome because it also promotes the view that people of advanced age are a burden to society, often generating negative attitudes and stereotypes that permeate different social realms. Nowhere else is it as blatant as it is in the work environment. McCann and Giles (2002) cogently stress this point:

> Although life span development theory ... suggests that aging is an individualized, unique process where universal patterns of growth cannot be expected during any one period of life, widely held perceptions that "the elderly" are cognitively deficient, physically unsuitable for work, unable to cope with change, poor performers at work, and pining for retirement still persist in society at large. Unfortunately, when extrapolated to a workplace context, these generalizations may play a part in stereotypical expectations by management and staff, which may serve as harbingers to ageist communication and discriminatory practices toward older adults. The repercussion of such age-laden discourse and practices can be devastating to both the older employee, who may suffer declines in self-esteem and mental health, as well as to corporations, which may be the recipients of declining older worker productivity and age discrimination lawsuits from older workers. (p. 167)

It is erroneous to believe that those advanced in age lack appropriate psychosocial resources, are less flexible in attitudes or personality styles, have

---

EXAMPLE **6.1**
Ageist Language

Examples of ageist language that refer to the decline in physical abilities and that are often heard in the workplace and other settings include the following:

1. "One foot in the grave"
2. "Over the hill by 50"
3. "We need young blood around here"
4. "Waiting for the gold watch"
5. "Marking time and fading fast"
6. "Having a senior moment"

Source: From R. McCann & H. Giles, "Ageism in the Workplace," in T. D. Nelson (Ed.). *Ageism: Stereotyping and Prejudice Against Older Persons.* Copyright © 2002 by Massachusetts Institute of Technology.

fewer coping resources, and are generally in poor health (Whitbourne & Sneed, 2002). On the contrary, the majority of older adults have what they call a "positive sense of subjective well-being" (p. 250), which is supported by extensive research (e.g., Diener & Suh, 1998; Rowe & Kahn, 1998). Moreover, older adults successfully adapt to the aging process and maintain a clear sense of who they are despite the proliferation of negative stereotypes directed at them. For example, the notion that aging can be viewed as a positive rather than a negative process was clearly evident among African Americans who had lived in a small town most of their lives, and who were able to maintain a sense of community and place despite their experiences with racism and discrimination (Taylor, 2001). However, we also underscore that many older adults can be adversely affected by exposure to negative images, attitudes, myths, and stereotypes, and may fall prey to self-fulfilling prophecies regarding ageist stereotypes. In other words, they may internalize these negative views, begin to devalue themselves, and withdraw, which prevents them from living a normal and active life (Meyers, 1998).

Ageism interacts with other forms of oppression (e.g., sexism, racism, heterosexism, and classism) that influence how individuals experience its effects. For instance, individuals who have low lifetime earnings and do not have the ability to save or invest in a pension plan not only receive less in Social Security benefits upon retirement but also are more likely to be economically dependent. When one adds gender, class, and race to this picture, the inequality becomes even more apparent:

> [W]hile a White, working class man will often have lower lifetime earnings than a similarly situated middle-class man, a White working-class woman will have even lower benefits, due to lower earnings, but, if lesbian, will not be able to collect a pension or Social Security as spouse. Similarly, because of the types of jobs that Black men are more likely to occupy, they are likely to suffer both more spates of unemployment and higher rates of disability than White men …. (Calasanti & Slevin, 2001, p. 22)

Likewise, gender differences in the perception of what constitutes being "old" based on physical characteristics are quite evident in the United States. If women have gray hair and facial wrinkles, for instance, they are perceived as less attractive than men of the same age with similar characteristics. Unfortunately, our society places a high value on youthfulness, so much so that women who age naturally are often critically viewed as "letting themselves go" whereas men's aging process is viewed more positively.

Because of societal pressure to remain youthful in appearance, women who have the financial resources may revert to costly surgical procedures. Clearly, there are class differences here as well. What about racial and ethnic differences? One could speculate that perhaps the cosmetic surgery craze to look younger is a phenomenon of the affluent European American population in contemporary U.S. society.

Ageism should also be understood in the context of history and culture. For example, Calasanti and Slevin (2001) conjectured that adult women in the 1950s were pressed to live up to a standard that embraced "motherhood and domestic life" (p. 26), which was quite evident in television programs like

CASE STUDY **6.2**

The Case of Jonathan

Jonathan is a 72-year-old Caucasian male who is in good health, lives in a modest home, and has a retirement pension that allows him to live a comfortable lifestyle. His wife passed away several years ago. At the time, he was diagnosed with mild depression, was prescribed medication, and attended counseling sessions on a regular basis. Recently, he colored his gray hair a dark shade of brown, bought new stylish clothes, and began dating a woman who is 15 years his junior. He met her at an event organized by his church. Even though Jonathan appears to be adjusting well to the loss of his wife, his adult children are concerned about the change in his appearance and new friendship with this woman. They are uncertain about the woman's intentions, and believe it is too soon for their father to have a relationship. They believe that this woman will be moving into Jonathan's house, and are all against it. Jonathan shares this information with his counselor and asks for help in getting his children to "let him be."

Case Discussion

Thinking About This Case

1. If you were Jonathan's counselor, how would you approach this issue?
2. Would your approach be different if this client was a woman who was dating a man 15 years her junior? If, so how?

This case is an example where a person appears to be adapting well from an external perspective, and the person believes that he is adapting well, but his current family support system does not react well to the changes that are happening. Part of what the counselor can do with the client is to try to uncover some of the pressures that are happening in the family. The family may want Jonathan to act a certain way based on their needs rather than his needs. This may involve their own difficulty with their mom having passed away. Transitions involve issues for both the main person involved and his or her support network.

---

the sitcom *Leave It to Beaver*. Accordingly, the result was a population of women who entered their senior years as economically and educationally disadvantaged compared to men. With respect to culture, Calasanti and Slevin also highlight that women in some cultures have considerable power as they age, such as Muslim Hausa women in Nigeria. However, the differential status of women in the United States is influenced by social class.

Views of Aging

Stuart-Hamilton (2000) states that there are at least seven different ways in which aging can be viewed: as proximal, distal, universal, probabilistic, primary, secondary, and chronological aging.

- **Proximal aging** effects are those that have happened recently, such as the recent development of back pain.
- **Distal aging** effects are those that have taken place over the life span, such as the gradual loss of hearing.
- **Universal aging** describes features that all will experience, such as wrinkled skin.
- **Probabilistic aging** describes features that are common with aging but not universal, such as arthritis.
- **Primary aging** describes changes in one's body due to age (e.g., bones become more brittle).

- **Secondary aging** describes processes that are influenced by aging but not the direct processes of aging (e.g., a weakened bone breaks from stress).
- **Chronological age** describes that which is literally related to the passage of time (e.g., growing older by one year every year).

In these ways, the process of aging can be described in a diversity of ways. These facets are valuable to consider, as they help us to remember that aging is a unique process for each person.

Effects of Ageism on Body Image

It is quite common to draw conclusions about how old someone is based on his or her physical appearance. Likewise, the social significance of the physical body in contemporary society as it relates to the aging process cannot be overlooked. In their landmark book *Gender, Social Inequalities and Aging*, Toni Calasanti and Kathleen Slevin (2001) offer important insight into the relationship between ageism and the physical body. First and foremost, contemporary U.S. society is focused on maintaining a youthful appearance. People have more options than they did a generation ago to transform their bodies through cosmetic procedures, exercise, and diet. Although the medical establishment advises the public that proper diet and exercise lead to overall better health outcomes for all ages, we still are fixated on slowing down the aging process. Second, the media play an important role in the increased attention given to the body and are replete with ageist language and images, particular toward women. The most obvious are ads marketing anti-aging creams and makeup with slogans such as "age defying," "fight the signs of aging," and "look younger—feel better." The message conveyed by such propaganda is that people in general and women in particular are in conflict with their aging bodies (Andrews, 1999). It is staunchly argued that the obsession with the body is also manifested in the youth culture through body piercing, tattooing, and dying hair in unusual colors (e.g., pink or green).

Another important issue addressed by Calasanti and Slevin (2001) is the notion that adolescent and early-adult women pay more attention to their physical appearance compared to men, and become increasingly dissatisfied with their bodies as they get older. Although there may be many contributing factors, one can speculate that women and girls are simply bombarded with messages that they must be thin, youthful, and attractive in order to be happy and successful. At the same time, there is a rise in men's and boy's dissatisfaction with their physical appearance; however, their perceptions center on physical strength and athletic abilities, whereas women focus on attractiveness.

Finally, important issues are raised concerning racial and ethnic, cultural, social class, and sexual orientation differences. With respect to race and ethnicity, for instance, Calasanti and Slevin (2001) state that the perceptions of body image for African American women tend to be more variable and positive compared to those of White women. In essence, the perception of beauty for African American women goes beyond physical characteristics and encompasses such aspects as "personality," "grooming," "how one moves," and a "sense of style" (p. 60). Likewise, African American women may be less likely to view themselves as overweight. Interestingly, Calasanti and Slevin also point out that other ethnic and cultural groups such as Asian and Hispanic women are more accepting of heavier body frames than White women. Furthermore, African American men may be equally invested as African American women in their physical appearance, more so than White men. One could hypothesize that this may be attributed to a strong motivational force to dispel persistent negative stereotypical images of African Americans. It is conceivable that many African Americans may focus on looking their best in public to dispel the negative, stereotypical images so pervasive in U.S. society. On the other hand, Calasanti and Slevin surmise that the role models for African Americans are heavily concentrated in the sports and entertainment industry "for whom physical attractiveness and physical fitness are important" (2001, p. 62). Regardless of the external forces, it is clear that role models influence body image. Although such differences are substantiated by research, the authors caution against overgeneralizing because one must consider other important intersecting factors, such as class, age, and level of acculturation.

In terms of sexual orientation, several studies conclude that physical appearance is more important for gay men than it is for heterosexual men, but when compared to heterosexual women, gay men are equally dissatisfied with their body image. Similar to heterosexual women, gay men may experience the same societal pressure to remain youthful; and, as controversial as it may be, gay men may be receiving ageist messages from their own communities. With respect to lesbians, Calasanti and Slevin (2001) note that the research on body image is scant and also mixed; however, some empirical work suggests that lesbians may have higher body satisfaction and give less importance to physical attractiveness compared to heterosexual women. Although the possible explanations for this perspective are complex, the authors conjecture that lesbians may have a different set of ideals that promote greater acceptance of the body. Once again, it is important not to generalize these perspectives because there may be considerable variability among gay, lesbian, and bisexual individuals.

Effects of Ageism in Young Children and Adolescents

Children and adolescents are victims of ageist attitudes and behaviors but in a different way than older adults. In particular, children are considered the most vulnerable population and unable to represent their own interests, and have virtually no power in society. Because of their low status, children are easy targets for discrimination and prejudice. There are numerous examples of how children and adolescents have been victimized through ageist acts. One of the classic examples is the exploitative nature of child labor that occurred during the 19th and early 20th centuries, when children as young as 6 years of age were forced to work long hours and in deplorable conditions because they were considered cheap and manageable (Westman, 1991). Interestingly, attempts to create laws to protect children from the oppressive nature of child labor were not focused on changing the work conditions, but rather these laws were created because society was producing a population of uneducated individuals. Later efforts did focus on improving work conditions, but these attempts were often met with resistance; and by 1938, the Fair Labor Standards Act was established, which set the minimum employment age at 14, particularly in the manufacturing industry. In fact, this law set the standard for all later legislation (Kerschner, 2000). Current federal child labor laws stipulate different minimum age requirements for nonagricultural and agricultural employment, list jobs that are prohibited for those under the age of 18, and mandate a wage structure.

Despite this heightened consciousness as evidenced in the creation of laws to protect children from this blatant form of discrimination and prejudice, we still see many forms of ageism that affect our children and adolescents in today's society. For instance, the rate of poverty among children under the age of 18 continues to increase and was estimated at 13 million in 2003, and the rate of poverty among children under the age of 18 is higher than the rate of any other age groups (U.S. Census Bureau, 2004). The rise in violence toward children such as sexual and physical abuse, including child pornography, and the low priority given to funding for children with special needs are all examples of the worst forms of ageist acts toward children (Westman, 1991).

Another, perhaps more subtle, demonstration of ageism is the way our society forces parents to segregate children in public places. Children are allowed to go to most, if not all, public recreational parks; however, they are not allowed in betting parlors or bars. Although the purpose is to restrict access in order to protect them from possible harm through exposure to such undesirable environments, Westman (1991) argued that "if our society respected its immature members, it would ensure public safety and support parents' efforts to foster the development of their children rather than accepting, and even promoting, influences that are inimical to the development of children" (p. 243). Furthermore, the notion of age segregation occurs in multiple institutional settings. We tend to segregate children by putting them in schools, where they spend a good part of their day, and recreational activities are often organized and targeted for specific age groups (e.g., "senior" fitness activities, or "youth" or "junior" activities). Unfortunately, this kind of separation perpetuated by our society, particularly for children and adolescents and for older adults, discourages cross-generational interaction (Hagestad & Uhlenberg, 2005).

REFLECTION QUESTIONS 6.4

- What are your experiences with ageism?
- If you've had direct experiences with ageism, how did you handle them?
- What are some of the words, phrases, and stereotypes that come to mind when you think about young people?
- What are some of the words, phrases, and stereotypes that come to mind when you think about older adults?
- How do your overall views of aging in terms of mental, physical, and spiritual aspects affect your views of young people versus older people as well as life in general?
- What can you do to challenge ageism in your work with clients and to continue to be more aware of any biases you may have about this phenomenon?
- What words or phrases do you tend to use that reinforce an ageist perspective, and how can you work to eliminate or reframe those?

REDUCING AGEISM FOR CHILDREN AND OLDER ADULTS

Confronting Ageism: What Counselors Can Do

As we have discussed, ageism is one of the most socially accepted forms of prejudice and discrimination in this country. As a result, it is highly probable that most of us have, to varying degrees, biases toward the very young and the very old. There is considerable evidence to suggest that many helping professionals such as psychologists and physicians have stereotypes and ageist attitudes that influence their approach to treatment. In particular, the treatment of older individuals tends to focus on disease management rather than prevention because many professionals in the medical field believe that older people will eventually become ill anyway. Likewise, older individuals are more likely to be prescribed medication and less likely to receive psychological services for mental health problems such as depression (Nelson, 2005).

Braithwaite (2002) noted that ageism is complex, consisting of negative stereotypes, prejudice, stigmatizing behaviors, and fear about the aging process. These aspects are interwoven to such an extent that combating it presents a formidable challenge. Nonetheless, she outlined a number of key points that can be used to confront ageism as well as increase counselor competencies in working with individuals of advanced age and the very young. Counselors must heighten their awareness of the pervasive nature of age segregation in our society and seek out opportunities for participation in age-integrated activities. With respect to older individuals, counselors should seek out opportunities to learn that they are valued contributing members of society. In addition, counselors are encouraged to take courses in aging and gerontology to further their understanding.

The importance of the advocacy role is underscored. Counselors should become knowledgeable about existing legislation on health and social care, employment, and education, as well as the laws governing children's rights (Herring, 2003; Meyers, 1998). Counselors can review such policies for evidence of discrimination and prejudice against older individuals and children. One of the most important ways of combating ageism is to promote intergenerational contact between young children and those of advanced age. The more contact among generations, the higher the probability of developing healthy attitudes about aging and reducing belief in stereotypes.

Braithwaite (2002) introduced a 10-step plan that can be used to increase counselor competencies in working with individuals of advanced age, and that can be applied to any age group. Here, we state the 10 steps in terms of older and younger individuals:

1. Heightening sensitivity to the stereotyping of older and younger people
2. Creating greater exposure to diversity in the personal characteristics of older and younger people
3. Having a greater commitment to recognizing and responding to diversity in dealing with older and younger people
4. Making deliberate use of perspective taking to see older and younger people as individuals
5. Seeking out opportunities for intergenerational cooperation

6. Taking advantage of opportunities to promote the social attractiveness of older and younger people
7. Strengthening institutional practices that promote the norm of human-heartedness
8. Desensitizing ourselves to the stigma of degeneration and dependency
9. Reviewing policies and practices for evidence of stigmatizing through disrespect, particularly the disrespect communicated through treating older and younger people as invisible groups
10. Mandating inclusiveness of older and younger people in policy planning and implementation (pp. 331–332)

Ageist Language

The way in which we communicate with individuals in particular age groups may have ageist aspects. Most of the research examining ageist communication patterns has focused on adults of advanced age. *Overaccommodation* and *baby talk* are terms often found in the literature describing a pattern of communication with older adults, stemming from the negative stereotype that they have cognitive deficits. For instance, we sometimes incorrectly assume that older individuals have diminished hearing ability, so we talk to them louder and slower. Another form of overaccommodation, viewed as patronizing and condescending, is the use of baby talk with an older adult. This kind of communication pattern is described as exaggerated, simplified, louder, and slower speech combined with a high-pitched sound, similar to speaking to a baby (Nelson, 2005). One can only imagine how disrespectful this could feel when one is on the receiving end of this type of communication.

SPECIAL TOPICS RELATED TO COUNSELING AND OLDER ADULTS

Cultural Context in Caring for Aging Adults

We all agree that aging is a universal process; however, the issue of who cares for those in advanced age may vary across cultures. For instance, in many Asian cultures the adult children provide care for their aging parents in poor health, due in part to the cultural tradition of *filial piety*—the expression of respect for and showing affection toward parents, as well as sacrificing for them in times of need (Sung, 2000). In Latino and Hispanic culture, it is common for family members to care for aging parents, especially those whose health is declining (e.g., Santiago-Rivera, Arredondo, & Gallardo-Cooper, 2002), because of a strong familistic orientation (i.e., *familismo*) manifested in a preference for maintaining close relationships and connections with immediate and extended family. Likewise, many Native American tribes value a supportive family network, hold elders in the highest esteem, and may be more likely to care for them as they reach advanced age (e.g., Herring, 1999). Extended family and strong kinship bonds are also important values in African American communities (e.g., McCollum, 1997). Can these cultural dimensions contribute to the underrepresentation of ethnic minorities in nursing homes? One could speculate that cultural differences between the care provider in a nursing home and an ethnic group member may be a contributing factor; thus, the family becomes the primary caregiver (Markides & Miranda, 1997).

On the other hand, the notion that African Americans, Latinos, Native Americans, and Asian Americans consider filial responsibilities important, and therefore are presumed to be more nurturing and willing to assume the role of the caregiver in the family (known as *informal care*), may be promoting the misconception that they are less likely to consider *formal care* such as a nursing home (Groger, 1999). The reality is that one must consider a variety of factors that may influence the desire and ability to assume the caregiver role as opposed to placing the person in a nursing home facility. These factors include the availability of family support, the age and life stage of the potential caregiver, the location of nursing home facilities, and the adequacy of health

CASE STUDY **6.3**

The Case of Sylvia

Sylvia, an African American woman who is 50 years old, has worked for the IRS for 29 years and expects to retire in 5 years. She intends to go back to school, cashing in on a deal she made with her son who agreed that he would help her finish college because she helped him become an electrical engineer. In the meantime, Sylvia has a second full-time job that is more taxing than her work for the IRS: She takes care of her 79-year-old mother, who suffers from Alzheimer's disease. Sylvia checks on her mother by phone several times during the day; runs by her house in the evening to do chores for her, and takes her to stores, medical visits, and visits with friends. To do all this, Sylvia gave up two part-time jobs she had taken to save money for a down payment on a house. Sylvia has taken care of her mother for 3 years. She has visited a number of nursing homes, interviewed staff, and chosen two facilities where her mother is on a waiting list. She feels that a nursing home would be the only place her mother would be completely safe. But her mother refuses to sign the papers. Sylvia is torn about the decision: She has already turned down one opportunity, and she thinks that when the next bed becomes available, she may well turn it down again because she believes one should take care of one's elders. In the meantime, she lives with the nightmare of imagining what might happen to her mother in a nursing home.

Case Discussion
Thinking About This Case
1. Consider the possibility that Sylvia is experiencing frustration and disappointment, and decides to see a counselor for help. What would you need to know, and how could you be culturally responsive to her needs?
2. What are some of the key questions to explore about Sylvia balancing her own needs with the needs of her mother?
3. As a counselor, what cultural biases do you bring about whether the mom's own home or a nursing home is a better place for her? How might you work toward not having this bias inappropriately influence your counseling?

Sylvia is an example of how cultural values can be important in people's lives. Here, there is the tension of her being individually fulfilled versus helping out family members. The consumer side of society would suggest that Sylvia should mainly look out for her own needs, and that the needs of her mother should be hired out to others (a nursing home). This may not be so simple both culturally and practically. On the cultural level, there can be a value of taking care of one's family members; and, on a practical level, hiring out these services can be very expensive. Furthermore, Sylvia may give better and more supportive care to her mother than someone who is hired to care for her. This factor may be very important to both Sylvia and her mother. Having said this, when Sylvia prioritizes her mother it makes it hard for her to look out for her own needs.

Source: From L. Groger "Relinquishing care," *Anthropology Newsletter*, 40(3), p. 19. Copyright © 1999 by the American Anthropological Association.

insurance coverage (Groger & Mayberry, 2001; Markides & Miranda, 1997). Furthermore, as people become more mobile, as more women enter the workforce in greater numbers, and as the aging population continues to grow, we are witnessing a shift in the degree to which families are capable of caring for older people. This phenomenon is affecting the structure of families, and the values of familism and filial responsibility (Bengtson & Putney, 2000). From a cultural perspective, an individual may be conflicted about placing an aging parent in a nursing home his or her cultural traditions are rooted in duty and obligation. This issue is more apparent today than in previous generations among adults who are challenged to make decisions about the care of their parents. As a result, this may create considerable stress and strain.

Women, Aging, and Caregiving

Although feminist scholars argue that we must not assume that caregiving is a "woman's job," in reality women do provide most of the informal care to family members (e.g., spouses, parents, and in-laws; see, e.g., Parrott, Mills, & Bengtson, 2000). Women's roles as caregivers are quite varied in that they may be the friend or companion of an aging person, provider of "hands-on" health care, care manager, and/or decision maker (Family Caregiver Alliance, 2003). As previously discussed, taking care of an older person may be so emotionally and financially draining that it can affect overall psychological and physical well-being. As illustrated in Sylvia's situation (see Case Study 6.3), women who work and are also providing informal care experience enormous demands on their time.

National survey results report that women who work full-time and provide informal care of older people are more likely to reduce their working hours; pass up a job promotion, training, or a work assignment; take a leave from their jobs; or switch from full-time to part-time employment. In turn, these changes in their employment status affect their future retirement financial stability such as pension contributions and Social Security benefits (Family Caregiver Alliance, 2003). It is also conceivable that women in the caregiver role of a loved one could develop psychological problems because of the physical and emotional demands placed on them.

There are other experiences in aging that are markedly different for women when compared to men. Demographic trends inform us that women outlive men by approximately 7 years and may live the last 11 or more years alone and in the care of other women. Also, it is highly probable that older women will experience a decline in financial resources following the death of a spouse. Furthermore, women are significantly less likely to receive a pension income; and, when they do, it is considerably less than what men receive (Parrott et al., 2000). In sum, these varying issues and circumstances may place women at risk for mental health problems.

OPENING THE DIALOGUE ON AGE AND AGEISM

With all of the topics discussed in this chapter, you are now challenged to think through how you would utilize this information in session with any number of clients from a variety of cultural backgrounds and worldviews.

Questions for reflection offered to you throughout this chapter also serve as excellent process questions for opening the dialogue with clients on issues of age and experiences with ageism. Some of these questions are listed here to assist you in terms of opening the dialogue with your clients:

- Who are you in terms of age? How important is this in your personal and cultural identity, and what impact do these dimensions have on how you view the world and live your life?
- Where did your concept of aging originate, and how has it been reinforced or challenged during your life?
- What does your culture say about age?
- What do your family and community say about age in terms of both beliefs and practice?
- How do issues of power and privilege influence your definition of age and concept of aging?
- How has your definition of age affected the way you define yourself now and at previous points in your life?
- How will your definition of age and aging continue to affect the way you define yourself and the way others see you or treat you?
- How has your definition of age and aging affected the way you interact with others who are similar in age to you versus different in age to you at different points in your life?
- How will your definition of age change as you grow older?
- When and how did you first become aware of ageism? What was your initial reaction, and how did that reaction change over time?
- What have your experiences with ageism been, and in what ways have those experiences shaped who you are as a person, as well as the issues you are dealing with now?
- What efforts have you made to work toward positive social change with regard to the ageism that exists in your own life at the individual, group, and societal levels, and what other kinds of efforts would you like to make?
- To what extent do you value a person's age as a sign of his or her worth?
- Have you ever stood up for someone being harassed or oppressed on the basis of age? If not, why not? Has anyone ever stood up for you in this way?
- How might the difference or similarity in age between you (client) and me (counselor) affect your experience in the process of counseling as well as the relationship between us?
- How does age play into the issues you are bringing to counseling, and how can we address this in a way that is most helpful to you?

CONCLUSION AND IMPLICATIONS

In this chapter, we have defined the concept of age, reviewed the history of the study of aging, discussed how there are important counseling life stages to be aware of, explored the problems of ageism, and considered other issues related to age. This has led to a broad exploration of a contextual understanding of age. To reinforce this understanding, we conclude with one final analysis of the poem at the beginning of the chapter. An important understanding of age can be seen in a key point of the poem. It points out that many choices in life change people considerably, but the choices made may not have been good or bad, only different. Sometimes people interpret the line "that has made all of the difference" as a triumphant call by Robert Frost (1946) that he has lived his life well. But that interpretation misses an important subtlety. Toward the beginning of the poem, Frost describes the second path as "just as fair," and toward the end he tells "with a sigh" about the first path. He is not triumphant about his choice, nor is he sad about it; he is merely pointing out the power that we have in life to

make choices, and that those choices make "all the difference." He is sad that he could not take both roads. However, powerfully, he is simply in awe of how the simple choices we make over time shape our lives. As counselors, we need to help people explore the power of the choices that they have made or that have been made for them, and help them to look at both the distance they've traveled and where they have yet to travel in terms of what may be next. Sometimes, that means making big changes, and sometimes it means simply being in awe of how one's life unfolds.

GLOSSARY

Age: The whole duration of a person since beginning.

Ageism: Negative perceptions and/or behaviors toward an individual exclusively based on age; this can be unintentional, operating at the unconscious level of awareness.

Chronological age: Describes age related to the passage of time.

Distal aging: Effects that have taken place over the life span, such as the gradual loss of hearing.

Probabilistic aging: Features that are common with aging but not universal, such as arthritis.

Proximal aging: Effects that have happened recently, such as the recent development of back pain.

Primary aging: Changes in one's body due to age (e.g., bones becoming more brittle).

Secondary aging: Processes that are influenced by aging but not the direct processes of aging (e.g., a weakened bone breaks from stress).

Universal aging: Features that all will experience with aging, such as wrinkled skin.

REFERENCES

Andrews, M. (1999). The seductiveness of agelessness. *Ageing and Society*, 19, 301–318.

Bengtson, V., & Putney, N. M. (2000). Who will care for tomorrow's elderly? Consequences of population aging East and West. In V. L. Bengtson, K. D. Kim, G. C. Myers, & K. S. Eun (Eds.), *Aging in East and West: Families, states and the elderly* (pp. 263–286). New York: Springer.

Birren, J. E. (1961). A brief history of the psychology of aging. *Gerontologist*, 1, 67–77.

Braithwaite, V. (2002). Reducing ageism. In T. D. Nelson (Ed.), *Ageism: Stereotyping and prejudice against older persons*. Cambridge, MA: MIT Press.

Butler, R. N. (1969). Age-ism: Another form of bigotry. *Gerontologist*, 9, 243–246.

Calasanti, T. M., & Slevin, K. F. (2001). *Gender, social inequalities, and aging*. Walnut Creek, CA: AltaMira Press.

Diener, E., & Suh, E. (1998). Age and subjective well-being: An international analysis. *Annual review of Gerontology and Geriatrics*, 17, 304–324.

Duncan, C., & Loretto, W. (2004). Never the right age? Gender and age-based discrimination in employment. *Gender, Work, and Organization*, 11, 95–115.

Erikson, E. (1950). *Childhood and society*. New York, NY: WW Norton and Company.

Erikson, E. (1997). *The life cycle completed*. New York: Norton.

Family Caregiver Alliance. (2003). Women and caregiving: Facts and figures. Retrieved from http://www.caregiver.org

Frost, R. (1946). *The poems of Robert Frost*. New York: Random House.

Greenberg, J., Schimel, J., & Martens, A. (2002). Ageism: Denying the face of the future. In T. D. Nelson (Ed.), *Ageism: Stereotyping and prejudice against older persons* (pp. 27–48). Cambridge, MA: MIT Press.

Groger, L. (1999). Relinquishing care. *Anthropology Newsletter*, 40(3), 19.

Groger, L., & Mayberry, P. S. (2001). Caring too much? Cultural lag in African Americans' perceptions of filial responsibilities. *Journal of Cross-Cultural Gerontology*, 16, 21–39. Retrieved from http://www.stpt.usf.edu/~jsokolov/Groger.htm

Hagestad, G. O., & Uhlenberg, P. (2005). The social separation of old and young: A root of ageism. *Journal of Social Issues*, 61, 21–39.

Hall, S. (1922). *Senescence, the last half of life*. New York: NY: D. Appelton and Company.

Herring, R. (1999). *Counseling with Native American Indians and Alaskan Natives*. Thousand Oaks: CA: Sage.

Herring, J. (2003). Children's rights for grown-ups. In S. Fredman & S. Spencer (Eds.), *Age as an equality issue* (pp. 145–173). Portland, OR: Hart.

Jonker, A. A. G. C., Comijs, H. C., Knipscheer, K. C. P. M., & Deeg, D. J. H. (2009). The role of coping resources on change in well-being during persistent health decline. *Journal of Aging and Health*, 21, 1063–1082.

Kerschner, A. (2000, June). Child labor laws and enforcement. In A. Herman (Ed.), *Report on the youth labor force* (pp. 3–13). Washington, DC: U.S. Department of Labor. Retrieved from http://www.bls.gov/opub/rylf/rylfhome.htm

Levinson, D. J., with Darrow, C. N., & Klein, E. B. (1978). *Seasons of a man's life*. New York: Random House.

Levinson, D. J., & Levinson, J. D. (1996). *Seasons of a woman's life*. New York: Knopf.

Levy, B., & Banaji, M. R. (2002). Implicit ageism. In T. D. Nelson (Ed.), *Ageism: Stereotyping and prejudice against older persons* (pp. 49–76). Cambridge, MA: MIT Press.

Markides, K.S., & Miranda, M. (Eds.). (1997). *Minorities, aging, and health*. Thousand Oakes, CA: Sage.

McCann, R., & Giles, H. (2002). Ageism in the workplace: A communication perspective. In T. D. Nelson (Ed.), *Ageism: Stereotyping and prejudice against older persons* (pp. 163–199). Cambridge, MA: MIT Press.

McCollum, V. J. C. (1997). Evolution of the African American family personality: Considerations for family therapy. *Journal of Multicultural Counseling and Development*, 25, 219–229.

McHugh, K. E. (Ed.). (2003). Three faces of ageism: Society, image and place. *Aging & Society*, 23, 165–185.

Meyers, J. E. (1998). Combating ageism: The rights of older persons. In C. C. Lee & G. R. Walz (Eds.), *Social action: A mandate for counselors* (pp. 137–159). Alexandra, VA: American Counseling Association.

National Academy for Teaching and Learning About Aging, Center for Public Service, University of North Texas. (N.d.). [Home page]. Retrieved from http://www.cps.unt.edu/natla

Nelson, T. D. (2002). *Ageism: Stereotyping and prejudice against older persons*. Cambridge, MA: MIT Press.

Nelson, T. D. (2005). Ageism: Prejudice against our feared future self. *Journal of Social Issues*, 61, 207–221.

Parkes, A., Wight, D., Henderson, M., & West, P. (2010). Does early sexual debut reduce teenagers' participation in tertiary education? Evidence from the SHARE longitudinal study. *Journal of Adolescence*, 33, 741–754.

Parrott, T. M., Mills, T. L., & Bengtson, V. L. (2000). The United States: Population demographics, changes in the family, and social policy challenges. In V. L. Bengtson, K. D. Kim, G. C. Myers, & K. S. Eun (Eds.), *Aging in East and West: Families, states and the elderly* (pp. 191–224). New York: Springer.

Piaget, J., & Inhelder, B. (1969). *The psychology of the child*. New York: Basic.

Rowe, J. W., & Kahn, R. L. (1998). *Successful aging*. New York: Pantheon.

Santiago-Rivera, A., Arredondo, P., & Gallardo-Cooper, M. (2002). *Counseling Latinos and la familia: A practical guide*. Thousand Oaks, CA: Sage.

Schlossberg, N. K. (2004). *Retire smart, retire happy: Finding your true path in life*. Washington, DC, US: American Psychological Association.

Siegler, I.C., Bastian, L.A., Steffens, D.C., Bosworth, H.C., & Costa, P.T. (2002). Behavioral medicine and aging. *Journal of Consulting and Clinical Psychology*, 70, 843–851.

Stuart-Hamilton, I. (2000). *The psychology of ageing: An introduction*. London: Jessica Kingsley.

Sung, K. (2000). An Asian perspective on aging East and West: Filial piety and changing families. In V. L. Bengtson, K. D. Kim, G. C. Myers, & K. S. Eun (Eds.), *Aging in East and West: Families, states and the elderly* (pp. 41–56). New York: Springer.

Taylor, S. P. (2001). Place identification and positive realities of aging. *Journal of Cross-Cultural Gerontology*, 16, 5–20.

Thornton, J. E. (2002). Myths of aging or ageist stereotypes. *Educational Gerontology*, 28, 301–312.

U.S. Census Bureau. (2004). *Poverty: 2003 highlights*. Retrieved from http://www.census.gov/hhes/poverty/poverty03/pov03hi.html

Webster, N. (1983). *Webster's new universal unabridged dictionary*. New York: Simon & Schuster.

Westman, J. C. (1991). Juvenile ageism: Unrecognized prejudice and discrimination against the young. *Child Psychiatry and Human Development*, 21, 237–256.

Whitaker, A. (2009). Family involvement in the institutional eldercare context: Towards a new understanding. *Journal of Aging Studies*, 23, 158–167.

Whitbourne, S. K., & Sneed, J. R. (2002). The paradox of well-being, identity processes, and stereotype treat: Agesim and its potential relationships to the self in later life. In T. D. Nelson (Ed). *Ageism Stereotyping and prejudice against older persons* (pp. 247–271). Cambridge, MA, US: The MIT Press.

Wilkinson, J. A., & Ferraro, K. F. (2002). Thirty years of ageism research. In T. D. Nelson (Ed.), *Ageism: Stereotyping and prejudice against older persons* (pp. 339–358). Cambridge, MA: MIT Press.

Woodruff-Pak, D. (1988). *Psychology and aging*. Englewood Cliffs, NJ: Prentice Hall.

CHAPTER 7

Gender and Sexuality

Using Russian nesting dolls as a framework suggests that history, culture, relationships, psyche, organism, and cell are each appropriate locations from which to study the formation and meaning of sexuality and gender. Developmental systems theory, whether applied to the assembled doll or to its subunits, provides the scaffolding for thought and experiment. Assembling the smaller dolls into a single large one requires the integration of knowledge derived from very different levels of biological and social organization. The cell, the individual, groups of individuals organized in families, peer groups, cultures, and nations and their histories all provide sources of knowledge about human sexuality. We cannot understand it well unless we consider all of these components. (pp. 254–255)

Source: A. Fausto-Sterling, *Sexing the Body: Gender Politics and Construction of Sexuality* (New York: Basic Books). Copyright © 2000 by Anne Fausto-Sterling. Reprinted with permission.

Across societies and cultures, one of the most fundamental ways that human beings make sense of themselves is through their gender and sexual identity. However, the idea of being a man or a woman is deceptively simple, and has many intricate layers of meaning buried below the surface. Using the Russian nesting doll, Anne Fausto-Sterling illustrates the complexity of conceptualizing and understanding the constructs of human sexuality and gender.

Because so much of our learning about these concepts is implicit rather than explicit, we typically don't attend to these complexities. However, counselors need to do so because gender and its accompanying construct of sexuality are deeply intertwined with gender identity, gender roles, and gender expression. This chapter provides you with an overview of these constructs including a discussion of essentialist, social constructionist, and feminist perspectives. In Chapter 8, we will explore the issue of sexual orientation more deeply.

REFLECTION QUESTIONS 7.1

- What's the first memory you have about your gender and what that meant?
- What messages did you receive as a child about what it meant to be a "boy" or a "girl"?
- What messages did you receive when you were a teen about what it meant to be male or female?
- Who did you receive those messages from (parents, teachers, coaches, other kids, etc.) at different points in your life, and what effect did they have on you?

We begin with a discussion on how gender and sexuality have been defined and examined in social arenas. For instance, **gender** has been referred to as the various expressions of a subjective sense of self as either male or female (Fausto-Sterling, 2000). One's gender identity is heavily influenced by what a given society designates as "appropriate" or "typical" male or female attitudes and behaviors (Savin-Williams & Cohen, 1996). From a feminist perspective, gender is often construed as the shaping of masculinity and femininity by society. However, some scholars from varying disciplines (including feminists) argue that this perspective excludes the human body's anatomy and physiology. On the other hand, **sexuality** can be viewed as a broader construct that encompasses gender, gender roles, and sexual orientation (D'Andrea & Daniels, 2001). Some note that it also includes sexual feelings (i.e., eroticism), as well as sexual practices, behaviors, and relationships (Jackson & Scott, 1996). Regardless of the differing views, most would agree that gender and sexuality are related and central to an individual's identity. However, notice that *male* and *female* are binary label assignments given in this society, whereas other cultures may allow for more than two gender designations. Gender differs from sexuality in that sexual behavior is not required for gender to be assigned. For instance, although celibate, monks and nuns are very definitely given gender identities as men and women.

The debate about sexuality and gender involves a variety of complex issues such as whether or not there are only two sexes based on biological differences (male and female) and whether or not gender and sexuality are socially constructed phenomena. Further fueling the debate are the contrasting essentialist and postmodernist ideologies on such topics as the construction of masculinity and femininity, and differentiated gender roles (Philaretou & Allen, 2001). Another dimension to the debate and controversy involves feminist thought that challenges male dominance, traditional gender roles, and power differentials between men and women. Jackson and Scott (1996) made this point very clear:

> The social distinction and hierarchical relationship between men and women profoundly affect our sexual lives. This is true not only by those of us who are heterosexual: lesbian and gay sexualities are also shaped by wider understandings of masculinity and femininity, as are heterosexual attitudes to other sexualities—for example, the idea that lesbians are not 'real women'. Gender and sexuality intersect with other social divisions such as those based on 'race' and class, so that we each live our sexuality from different locations within society. (p. 3)

To paraphrase Bullough (2002), the term *gender* was and continues to be widely used in linguistics to label nouns as masculine, feminine, or neuter (neither masculine or feminine); however, it entered the realm of the social sciences in the mid 1950s when John Money, well known for his research on hermaphrodites, used the term to differentiate between feminine and masculine behaviors, and for the first time distinguished it from the biological and physiological characteristics of the male and female sex. Money also coined the term **gender identity**, defined as "the total perception of the individual about his or her own gender, including a basic personal identity as a man or woman, boy or girl" (p. 4). In essence, gender was conceptualized as social and psychological phenomena, and captured both the public and personal manifestations of masculinity and femininity (Bullough, 2002).

REFLECTION QUESTIONS 7.2

- What are sexuality and gender, and are they different?
- How has your culture influenced the way you define these two constructs?
- How have your definitions of sexuality and gender changed over time, if at all, and why?
- How does one's gender influence the way in which we think and behave?

MASCULINITY AND FEMININITY

As noted above, when discussing gender, the concepts of *masculinity* and *femininity* are at the forefront. Essentially, these concepts are about the content of the roles assigned to each gender and the characteristics deemed socially appropriate that go along with each gender role. One could ask, What constitutes masculine and feminine ways of being, and how are they shaped by society? Scholars have consistently pointed out that gender-specific masculine and feminine behaviors (e.g., boys wear blue and girls wear pink, and boys play with trucks and girls play with dolls) are differentiated at an early age through the socialization process (e.g., McLean, Carey, & White, 1996; Thompson, 2000). You may notice that one of the first questions asked of a newborn infant's parents is about the gender of the child. Because a newborn has no need of a gender identity at this stage in its life, it follows that the question is asked more to shape the perceptions of the questioner. We receive messages from an early age about what are acceptable and preferred masculine and feminine behaviors. Historically, individualism, rationality, and militaristic behaviors have been highly valued and attributed to males, whereas emotions, emotional behavior, virtues, and interdependence are less valued and attributed to women (Smith, 1996). How often have we heard statements like "Girls socialize and talk more than boys in school settings"; "Boys excel in math, whereas girls excel in verbal expression"; "Women are emotional"; "Men are more competitive than women"; "Men are not suppose to show emotions"; and "Boys are more aggressive than girls". Such statements and countless others create and perpetuate prescribed gender-specific roles that become so much a part of our personal identities.

In chapter 4, the cycle of oppression demonstrated how we learn social roles and information about members of a group. The process described in that chapter applies equally to the process of gender socialization.

Gilbert and Scher (1999) present a model on how gender can frame different aspects of lived experience, including discourse, structure, difference, and process. **Gendered discourse** refers to the ways in which our expectations of gender affect how we structure our language and assumptions; **gendered structure** focuses on the differential opportunities, accesses, and policies that impact men and women; **gendered difference** is about how we view men and women as different; and **gendered process** focuses on the ways we interact. As an example, let us look at the notion of women who are working parents. Gendered discourse refers to such women as *working mothers*, whereas there is no similar term for men who are also parents. Their identity as fathers does not subsume their other identities as it tends to do for mothers. Gendered structure assumes that there are maternal leave policies but no corresponding paternal leave policies, because as gendered difference shows, women are

REFLECTION EXERCISE **7.1**

What does it mean to be masculine or feminine? Think about different adjectives that characterize masculinity and femininity, and make a list. Here are a few examples to get you started:

To be a "Real Man" is to be:	To be a "Real Woman" is to be:
1. Physically strong	1. Nurturing
2. Independent	2. Emotional
3. The breadwinner	3. Interdependent
4. Aggressive	4. Cooperative

Once you have generated your list, go back and look at which ones are positive characteristics and which ones are negative. How do these attributes influence gender-specific behaviors?

considered the primary nurturers whereas men are providers. Finally, gendered process shows how women give care whereas men take care.

Thompson (2000) argued that patriarchal societies in which authority and privilege are accorded to men essentially reinforce the idea that men must act, behave, and think in certain ways. In turn, men internalize certain behaviors and ways of thinking that are conveyed in the characteristics and attributes as outlined in the exercise above. Similarly, women internalize messages like the following: Women are less decisive, less sexual, and more appearance conscious, thus contributing to what Thompson calls the "framework for making sense of the world" (p. 30).

Although the perceptions of males as dominant, aggressive, and sexually powerful and females as submissive, nurturing, and emotional prevail in contemporary society, the reality is that there is no single lens with which to view masculinity and femininity because of varying social, political, historical, and cultural contexts (Philaretou & Allen, 2001), including class and race differences (e.g., White, Bondurant, & Travis, 2000). There truly is a wide range of conceptions about these constructs when one looks at them this way. For instance, in exploring the intersection of gender and culture among a group of working-class young Puerto Rican men (between the ages of 23 and 35) who were born on the island of Puerto Rico and had migrated to the United States at an early age, Weis, Centrie, Valentin-Juarbe, and Fine (2002) reported that they strongly adhered to a construction of masculinity that was associated with a highly valued traditional patriarchal family structure in which a man works to support the family, and a woman stays home to take care of children. In this case, maintaining this cultural tradition, which reinforces their identity as Puerto Rican men trying to successfully navigate in an often hostile Eurocentric society, appeared to be the driving force for adhering to prescribed gender roles. In essence, maintaining a patriarchal family structure for fear of losing their cultural identity defined their masculinity.

Another example of the intersection of race and gender is a historical one in the African American community. Although one of the idealized traditional roles assigned to women has been to stay home and take care of the children, it has been considered one of the benefits of the feminist movement that women were able to go out to work. However, note that since the beginning, African American women were always expected to work away from their children, first as enslaved persons who were assigned to the plantation fields or the plantation house, and then, afterward, often to support their family. In an ironic twist, the stereotype of the "Mammy" is about African American women having to leave their own children to take care of and raise the children of their White employers.

Similarly, the notion of power differential also adds to the complexity of the issue. Most of us would agree that, as a group, men historically have had higher status and power relative to women in U.S. society. This structure of power and division of labor between males and females is exemplified in known facts such as the following: (a) With similar education levels, men earn more money than women; (b) more men are represented in political arenas than women; and (c) employed women still do most of the activities

---

EXAMPLE **7.1**
John and Jill

John, a well-established businessman, sometimes puts in 12-hour days, and therefore he believes that he deserves to go out for a drink after work with his colleagues or play golf on the weekends. Because of his substantially large six-figure salary, Jill, his wife who has a successful career herself, was encouraged to cut back on her hours to spend more time with their 3-month-old son, and 2-year-old daughter. Jill felt ambivalent about doing this because she really enjoyed and derived much satisfaction from her work. However, Jill eventually conceded because she believed she had no choice.

---

associated with running a household compared with employed men. The notion of power differentials is an interesting one because it, too, has to do with context. For example, in certain arenas, women may have more "decision-making power" than men when it relates to the care and nurturance of children, and may exercise it without repercussion; however, in other contexts, they may be rendered powerless. Essentially, men's higher status position as main providers of the household income is often equated with entitlement.

Are there class differences in entitlement? Some scholars believe that there are distinct class differences in ways that men exercise their power. For instance, Pyle (1996) found that husbands from higher socioeconomic strata were more likely to discourage their wives from seeking employment and a career because they earned enough to support the family, and use their careers as a "cover-up" for leisure activities. In contrast, the men from working-class backgrounds were more direct and overt about pursuing leisure activities. These men were also more explicit about using their masculinity as a right to exercise power and control in their marriage. Interestingly, all men, regardless of class, did fewer household chores than their wives. Popular books like *Men Are From Mars and Women Are From Venus* by John Gray have had wide appeal because of their endorsement of traditional gender roles (Trigiani, 1999).

Another aspect of class differences has been between women. For women, to be able to work outside the home has meant that a whole labor force of child care providers has arisen. Typically, such helpers are largely female and poor, and often of color. Thus, even when women are not forced to stay at home to look after children, it is still women who provide child care, and it is still undervalued and poorly paid.

Identity, Gender, and Sexuality

One way to examine the complex layers that underlie gender and sexuality is to break down the various aspects of identity that form them. In Figure 7.1, the various aspects of biological identity, gender identity, gender expression, and sexual orientation are laid out. Notice that where a person might be in each of these identities, it is not so much a category as a place on a continuum.

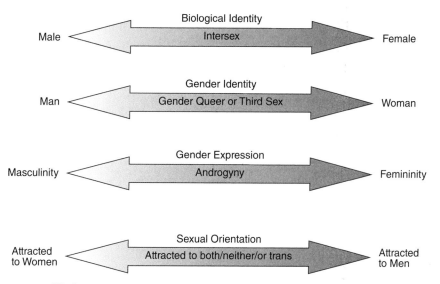

FIGURE **7.1** Dimensions of Gender Identity

Source: Diagram of Sex and Identity (August, 2001). Center for Gender Sanity. Retrieved from http://www.gendersanity.com/diagram.shtml

Biological identity is the extent to which chromosomes, internal reproductive structures, external genitalia, as well as primary sexual characteristics align themselves. Although women are associated with breasts, there are many women who have very small breast sizes and also men who have breasts. On a chromosomal level, there can be various pairings of chromosomes beyond the usual xx and xy, including xxx and xxy. These do have different influences on the physical and psychological levels. For example, individuals with xxx pairing are females with possible sterility problems and males with xxy pairing may also be sterile. However, without genetic testing, it is unlikely that persons may know their "true" biological identity while assuming it to be what the secondary sexual characteristics indicate.

Gender identity focuses on the degree to which one identifies oneself by a gender. It is possible to perceive oneself as a man or a woman, and also to perceive oneself as externally one gender while internally feeling more identified with the other gender. There is also a growing number of people who prefer to identify themselves as belonging not to one of the dual genders, but betwixt and between them; they are termed *gender queer* or third sex, which takes on components of both. Gender expression depicts the degrees to which we express ourselves in gendered behaviors, preferences, and values. Finally, sexual orientation is the degree to which we are attracted to others based on their gender, and of course it is possible to be attracted to one's own gender, the other gender, both genders, or neither.

Normatively we tend to expect the attributes to line up in the ways shown on either end of each continuum. Therefore, a "proper" man is male in his biological identity with a y chromosome, experiences himself as a man in his gender identity, expresses himself in socially normed masculine ways (for examples, just look at ways in which gifts for Father's Day are narrowly organized into masculine attire, such as ties and wallets, or masculine interests, such as sports memorabilia or technological gadgets), and is sexually attracted to women. However, there are more exceptions to these rules than there are examples. For instance, there may be a woman who has the requisite double x chromosome as well as secondary sexual characteristics to appear female, feels herself a woman, is attracted to men, but dresses exclusively in pants, wears no makeup, and works as a carpenter. Or what about the person who walks into a bar with long, groomed hair and skilled makeup, wearing a pink silk dress, looking flirtatiously at the men present, and ordering a cocktail, who actually is a gay male transvestite? We like to think that gender comes in only two definable categories, but it may in fact be much more multiple and complicated.

REFLECTION QUESTIONS 7.3

- What does it mean to be a "woman" in our society; what does it mean in your culture?
- What does it mean to be a "man" in our society; what does it mean in your culture?
- How does the feminist critique of gender help us to work more effectively with clients?
- How might contemporary perspectives on masculinity ideology help us to work more effectively with male clients?
- To what extent do you value a person's gender as a sign of his or her worth?
- Have you ever stood up for someone being harassed or oppressed on the basis of his or her gender? If not, why not? Has anyone ever stood up for you in this way?

INFLUENCE OF FEMINISM IN RECONSTRUCTING GENDER AND SEXUALITY

The women's movement of the late 1960s and beyond has had a tremendous impact on how we currently think about gender and sexuality in western society. This movement triggered an explosion of new theories in psychology that essentially challenged traditional views about men and women (e.g., Collins, Dunlap, & Chrisler, 2002; McLean, Carey, & White, 1996; Rider, 2004). Particularly important, Worell (1986) and Worell and Remer (1992) offered compelling evidence for the lack of attention given to women's psychological health and well-being.

1. Traditional theories of female and male development and behavior describe male traits as normative and female traits as deficient.
2. There is a preponderance of sex stereotyping and sex role bias in the diagnosis of psychopathology.

3. Women are blamed for their experiences of sexual and physical abuse.
4. Women's psychological problems have been overpathologized, resulting in an alarming increase in prescriptive drugs.

Worell and Remer (1992) asserted that the need for change regarding the above issues and others resulted in the creation of a psychology of women as a specialty within the profession that has made substantial contributions to feminist theory, the development of alternative intervention approaches, and new research areas that are endorsed by the broader professional community. The emergence of a psychology of women cannot be understated because it paved the way for new perspectives on gender and sexuality. Specifically, the focus shifted from viewing behaviors as internally predetermined by virtue of one's sex as either male or female to examining behaviors in the context of societal forces. From this perspective, behaviors that are typically ascribed to men and women may be explained, in part, by power, domination, and unequal status. As Kimball (2003) claimed, "men behave differently than women because they hold more power and are supported in their power by institutional sexism" (p. 133). Along these lines, the manifestations of power differentials between men and women are exemplified as follows:

1. Historically, women have occupied subordinate positions in organizations because of prescribed gender roles and expectations (Fain & Anderton, 1987).
2. Sexual harassment in the workplace is most often reported by women (e.g., Kurth, Spiller, & Travis, 2000).
3. With respect to interpersonal styles, women are often judged as less competent when using styles of communication that are perceived as tentative (Carli, 1989).

Feminist scholars also took the lead in challenging theories of human development. In particular, Sigmund Freud's theory of human sexuality has been the subject of much attention and criticism. Although it is not our intent to provide a comprehensive review of Freud's theory on sexuality,[1] a brief description of key factors is described herein.

One of the most critiqued aspects of Freud's theory of sexuality centers on his conceptualization of the development of the libido, considered an innate sexual drive and "masculine force" (Jackson, 1996). According to the theory, males and females undergo different sexuality developmental processes that influence their personalities as adults. In essence, Freud postulated that the so-called penis envy phenomenon associated with young girls as they experience the oedipal stage is the driving force for their lack of healthy superego development as adult women. Jackson (1996) powerfully describes the process:

> Freud makes much of the ideas that in the course of her psychic development a girl has to change her object choice—from her mother to her father, and her leading erotic zones—from the clitoris to the vagina. The energy absorbed in this

---

[1] For a thorough review of Freud's perspective on sexuality, refer to Freud (1903, 1948).

process is supposed to lead to an arrest of psychic development, and hence to a psychic rigidity and lack of creativity. Furthermore, because the girl[,] lacking a penis to begin with, has no castration fears, she remains in the Oedipal situation indefinitely. In not being forced to abandon it, she fails to develop the strong superego characteristic of the male and her mental life therefore remains closer to the instinctual level: she is somehow less civilized than the male. (p. 66)

In turn, the personality traits associated with adult women are "passivity, masochism, and narcissism" (Jackson, 1996; Ruderman, 2003). In contrast to the sexual development of females, the male's identification with the father and his fear of castration propel him to develop a healthy superego. Essentially, Freud postulated that one's sexuality determined all areas of personality development and that these processes were markedly different for men and women. Whether one endorses these beliefs or not is not the subject of debate here, but rather the purpose of describing this perspective is to point out that Freud's theories about human sexuality have had tremendous impact on current theories about psychosocial development. A classic example is Erik Erikson's description of identity development, which is considered "male-oriented." Specifically, Erikson (1950) postulated that achieving a secure identity for adolescent males requires choosing a career and identifying a purpose in life, whereas for adolescent females identity is achieved through their potential role as wife and mother (Worell & Remer, 1992).

Developmental theories have been challenged and reframed by renowned scholars, such as Chodorow (1978), who proposed that the differences in masculine and feminine gender roles and personality development are primarily due to differences in early socialization experiences, and not by their anatomy. Furthermore, Carol Gilligan's (1982) pioneering work on the moral development of women challenged Kohlberg's (1969) biased position, which did not take into account gender differences. Essentially, her theory postulates that women, in particular, focus on relationships with and involving the care of others, whereas men's view of morality focuses on rules and regulations.

Essentialist and Social Constructionist Perspectives on Sexuality and Gender

It is important to consider essentialist and social constructionist views that have guided the development of theories about gender and sexuality. **Essentialism** is a general term used to describe theoretical perspectives that focus on differences between men and women based on genetics and physiology, and a number of scholars note that it promotes biological determinism (Fuss, 1990). From this perspective, heterosexuality is supposedly the norm in which sex is an instinctive drive (Philaretou & Allen, 2001). Essentialism also endorses rigid gender roles and places the heterosexual male at the top of the hierarchy. For instance, Jackson (1996) argued that essentialist thinking has been the driving force for the development of distinct and prescribed masculine and feminine gender roles in our country with the male achieving a superior status, and others such as White (1996) claim that essentialism perpetuates the marginalization of gay, lesbian, and minority groups.

On the other hand, **social constructionism**, a postmodern ideology, focuses on the contextual, incorporating culture, social, and historical perspectives. In many respects, it centers on the individual in relation to the environment. Philaretou and Allen (2001) cogently articulate that it is "ecologically oriented and moves the focus of concern from the sexual actions of specific bodies—male or female, heterosexual, white or black, Christi[a]n or Muslim, Hispanic or Caucasian—to the greater cultural, social, historical contexts in which sexuality occurs" (p. 302).

Janis Bohan (1993) claimed that essentialist ideology defines gender as characteristics and traits that are *within* the individual, largely uninfluenced by the external environment, whereas constructionism focuses not on individual traits, but rather on what she envisions as social "transactions" or interactions we have with others. Gender, construed in this way, is "the meaning we have agreed to impute to a particular class of transactions between individuals and environmental contexts" (p. 13). These social transactions are what produce differences between masculine and feminine behaviors.

An example of essentialism is the belief that specific pathology is related to predetermined biological differences between the sexes. Specifically, the beliefs that women are biologically predisposed to anxiety and mood disorders because of fluctuations in their hormones, and men are inclined to develop antisocial personality disorders as a result of changes in the male hormone, testosterone, are examples of essentialist thinking (Yoder, Fischer, Kahn, & Groden, 2007).

Although feminist perspectives have been the driving force in reconstructing the concept of gender, they, too, have recently been criticized as essentialist in nature. In a critique, Bohan (1993) outlined important ways in which feminist theories promote essentialist thought:

1. Some theories focus on universality, generalizing ideas, perspectives, and approaches, and do not take into consideration the diversity of experiences among women, especially cultural and ethnic differences. Equally important, such generalizing also fosters stereotyping.
2. Addressing issues of oppression, institutional barriers, and the social forces that shape women's lives is often overlooked in these theoretical perspectives.
3. Referring to gender differences in "ways of knowing, or moral judgment" leads one to reach the erroneous conclusion that only women have these traits, and do not have access to other ways of being. Bohan points out that whereas feminists argue that is important to acknowledge that there are alternate ways of viewing the world and defining moral judgment, we still live in a male-dominated society and, therefore, such traits are often seen as not as important or highly valued compared to the traits ascribed to men.
4. The research has been plagued with inconsistencies in theory and methodology, and thus has been unable to replicate studies.

Bohan (1993) goes on to affirm that viewing gender from a constructionist perspective attempts to address some of the shortcomings associated with

CASE STUDY **7.1**

The Case of Margaret

Margaret is a new client who comes to you in some distress. She is a second-generation Irish American woman in her mid-40s; is married to Michael, a first-generation Irish American man; and has two children who are currently in high school. She tells you that she married Michael when she was in her late 20s.

She says to you, "I don't know what it is, but I just feel so sad. Nothing's wrong, nothing's happened, but it's like I can't sleep, I find myself crying, I just don't know.... I wouldn't have thought of coming to a counselor, but this girl at work said that I should try it, and maybe you can help me feel better."

About her marriage, she says, "We've been together about 18 years, and I guess that's impressive these days. But Michael, I think he drinks a lot. He goes out with his friends to the bars after work almost every day, and when he comes home there's nothing to talk about. He's provided for me, and I'm grateful, but I don't know what I am to him other than his wife and the mother of his children."

Regarding her children, she says, "When they were little, I thought I would go crazy. I had to quit work, and there I was in the house alone all day with these two kids. I felt like my brains turned to mush. But now, they are so grown up—Emily has started dating, and she's never home. I miss that time when I had them to myself—but I let it slip by."

She also tells you, "I tried going to my priest for help. But I don't know... there's not much comfort there. Somehow these days, the Church doesn't seem to offer me as much. I feel empty, and my faith used to be a strong part of me."

About her work, she tells you, "Before I got married and had kids, I used to work as a fashion buyer. I was pretty good at it. Now, because I took all that time off, I'm just working as an assistant. Its OK money, and I get to meet people other than Michael's friends. But I see the other women my age in the business, and they're directors and managers, and you know, I wonder where I could have been."

Case Discussion
Thinking About This Case:
1. What are the factors that contribute to Margaret's distress?
2. Based on your understanding of feminism, how would you reframe her concerns from intrapersonal to societal? That is, identify factors in the environment that might contribute to her problems.
3. What are some of the ways to increase Margaret's personal power?

Margaret is exhibiting symptoms of distress. She is concerned about her relationship with Michael, her spouse, and is questioning her role as a mother and wife. For example, now that the children are older and more independent, Margaret is experiencing a void, believing that she gave up a career to raise her children. She seems to regret that decision. She is comparing herself with other women who have advanced in their careers. She also reports that her faith is wavering, and her religious affiliation no longer serves as a source of support. From a strength-based approach, the counselor can help her to reframe her concerns. For example, the counselor can work with her to identify positive aspects of her life. It might be important to explore the messages she received from the external environment (i.e., expectations from others about the role of women in today's society) that could be contributing to a belief about being devalued. Margaret seems to be feeling disconnected from her husband and children, and she is expressing it as sadness. The counselor can work with Margaret to increase her positive self-worth, including a sense of control and empowerment, by identifying aspects of her life where she has made a difference. What has brought her joy and happiness? In addition, the counselor can help Margaret to explore new job opportunities. Because Margaret stated, "I wonder where I could have been," with respect to career advancement, this might be an important area to explore with her.

essentialism in feminist models. Interpreting gender as influenced by social interactions and particular settings, it allows us to see that one's behavior is determined not by the sex of the person, but rather by the context of the situation or the environment in which the interchange is taking place. A number of research findings support this idea, such as that women and men who work in similar occupations hold similar values about the work environment (Major, 1987), and single fathers engage in what are considered traditional female behaviors when needing to respond to the challenges of raising children by themselves (Risman, 1987).

THE MEN'S MOVEMENT

The rise of the "men's movement" is a response to the widespread criticism of traditional masculine roles and their position of power in society as evidenced in the previous discussions. However, there are wide variations in these responses. For example, there are men who are profeminist and antisexist, working toward gender equality and gay rights, and there are those who want to reclaim their power (Carey, 1996). Nonetheless, the movement has served as the impetus for the self-examination and redefinition of men and their experiences in contemporary society. The emerging field of men's studies is a good example. Men are seriously examining the causes of what Brooks (2003) calls their "dark side" such as male violence, rape and sexual assault, alcohol and drug use, and homelessness. These and other important issues are being reframed so that the focus is on empowering men to change, learn new roles, and actively participate with women for social justice on issues of inequality (e.g., Connell, 2008). Likewise, more attention is being given to ethnic and cultural variations in masculinity, its meaning, and its manifestations such as in African American (e.g., Hammond & Mattis, 2005), Mexican (Arciniega, Anderson, Tovar-Blank, & Tracey, 2008), and Asian American (Shek, 2006) men.

Although these issues have been widely acknowledged with concerted efforts to address them, there has been a shift toward increasing our understanding of men and their experiences as well. The development of the "gender role strain paradigm" is an example of this shift (e.g., Brooks, 2003; Levant, 1996; Levant & Richmond, 2007). Its premise is that men may experience a great deal of stress because of the powerful gender role socialization processes that promote masculine normative behaviors, such as being strong and confident. According to Addis and Mahalik (2002), these behaviors will discourage men from seeking help. Interestingly, contemporary perspectives on men's issues also emphasize that mental health problems, such as anxiety and distress may be associated with their prescribed gender role expectations, such as being tough, independent, and unable to show intense emotions (Philaretou & Allen, 2001). Specifically, Levant et al. (2003) found that there were some cultural differences in the endorsement of traditional **masculinity ideology**, defined as the "endorsement and internalization of cultural belief systems about masculinity and male gender, rooted in the structural relationship between the two sexes (Pleck, Sonenstein, & Ku, 1993, p. 88)" among the men in the sample. For instance, they found that African American and Latino males tended to endorse a more traditional masculinity ideology compared to European Americans, although there were variations according to geographic location (e.g., urban versus rural communities). In addition, Pleck

CASE STUDY **7.2**

The Case of Henry

Henry is a new client in his mid-40s who was referred to a counselor by his employer's department of human resources. His immediate supervisor referred him because his productivity has declined in the last 6 months. Henry has been experiencing severe headaches and stomach problems during the last several months. He has not been eating or sleeping well, and has lost 10 pounds. Due to the economic downtown, he is worried about losing his job and the impact that would have financially on his family. He comes home tired and upset, but does not share his troubles with his wife. He has lost interest in intimacy and sexual activity with his wife. On his first visit to see you, the counselor, he tells you that he doesn't "need therapy" and only came because he was forced to by his boss. Henry states that what he needs is to "get back on track with work and all will be fine."

Case Discussion

Thinking About This Case:
1. What might be the source of Henry's distress?
2. What might be the issues Henry is facing, and how is he manifesting them?

3. Henry tells you that he "does not need to see a counselor." How do you engage him in counseling?

As a counselor, it is important to determine Henry's comfort level in seeking help at the onset. The counselor can explore the extent to which the gender of the counselor plays a role in his resistance to seek help. Because he reports being "forced" to see a counselor and "doesn't need therapy," it would be important to explore this issue with him, Henry could be endorsing prescribed gender role expectations such as being strong, successful, and self-reliant. This is evident in his statement about not needing to seek help from a counselor. Likewise, Henry could be experiencing "gender role strain" but may be unaware of its manifestations. His physical symptoms could be a function of this strain; however, it would be wise to recommend a thorough health exam to rule out a biological basis for his physical ailments. A counselor can help Henry explore the extent to which his identity matches traditional male roles and whether this is a source of the concerns.

---

et al. found that **alexithymia,** defined as the "inability to put emotions to word" (p. 92), was highest among the men who endorsed traditional masculinity ideology.

OPENING THE DIALOGUE ON GENDER

With all of the topics discussed in this chapter, you are now challenged to think through how you would utilize this information in session with any number of clients from a variety of cultural backgrounds and worldviews. Questions for reflection offered to you throughout this chapter also serve as excellent process questions for opening the dialogue with clients on issues of gender and sexuality. Some of these questions are listed here to assist you in terms of opening the dialogue with your clients:

- How important is your gender in terms of your personal and cultural identity, and what impact does this have on how you view the world and live your life?
- How did your gender-based definition of yourself develop, and who were some significant people in your life that helped to shape this definition?
- How has your view of gender and sexuality been reinforced or challenged during your life?

- What does your culture say about gender and sexuality?
- What do your family and community say about gender and sexuality in terms of both beliefs and practice?
- What does it mean to be a "woman" in our society; what does it mean in your life specifically? In your family? In your culture?
- What does it mean to be a "man" in our society; what does it mean in your life specifically? In your family? In your culture?
- How do issues of power and privilege influence your view of gender and sexuality and your concept of sexism?
- How has your view of gender and sexuality affected the way you define yourself now and at previous points in your life?
- How will your view of gender and sexuality continue to affect the way you define yourself and the way others see you or treat you?
- How has your view of gender and sexuality affected the way you interact with others who are similar versus different to you in age at different points in your life?
- Who are some people of your own gender and sexuality who you look up to, and why?
- How might the difference or similarity in gender between you (client) and I (counselor) affect your experience in the process of counseling as well as the relationship between us?
- When and how did you first become aware of sexism? What was your initial reaction, and how did that reaction change over time?
- What have your experiences with sexism been, and in what ways have those experiences shaped who you are as a person, as well as the issues you are dealing with now?
- What efforts have you made to work toward positive social change with regard to the sexism that exists in your own life at the individual, group, and societal levels, and what other kinds of efforts would you like to make?
- To what extent do you value a person's gender and sexuality as a sign of his or her worth?
- Have you ever stood up for someone being harassed or oppressed on the basis of gender? If not, why not? Has anyone ever stood up for you in this way?
- How do gender and sexuality play into the issues you are bringing to counseling, and how can we address this in a way that is most helpful to you?

CONCLUSION AND IMPLICATIONS

As a counselor you might ask: How are gender and sexuality related to psychological health? Given the previous discussion, it is clear that there are, indeed, mental health implications. For instance, we discussed gender role stereotypes, power differentials between men and women, as well as biased perspectives on human sexuality. It is reasonable to conclude that these issues and circumstances have profound effects on one's psychological well-being and sense of personal worth.

As noted earlier, more women are diagnosed with, treated for, and prescribed medications for mental illness than men. There are numerous societal forces that affect women's psychosocial well-being such as disproportionately higher rates of poverty, frequent acts of violence and abuse, and gender segregation in the labor market combined with lower wages, all of which create stress and strain (Worell & Remer, 1992). Men, too, experience stress and strain with conflicting gender roles and expectations in contemporary society. In addition, men may not seek counseling services if they highly endorse traditional masculinity ideology (Levant & Richmond, 2007). Counselors need to be knowledgeable of the ways in which clients' sexuality and gender affect psychological well-being. This includes understanding how gender roles affect a client's sense of personal worth, psychological well-being, and physical health.

In this chapter, we discussed the complex nature of gender, including the related constructs of masculinity and femininity. We briefly presented a historical perspective on how feminist thought has influenced the reconstruction of gender and sexuality as well as how the essentialist and social constructionist points of view have helped to shape the theories associated with these concepts. The impact of the both the women's and men's movements in our society was presented, which has challenged our thinking about the lack of attention given to women's psychological health and well-being, and, for men, a redefinition of their roles including a reexamination of what constitutes masculinity.

GLOSSARY

Alexithymia: The inability to describe emotions in words.

Essentialism: A theoretical perspective focusing on differences between men and women based on genetic, biological, and physiological differences.

Gender: An expression of self as female or male, including socially constructed roles, behaviors, and characteristics that define men and women in a given society. The definition may include the human body's anatomy and physiology.

Gender identity: The perception of self about one's gender that may or may not be related to the person's biological characteristics. It may incorporate personal manifestations of masculinity and femininity and sexual orientation.

Gendered difference: An aspect of Gilbert and Scher's (1999) model of gender, which is defined as how we see men and women as having different roles (e.g., women as nurturers and men as providers).

Gendered discourse: An aspect of a model proposed by Gilbert and Scher (1999), which refers to the ways in which gender expectations influence what we talk about, the language we use, and our assumptions about men and women.

Gendered process: An aspect of Gilbert and Scher's (1999) model, in which there are specific ways in which men and women interact with others.

Gendered structure: An aspect of Gilbert and Scher's (1999) model that focuses on the differences between men and women in opportunities, access to resources, and policies.

Masculinity ideology: The endorsement of beliefs, attitudes, and behaviors about masculinity and the male gender that socially constructed and grounded in the differences between males and females. It may be viewed as the extent to which males endorse traditional male roles in society.

Sexuality: The way in which individuals express themselves as sexual beings, including practices, behaviors, and relationships.

Social constructionism: A postmodern ideology perspective emphasizing that individuals are influenced by the social environment. It focuses on contextual, historical, and historical perspectives.

REFERENCES

Addis, M., & Mahalik, J. R. (2002). Men, masculinity, and the context of help seeking. *American Psychologist, 58,* 5–14.

Arciniega, G. M., Anderson, T. C., Tovar-Blank, Z. G., & Tracey, T. J. G. (2008). Towards a fuller conception of machismo: Development of a Traditional Machismo and Caballerismo Scale. *Journal of Counseling Psychology, 55,* 19–33.

Bohan, J. (1993). Regarding gender: Essentialism, constructionism and feminist psychology. *Psychology of Women Quarterly, 17,* 5–22.

Bullough, V. (2002). Transgenderism and the concept of gender. *International Journal of Transgenderism, 4*(3). Retrieved from http://www.symposion.com/ijt/gilbert/bullough.htm

Carey, M. (1996). Perspectives on the men's movement. In C. McLean, M. Carey, & C. White (Eds.), *Men's ways of being* (pp. 153–162). Boulder, CO: Westview Press.

Carli, L. L. (1989). Gender differences in interaction styles and influence. *Journal of Personality & Social Psychology, 56,* 565–576.

Chodorow, N. (1978). *The production of mothering: Psychoanalysis and the sociology of gender.* Berkeley: University of California Press.

Collins, L. H., Dunlap, M. R., & Chrisler, J. (Eds.). (2002). *Charting a new course for feminist psychology.* Westport, CT: Praeger.

Connell, R. W. (2008). Change among the gatekeepers: Men, masculinities, and gender equity in the global arena. In J. Z. Spade & C. G. Valentine (Eds.), *The kaleidoscope of gender: Prisms, patterns, and possibilities* (pp. 531–547). Thousand Oaks, CA: Pine Forge Press.

D'Andrea, M., & Daniels, J. (2001). Respectful counseling: An integrative multidimensional model for counselors. In D. B. Pope-Davis & H. L. K. Coleman (Eds.), *The intersection of race, class, and gender in multicultural counseling* (pp. 417–466). Thousand Oaks, CA: Sage.

Erikson, E. (1950). *Childhood and society.* New York, NY: WW Norton and Company.

Fain, T. C., & Anderton, D. L. (1987). Sexual harassment: Organizational context and diffuse status. *Sex Roles, 17,* 291–311.

Fausto-Sterling, A. (2000). *Sexing the body: Gender politics and construction of sexuality.* New York: Basic.

Freud, S. (1903). *Three essays on sexuality.* In *Standard edition* (Vol. 8). London: Hogarth Press.

Freud, S. (1948). Some psychological consequences of the anatomical distinction between the sexes. In *Collected papers* (Vol. 5). London: Hogarth Press.

Fuss, D. (1990). *Essentially speaking: Feminism, nature and difference.* New York; Routledge.

Gilbert, L., & Scher, M. (1999). *Gender and sex in counseling and psychotherapy.* Boston: Allyn & Bacon.

Gilligan, C. (1982). *In a different voice: Psychological theory and women's development.* Cambridge, MA: Harvard University Press.

Gray, J. (1992). *Men are from Mars and women are from Venus.* New York, NY: HarperCollins Publishers.

Hammond, W. P., & Mattis, J. S. (2005). Being a man about it: Manhood meaning among African American men. *Psychology of Men & Masculinity, 6,* 114–126.

Jackson, S. (1996). The social construction of female sexuality. In S. Jackson & S. Scott (Eds.), *Feminism and sexuality: A reader* (pp. 62–73). New York: Columbia University Press.

Jackson, S., & Scott, S. (1996). *Feminism and sexuality: A reader.* New York: Columbia University Press.

Kimball, M. (2003). Feminist rethink gender. In D. B. Hill & M. J. Kral (Eds.), *About psychology: Essays at the crossroads of history, theory, and philosophy* (pp. 127–146). Albany: State University of New York Press.

Kohlberg, L. (1969). Stage and sequence: The cognitive-developmental approach to socialization. In D. A. Goslin (Ed.), *The handbook of socialization theory and research.* Chicago: Rand McNally.

Kurth, S. B., Spiller, B. B., & Travis, C. B. (2000). Consent, power, and sexual scripts: Deconstructing sexual harassment. In C. B. Travis & J. W. White (Eds.), *Sexuality, society, and feminism* (pp. 323–354). Washington, DC: American Psychological Association.

Levant, R. F. (1996). The new psychology of men. *Professional Psychology: Research and Practice, 27,* 259–265.

Levant, R. F., & Richmond, K. (2007). A review of research on masculinity ideologies using the Male Role Norms Inventory. *Journal of Men's Studies, 15,* 130–146.

Levant, R. F., Richmond, K., Majors, R. G., Inclan J. E., Rossello, J. H., Heesaker, M., et al. (2003). A multicultural investigation of masculinity ideology and alexithymia. *Psychology of Men & Masculinity, 4,* 91–99.

Major, B. (1987). Gender, justice, and the psychology of entitlement. In P. Shaver & C. Hendrick (Eds.), *Review of personality and social psychology: Vol. 7. Sex and gender* (pp. 124–148). Beverly Hills, CA: Sage.

Philaretou, A. G., & Allen, K. R. (2001). Reconstructing masculinity and sexuality. *Journal of Men's Studies, 9,* 302–321.

Pleck, J. H., Sonenstein, F. L., & Ku, L. C. (1993). Masculiity ideology and its xorrelates. In S. Oskamp and M. Costanzo (Eds.). *Gender issues in contemporary society.* (pp. 85–110), Thousand Oaks, CA: Sage.

Pyle, K. D. (1996). Class-based masculinities: The interdependence of gender, class, and interpersonal power. *Gender and Society, 10,* 527–549.

Rider, E. A. (2004). *Our voices: Psychology of women* (2nd ed.). Hoboken, NJ: John Wiley.

Risman, B. J. (1987). Intimate relationships from a microstructural perspective: Men who mother. *Gender and Society, 1,* 6–32.

Ruderman, E. G. B. (2003). Plus ca change, plus c'est la même chose: Women's "masochism" and ambivalence about ambition and success. In J. B. Sanville & E. B. Ruderman (Eds.), *Therapies with women in transition: Toward relational perspectives with today's women* (pp. 1–26). Madison, CT: International Universities Press.

Savin-Williams, R. C., & Cohen, K. M. (Eds.). (1996). *The lives of lesbians, gays and bisexuals: Children to adults.* Fort Worth, TX: Harcourt Brace.

Shek, Y. L. (2006). Asian American masculinity: A review of the literature. *Journal of Men's Studies, 14,* 379–391.

Smith, G. (1996). Dichotomies in the making of men. In C. McLean, M. Carey, & C. White (Eds.), *Men's ways of being* (pp. 27–49). Boulder, CO: Westview Press

Thompson, N. (2000). The ontology of masculinity—the roots of manhood. In D. A. Lund (Ed.), *Men coping with grief* (pp. 27–36). Amityville, NY: Baywood.

Trigiani, K, (1999). Masculinity-femininity: Society's difference dividend. Retrieved from http://web2. airmail.net/ktrig246/out_of_cave/mf.html

White, M. (1996). Men's culture, the men's movement, and the constitution of men's lives. In C. McLean, M. Carey, & C. White (Eds.), *Men's ways of being* (pp. 163–193). Boulder, CO: Westview Press.

White, J. W., Bondurant, B., & Travis, C. B. (2000). Social constructions of sexuality: Unpacking hidden meaning. In C. B. Travis & J. W. White (Eds.), *Sexuality, society, and feminism* (pp. 11–33). Washington, DC: American Psychological Association.

Weis, L., Centrie, C., Valentin-Juarbe, J., & Fine, M. (2002). Puerto Rican men and the struggle for place in the United States: An exploration of cultural citizenship, gender, and violence. *Men and Masculinity, 4,* 286–302.

Worell, J. (1986, November). The DSM IIIR: Controversies in gender bias. Invited paper presented at the annual meeting of the Association for the Advancement of behavior Therapy, Chicago.

Worell, J., & Remer, P. (1992). *Feminist perspectives in therapy: An empowerment model for women.* New York: John Wiley.

Yoder, J., Fischer, A. R., Kahn, A.S., & Groden, J. (2007). Changes in students explanations for gender differences after taking a psychology of women class: More constructionist and less essentialist. *Psychology of Women Quarterly, 31,* 415–425.

CHAPTER 8

Sexual Orientation

Because much stress has been placed here on heterosexuality as word and concept, it seems important to affirm that heterosexuality (and homosexuality) came into existence before it was named and thought about. The formulation of the heterosexual idea did not create a heterosexual experience or behavior; to suggest otherwise would be to ascribe a determining power to labels and concepts. But the titling and envisioning of heterosexuality did play an important role in consolidating the construction of the heterosexual's social existence. Before the wide use of the word "heterosexual," I suggest, women and men did not mutually lust with the same profound, sure sense of normalcy that followed the distribution of "heterosexual" as universal sanctifier.

According to this proposal, women and men make their own sexual histories. But they do not produce their sex lives just as they please. They make their sexualities within a particular mode of organization given by the past and altered by their changing desire, their present power and activity, and their vision of a better world. That hypothesis suggests a number of good reasons for the immediate inauguration of research on a historically specific heterosexuality.

The study of the heterosexual experience will forward a great intellectual struggle still in its early stages. This is the fight to pull heterosexuality, homosexuality, and all the sexualities out of the realm of nature and biology [and] into the realm of the social and historical. Feminists have explained to us that anatomy does not determine our gender destinies (our masculinities and femininities). But we've only recently begun to consider that biology does not settle our erotic fates. The common notions that biology determines the object of sexual desire, or that physiology and society together cause sexual orientation, are determinisms that deny the break existing between our bodies and our situations and our desiring. Just as the biology of our hearing organs will never tell us why we take pleasure in Bach or delight in Dixieland, our female and male anatomies, hormones, and genes will never tell us why we yearn for women, men, both, other, or none. That is because desiring is a self-generated project of individuals within particular historical cultures. Heterosexual history can help us see the place of values and judgments in the construction of our own and others' pleasures, and to see how our erotic tastes—our aesthetics of the flesh—are socially institutionalized through the struggle of individuals and classes.

From Katz, J. N., "The Invention of Heterosexuality," in P. S. Rothenberg (Ed.), *Race, Class, and Gender in the United States, 6th ed.* (New York: Worth) Reprinted with permission.

Sexual orientation is probably one of the most heated issues in society today, generating strong opinions. On the other hand, a range of sexual orientations are also much more visible in today's society. In this chapter, we consider this construct and its meanings across history and in terms of counseling. Notice as you read this chapter that although we automatically think of gays, lesbians, and bisexuals in terms of sexual orientation, **heterosexuals**, too, have a place in the discussion. However, rather than being the norm from which other sexual orientations are deviations, we will consider the possibility that particular orientations fall along a continuum. In chapter 7, we considered the notion of gender; now we focus our attention on sexual orientation.

REFLECTION QUESTIONS 8.1

- How do you define sexual orientation and sexual identity?
- How do you know your own sexual orientation?

We begin this chapter with a discussion about the terminology in this area, which is unsettled and can often lead to confusion among those who are not an integral part of the particular community. It also tends to vary across geographical areas, cultures, and time periods (American Psychological Association, 1991). One of the most familiar terms in referring to those who are attracted to others of their gender is **homosexual**. According to Herzer (1985), the term was invented in the late 1860s, and popularized by later scholars, such as Krafft-Ebbing and Havelock Ellis in the field of sexuality. In the last few decades, however, as there has been increasing self-identification by members of this community, the term *homosexual* is often rejected because of its links to negative stereotypes and a diagnosis of pathology (American Psychological Association, 1991). In addition, many persons find the focus of the term on sexuality to be minimizing of the range of attraction and affiliation that characterize relationships. The alternate term **gay**, which has unknown origins, has been increasingly used since the late 1960s. The term **lesbian** has a much older history, and appears to be sourced in the name of the Greek poet Sappho, who lived on the island of Lesbos around 600 B.C. and celebrated same-sex love in her poetry (Money, 1998). Though *gay* was often used to describe all persons attracted to their own gender, it became increasingly significant to have a name that represented women's separate and unique experiences with same-gender attraction. On the other hand, many persons who consider themselves attracted to men and women find it acceptable to be termed **bisexual,** and this has gained currency as a descriptive label. Within the community, persons may shorten it to *bi.* **Straight** was a term that was developed by the gay community to describe heterosexual persons, to reference their own sense of themselves as deviating from the norm of society's acceptable sexuality. Finally, **transgender** began to be used in the 1990s as a new way to think about the intersection between sex and gender. Originally applied as *transsexual* to describe those persons whose sexual identity transgresses sex–gender norms (such as a person identified as male at birth who considers that he is actually female born into the wrong body), it became quickly used to describe almost anyone who resisted gender norms. For instance, women who were not stereotypically feminine, even if they were attracted to men, could use the term (Denny, 1997).

Although issues of sexual orientation are present in every culture and group, there is less open discussion in many cultures about it. However, there have been terms used within cultures to describe the sexual orientation of members of that culture. For instance, some Native Americans may sometimes use the term *two-spirited* to describe an integration of the spiritual and social aspects of alternative sexuality (Tafoya, 1997). In referring to members of populations considered "alternate" in their sexuality, the acronym LGBT (for *lesbian, gay, bisexual, and transgender*) has often been used as a grouping label. An emerging term that is increasingly popular is *queer*, applied generically to any LGBT person. It is somewhat controversial because of past connotations as a derogatory taunt, as well as current associations with radical politics (Rust, 1996). The issue of using a particular label or name is sensitive because of the historical powerlessness associated with being labeled or named by others outside the community.

HISTORICAL PERSPECTIVES

Although many may feel that the issues of sexual orientation and alternate sexualities are exploding into public consciousness only recently, there has been a long history of diverse responses to these issues. As Katz (2003) points out, the division of sexuality into abnormal and normal (along the lines of portraying heterosexuality as normal and all other sexualities as abnormal) has not been a historical constant. Early Greek societies saw male bisexuality as normal and preferred. The Sacred Band, a group of elite warriors, was composed of male lovers, with the idea being that men would fight fiercely in protection of their lover. Several of the Greek myths deal with the issue of same-gender attraction. Medieval Persian poetry has examples of romantic love between men. Other periods and contexts in history, however, have not been as tolerant or accepting. In the medieval period in Europe, people would be burned to death for their sexuality. The derogatory term *faggot* comes from this origin, because it was originally meant a bundle of twigs to be used for kindling. In early 19th-century Europe and the United States, there existed ideals of true womanhood, manhood, and love that were characterized by purity, and the only legitimate natural desire was for the purposes of procreation (Katz, 2003). It was only in the late 1800s to early 1900s that the ideas of heterosexual and homosexual were formulated, primarily by the medical establishment. Dr. Krafft-Ebbing published the influential *Psychopathia Sexualis*, where "hetero-sexual" was used to refer to an erotic feeling for a different sex, whereas "homosexual" referred to erotic feelings for the same sex. There was also a third category of *psycho-sexual hermaphroditism*, defined by impulses toward both sexes (Katz, 2003). In the same period, women living in same-gender relationships often escaped social notice or disapproval because of the lack of perceiving such relationships, often known as "Boston marriages," as sexual (Broido, 2000).

During the Nazi period in Germany, gays and lesbians were forced to wear pink triangles or a patch marked "175" on their clothes. During the Nazi regime, an estimated half a million gays and lesbians were sentenced because of their sexual orientation and ended up in concentration camps, where they were often brutalized and killed. After liberation, when other prisoners were released, those who wore the pink triangle remained in German prisons to serve out the rest of their sentence (Rector, 1981). Moreover, in the United States, no community provided contacts, support, resources, role models, or legal protection for same-gender attraction. "Homosexuality" was illegal in every state, and police often raided bars that were known to be frequented by lesbian and gay populations, subjected persons to verbal and physical abuse, arrested them, and gave their names to the media. Parents disowned children, and other losses of jobs, custody of children, visitation rights, and/or housing were a constant threat. The McCarthy period of the 1950s targeted not only suspected communists but also those suspected to be homosexual, and they were barred from federal jobs (D'Emilio, 1983).

Harassment and isolation continued, but after World War II, when overseas travel through military service allowed LGBT persons to meet and connect with others like themselves, communities began to form, often in the larger port cities such as New York and San Francisco. The Mattachine Society for gay persons, formed in 1951, appears to be the first "gay rights" group in the United States (Bohan, 1996).

One of the most significant turning points in the political and social climate occurred on June 28, 1960. The Stonewall Inn bar in Greenwich Village, New York City, was undergoing a routine police raid, but instead of

---

EXAMPLE **8.1**

The Times of Harvey Milk

In 1978, Harvey Milk was elected to the San Francisco City Council, becoming the first openly gay person to be elected to public office in California. Through tireless coalition building, campaigning, and good humor, Milk successfully integrated people and politics across diverse boundaries. Barely 11 months later, he and Mayor George Moscone were shot and killed by Milk's fellow council member, former police officer and firefighter Dan White, on November 27, 1978. The tumultuous story of Milk's grassroots political organizing and election, through the shocking murders and their repercussions—including the eloquent candlelight memorial joined by tens of thousands of San Franciscans on the evening of the assassinations, and the angry mobs who stormed City Hall, breaking windows and torching police cars in the aftermath of White's lenient sentencing at his murder trial—is chronicled in an award-winning documentary as well as portrayed in a feature film starring Sean Penn called *Milk* (Van Sant, Jinks, & Cohen, 2008).

---

submitting to the usual harassment and arrests, patrons fought back. Hundreds of protestors gathered to support the resistance and battle the police, which went on for several days. Inspired by this event, a mass liberation movement began to form that drew from strategies by the civil rights movement, which had fought against stigmatization, and the women's liberation movement, which provided political analysis of sexism and gender roles. In June 1970, a march in New York City to commemorate Stonewall drew 5,000 participants, the largest demonstration up to that point (D'Emilio, 1983).

The burgeoning political solidarity of the 1970s continued in the face of the great threat in the 1980s of the HIV/AIDS epidemic. The medical and social crises of illness, deaths, losses of friends and partners, and fear of diagnosis pervaded people's lives. In the early years, the epidemic was viewed as something that affected only a despised portion of the population, resulting in the seeming indifference of the government and social agencies and the simultaneous energizing of the AIDS-affected community to care for their own as well as organize to seek more funding for services and for research toward a cure. HIV/AIDS continued to consume much of the energy of the communities into the 1990s. In recent years, the focus has broadened to include the lack of legal protection for LGBT people across many areas and the need for civil rights at all levels in the society. The rise in gay and lesbian unions, the debates about the heterosexualization of the institution of marriage, and the increased visibility of the "gay baby boom" are on the forefront of the issues (Hunter & Hickerson, 2003). Polls show that more people accept gays and lesbians than before, with 52% considering it acceptable in 2001 as opposed to 24% in 1983. However, this change is due to a

EXAMPLE **8.2**
The Murder of Matthew Shepard

Matthew was a 22-year-old political science student at the University of Wyoming in Laramie. On October 6, 1998, Aaron McKinney and Russell A. Henderson entered a Laramie bar that was known as a place where gays often hung out. The two men left the bar in the company of Matthew Shepard, who they drove to an open field. After being tied to a fence and beaten within an inch of his life, Shepard was left for dead in the near-freezing temperatures. The two men had also stolen his wallet and shoes. Eighteen hours later, he was found by two passing motorcyclists who thought at first that Shepherd was a scarecrow because of the way he was positioned on the fence. Shepherd was flown to a hospital, where he remained in critical condition for several days before dying on October 12. Rev. Fred Phelps of the Wesboro Baptist Church (Topeka, Kansas) started organizing a protest over Shepherd's funeral, urging people to arrive with signs containing hate messages. He also started a website, godhatesfags.com.

Whereas Russell A. Henderson pleaded guilty to felony murder, Aaron McKinney's defense strategy planned on introducing the "gay panic" defense, stating that Shepard could have been responsible for his own death. The defense was rejected by the judge; McKinney was convicted on two counts of felony murder charges and was sentenced to two consecutive life sentences for his involvement.

solidification of attitudes with much fewer people having no opinion. Thus, the 42% of Americans who believe homosexuality should be illegal has stayed the same since the 1970s (Brammer, 2004). Such polarization and hardening of attitudes have also led LGBT individuals to be significantly overrepresented among victims of violence (Kantor, 2009).

With respect to mental health, gay, lesbian, bisexual, and transgender persons continued to make strides. Even though Freud himself did not consider homosexuality as an illness, the psychoanalytic tradition fueled this perception (Isay, 1989). Explicitly linked to homosexuality was the notion of mental disorder, unhappiness, lack of fulfillment, and an inability to maintain relationships (Broido, 2000). In the United States, it was treated as such until 1972, when the American Psychiatric Association listed only *ego-dystonic homosexuality* as a disorder in the second edition of the *Diagnostic and Statistical Manual of Psychiatric Disorders* (DSM-II; American Psychiatric Association, 1972). This framed such clients as those who refused to accept their sexual orientation and suffered guilt and shame regarding their sexuality. Notice that such a definition shifts the focus of the disorder from being LGBT to feeling shame and guilt about it. By the late 1980s, this reasoning was also challenged with the argument that discomfort or denial of one's sexual orientation might have more to do with discrimination by society than with the mental health of the individual. In 1987, the revised third edition of the DSM (American Psychiatric Association, 1987) removed the category of homosexuality completely as pathology.

In the field of psychology, attempts have been made over the years to explain the etiology and roots of being gay, lesbian, or bisexual. Freud (1905) believed that all human beings were born bisexual with latent homosexual impulses. He traced developing a gay sexual orientation to an unresolved oedipal complex, in which a young boy took on the sexual orientation of his mother after failing to identify with his father. Stoller (1968) reiterated this psychoanalytic position of sexual orientation being dependent on early interactions with parents, based on research where he concluded that domineering mothers and distant fathers caused the development of sexual confusion in boys. This research followed a familiar course of blaming the primary caretaker, who was the mother. Later researchers tended to look for biological explanations that included levels of maternal testosterone to which the fetus was exposed, environmental stressors, and genetic predispositions (Turner, 1995).

DEVELOPMENT OF SEXUAL ORIENTATION IDENTITY

Much of the work on identity development has focused specifically on lesbian, gay, bisexual, or heterosexual identity development rather than on overall sexual orientation identity development. The normative process has been understood to be the development of heterosexual identity, and therefore work has tended to focus more on examining the processes undergone in developing a sexual identity in individuals considered part of a "minority group." This is similar to the work on racial identity development, described in chapter 4, where a racial minority group's identity development (e.g., that of Blacks or African Americans) has received more attention than that of a majority group (e.g., Whites). A problem with this focus is that it can continue to perpetuate minority group status as "other," as well as reinforce the belief that majority group identity development is normative and universally understood.

REFLECTION QUESTIONS 8.2

- At what point in your life did you become aware of your sexual orientation and sexual identity?
- What role did your family, peers, and the larger society play in your decision making about your sexual identity?
- Has your understanding of your own sexual identity changed over time, and if so, how? If not, why not?
- Do you recall a period of exploration and coming to a decision, or was your sexual orientation something you took for granted?

Heterosexual Identity Development

One model developed by Worthington, Savoy, Dillon, and Vernaglia (2002) is a multidimensional one, defining heterosexual identity development as the individual and social processes by which heterosexually identified persons acknowledge and define their sexual needs, values, sexual orientation and preferences for sexual activities, models of sexual expression, and characteristics of sexual partners ... to this definition the assumption that heterosexual development entails an understanding (implicit or explicit) of one's membership in an oppressive majority group, with a corresponding set of attitudes, beliefs, and values with respect to members of sexual minority groups. (p. 510)

The model incorporates six biopsychosocial influences and six dimensions of individual identity that interact with aspects of group membership identity and attitudes toward sexual minorities, and is shown in Figure 8.1. The authors distinguish between sexual identity as a comprehensive process regarding one's identity as a sexual being versus sexual orientation identity regarding the acceptance and recognition of one's sexual orientation. Of the biopsychosocial context, the authors describe (a) the influence of *biological factors* encountered by individuals during critical points in development in physical maturation; (b) the *microsocial context* influencing sexual identity by the values and beliefs espoused through relationships with family, peers, and community; (c) *gender norms and socialization*, where individuals internalize constructions of gender and act according to these prescribed roles and norms in their interpersonal interactions; (d) *culture* influencing the

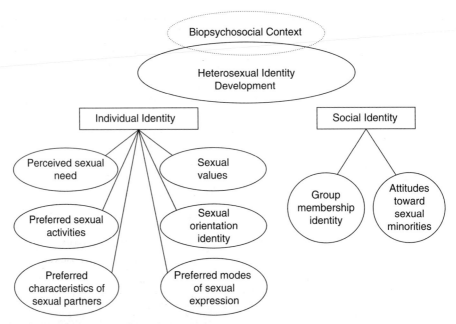

FIGURE **8.1** Dimensions of Heterosexual Identity Development

From R. L. Worthington, H. B. Savoy, F. R. Dillon, & E. R. Vernaglia, "Heterosexual Identity Development: A Multidimensional Model of Individual and Social Identity," *The Counseling Psychologist*, 30, p. 513. Copyright © 2002 by Sage. Reprinted with permission.

construction and variation in socially acceptable sexual practices, values, and beliefs; (e) *religious orientation* intertwining with sexual identity because the majority of religions regulate sexual behavior and dictate moral values and convictions regarding sexuality; and (f) *systemic homonegativity, sexual prejudice,* and *privilege,* which flood society with images, role models, and stereotypes that depict LGBT populations negatively and implicitly sanction discrimination and even violence toward individuals identified as LGBT.

In addition, this model also describes an interactive developmental process that can occur both consciously and unconsciously at all stages in the model, and is not linear in progression through stages: (a) *Unexplored commitment,* describing the acceptance of microsocial and societal mandates for prescribed gender and sexual behavior roles and the avoidance of sexual self-exploration; (b) *active exploration,* where there is purposeful exploration, evaluation, or experimentation (cognitive, affective, or behavioral) of sexual needs, values, orientation, or preferences for activities, characteristics in partners, or sexual expression; (c) *diffusion,* which may resemble the active exploration but lacks goal-directed intentionality, is more likely to be chaotic or reactive, and often arises from crisis; moving to (d) *deepening and commitment* as needs, values, modes, and expressions of sexual preferences and characteristics are identified; and to (e) *synthesis,* characterized by congruence and consistency between individual identity and development process.

Lesbian, Gay, and Bisexual (LGB) Identity Development

The process heterosexual identity development is often referred to as **coming out,** with the starting point of first recognition of one's sexual minority orientation. This process typically consists of two intersecting but separate levels of coming out to oneself and coming out to others. A wide range of gay and lesbian identity models have been proposed, with some of the most popular being the models proposed by Cass (1979) and Troiden (1989) (as cited in Reynolds & Hanjorgiris, 2000).

In the best known of these models, Cass (1979) identified six stages of a common gay and lesbian identity formation that moved from a pregay to a gay identity through the stages of confusion, comparison, tolerance, acceptance, pride, and synthesis. This model was derived from clinical and empirical data and grounded in interpersonal congruency theory, assuming that identity was acquired through a developmental process, and that the locus lay in the interaction process between persons and their environment.

In Stage 1 of *identity confusion,* heterosexual identity is called into question with increasing awareness of feelings of intimate and physical attraction toward others of the same sex, and the individual wonders, "Could I be gay or lesbian?" It becomes personally relevant to have gay and lesbian information or awareness, and the normative assumption of heterosexuality begins to be undermined. At this stage, confusion is great and denial is usually the primary coping strategy.

In Stage 2, *identity comparison* begins with accepting the idea that same-sex feelings are a part of the self. The realization that one might be gay or lesbian may cross the individual's mind. Alternately, reframing of same-gender sexual attraction as a special case that only occurred with one specific person may occur. In addition, in some cases the notion that one may be bisexual may serve as a strategy to allow for potential heterosexuality. Essentially, the individual seeks to reduce the incongruence between same-sex attractions and a view of one's self as heterosexual. As individuals become increasingly aware of their difference from the larger, aggressively normative heterosexual society, they may experience social alienation and isolation.

Stage 3 of *identity tolerance* is characterized by an increasing inner acceptance of one's gay or lesbian identity. This helps dispel the sense of confusion and turmoil of prior stages, but creates a greater distance in the comparison between self and others, with a resultant need to be secretive or mask one's identity socially. Masking involves being able to convincingly come across to others as heterosexual despite grappling internally with one's identity. Although this creates some safety for the individual to deal with his or her sexual orientation, the price includes maintaining a high level of vigilance and a constant struggle to separate the private and public selves. A further consequence is that intimate relationships with family and friends may be experienced as deceptive and illusory. Positive experiences are crucial to developing a degree of self-acceptance (versus self-hatred) during this period. Contact with gay-affirmative people becomes a more pressing issue to alleviate a sense of isolation and alienation and to provide the individual with the experience of being accepted for his or her whole being and not just for a "mask."

In Stage 4 of *identity acceptance*, there is a progressively well-developed gay or lesbian identity that usually involves increasing contact with other gays and lesbians. Finding other gay and lesbian teens is difficult at best for many adolescents. At this point, individuals have a full inner acceptance of their sexual orientation identity, though they may well be selective about disclosing it externally. The struggle continues to now determine, given one's sexual orientation, how and where to fit in.

In Stage 5 of *identity pride*, individuals may move into a strong identification with and immersion in gay or lesbian culture and a corresponding devaluation and repudiation of heterosexuality and its institutions. Social activism and advocacy movements become important, and many individuals in this stage may live and work in communities where they socialize and interact as exclusively as possible with other gay or lesbian folks. This stage is also characterized by an increasing disclosure of identity.

Finally, Stage 6 of *identity synthesis* describes a coherent sense of self where sexual orientation is incorporated as part of a complex identity, with a concurrent softening of the "us versus them" attitude toward heterosexuals and more inclusive and cooperative approaches. Individuals may be cognizant of **heterosexism** and **homophobia** while focusing less on anger.

Troiden (1989) developed a similar model, but with the underlying assumption that the process of gay and lesbian identity development began prior to puberty, and worked through the stages with some relevance to chronological age. There are four stages, starting with (a) *sensitization*, occurring before puberty and characterized by a sense of feeling different, typically through gender-neutral or gender-atypical behavior; (b) *confusion* in the postpubertal period, where the adolescent becomes increasingly aware of homoerotic thoughts and feelings, as well as aware of the stigmatization and negative messages of society; (c) *identity assumption*, where the late adolescent may begin to try out a gay identity, characterized by more contact with the gay community, and sexual experimentation and exploration; and ending with (d) *commitment* characterized by self-acceptance and comfort with a gay identity.

Although these earlier models presented an overall model of identity development for sexual minorities, they were critiqued for subsuming lesbian identity development under the rubric of gay identity, based primarily on data from White, middle-aged males (Barret & Logan, 2002; Sophie, 1985). McCarn and Fassinger (1996) developed a model of lesbian identity development that incorporated the effects of multiple minority status and multiple oppressive environments, and focused on the tendency of women to develop and come out in the context of a relationship. Similar to the racial identity work of William E. Cross (1995) described in chapter 5, their model described a dual-identity process of both personal identity and reference group orientation that allows lesbians to incorporate the reality of factors such as work environment, geographic location, and ethnicity that affect disclosure.

Bisexual Identity Development

Limited scholarship has focused on specific bisexual identity development, even though as far back as 1948, the groundbreaking Kinsey et al. study suggested that bisexuality was much more common than previously understood (Reynolds & Hanjorgiris, 2000). Paul (1985) theorized that due to the fluidity of sexuality, many bisexuals may define their sexual orientation by their current partner rather than by an independent orientation. Bisexuality also tends to be perceived unsupportively by lesbians, gays, as well as heterosexuals based on different assumptions that include the beliefs that bisexuals are promiscuous, just going through a phase, or experimenting, as well as beliefs that individuals cannot be simultaneously attracted to men and women. Lesbian and gay communities see bisexuals as hiding behind heterosexual privilege. Together, the resultant biphobia implies that bisexuals have restricted spaces where they are welcomed. Weinberg, Williams, and Pryor (1994) proposed a model of bisexual identity development based on three stages.

In Stage 1 of initial confusion, the individual experiences attractions to both sexes. This experience may be disorienting, and the individual may not be able to categorize him or herself into a definable gay or heterosexual identity. In Stage 2, the individual begins to label behavior as bisexual and begins to make sense of having feelings for both sexes. In Stage 3, the individual settles into the identity, becoming more self-accepting and less concerned about the perceptions of others.

Transgenderism

In recent years, *transgenderism* has been used as a broad umbrella term to capture a wide variety of behaviors that are associated with individuals who prefer to identify with a sex they may not have been assigned to them at birth. The direction of the change across genders is often referred to as **male** to female (MtF) or female to male (FtM); however, it has been argued that there is another category reflecting an integration of the two genders so that gender, itself, ceases to exist (Kessler & McKenna, 2000); this is discussed in the next paragraph.

One way to think about the possible permutations is to examine the word *trans*, which has different meanings as a prefix. *Trans* can mean change, as in the word *transform*. In this sense, transgendered people change their bodies to fit the gender they feel they always were. They change from MtF or from FtM. Transgender in this sense is synonymous with what is typically meant by the term **transsexual**. *Trans* can also mean across, as in the word *transcontinental*. Here, a transgendered person is one who moves across genders. This meaning does not imply being essentially or permanently committed to one or the other gender, and therefore it has a more social-constructionist connotation. Nevertheless, the transgendered person in this meaning does not leave the realm of two categories of gender. Persons who assert that although they are "really" the other gender, they do not need to change their genitals, are transgendered in this sense of *trans*. The emphasis is on the crossing and not on any surgical transformation accompanying it. Such a person might say, "I want people to attribute the gender 'female' to me, but I'm not going to get my genitals changed. I don't mind having my penis." This type of identity is relatively recent as an open, public identity, but it does not seem to be an identity separate from male and female. It is more like a previously unthinkable combination of male and female. The third meaning of *trans* is beyond or through, as in the word *transcutaneous*. In this third sense, a transgendered person is one who has gotten through gender, beyond gender. No clear gender attribution can be made, or is allowed to be made. Gender ceases to exist, for both this person and those with whom they interact. This third meaning is the rarest and most radical.

Other terms and descriptors used by and about transgendered individuals include **cross-dressers**, *transsexuals*, and *transvestites*. In addition, *intersex* individuals (individuals with ambiguous genitalia) are often considered part of this group.[1] The behaviors associated with *transgenderism* vary as much as the descriptors themselves (Bullough, 2002). See the glossary of terms at the end of this chapter for definitions.

Transgenderism continues to be associated with pathology. For instance, the DSM-IV (American Psychiatric Association, 1994) has a classification called *gender identity disorder*, referring to a persistent psychological identification with the opposite sex. However, the emerging transgender community is challenging current beliefs, stereotypes, and misconceptions that denigrate their presence (Hird, 2003).

---

[1] There is considerable controversy about genital surgery being performed on children who are born with ambiguous genitalia. Our society continues to have a dichotomous view of sexuality: One is either a male or a female. This is clearly reflected in our medical establishment's push to surgically alter intersex children and/or give them hormonal treatments, known as *sex reassignment* (Fausto-Sterling, 2000; Hird, 2003).

As counselors, it is important to understand and appreciate the transgendered community's experiences. In particular, Stern (2009) notes that there is a long history of *transgenderism* in different societies, as well as significant cultural differences in its expression and how societies embrace it. In addition, there are distinct cultural differences in the development of sexual identity and sexual orientation. For instance, the Sambia of Highlands Papua New Guinea allow and encourage young males to have erotic sexual contact with other males, whereas adolescents are forbidden to have contact with the opposite sex until they marry, and married men are allowed to engage in homosexual activities until their wives give birth (Herdt, 1991, cited in White, Bondurant, & Travis, 2000). The process for transgender persons is historically circumscribed by the Harry Benjamin standards. Dr. Harry Benjamin (1885–1986) was one of the first doctors to work with transgender individuals. In the course of his work, he developed standards of clinical care that laid out the process and activities by which transgender individuals could transition across gender, as well as the psychological and medical stages and tasks. The sixth and most recent version, released in 2001 (World Professional Association for Transgender Health, 2001), lay out the clinical guidelines for working with transgender individuals, including required competencies and tasks for mental health professionals. For instance, many clients are required to have supportive and insight-oriented psychotherapy prior to presenting themselves for hormone therapy or sexual reassignment surgeries. They are required to have some real-life experience in "passing" in the gender to which they seek to cross, including going out in public in appropriate clothing, participating in recreational activities, as well as functioning in employment or as a student in the desired gender identity.

Special Challenges

Swann & Anastas (2009) described the challenge facing many LGBT persons of having to create themselves in terms of identities, relationships, and communities because of falling outside the heterosexual norm. In this section, we describe some of the challenges of conceptualizing and creating a minority sexual orientation identity, given both the notion that it can be a central part of identity while acknowledging the ways in which other aspects of identity such as race, gender, class, age, and religion can impact and influence one's self-creation.

Social images and roles

Society is filled with images of heterosexual, lesbian, gay, and bisexual persons. Often young people growing up base much of their information and understanding of sexual orientation on media portrayals. Gay men are often portrayed as unable to commit, having difficulty with long-term relationships, shallow, obsessed with fashion, and always demonstrating effeminate characteristics. Lesbians, on the other hand, are often rendered invisible or portrayed as witches, emasculating bullies, as well as tomboys with masculine characteristics (Barret & Logan, 2002). Notice the impact of gender roles on these stereotypes, where those who are attracted to men are considered effeminate or playing the "woman's role," whereas lesbians are portrayed as secondhand men. Heterosexual women are portrayed as competing for male attention, sexually restricted if they are "good," and "sluts" if they are sexually active. Heterosexual men are portrayed as players who would rather score in the sexual game than develop a monogamous, long-term relationship. These restrictive images also mean that as heterosexuals, gay men, lesbians, and bisexuals develop intimate relationships, much of these messages and stereotypes impact them through internalized oppression.

Lesbians, as mentioned earlier, are more likely to come out in the context of a relationship. So, it is quite likely that simultaneously as a woman is dealing with the uncertainty of a new relationship, she may be simultaneously struggling with her sexual orientation and identity. Social messages condition women to develop intense emotional bonds with intimate others. Whereas in heterosexual relationships, this is offset by stereotypical depictions of male independence and isolation, in lesbian relationships, both partners may emotionally fuse in a high-drama, roller-coaster journey that falls apart under its own pressures (Barret & Logan, 2002). Among gay men, the challenge is to move beyond sex and develop lasting intimacy. The old joke that the second date for lesbians involves bringing a moving truck, whereas for gay men, the joke goes, there is no second date, may sometimes ring true as both groups struggle with learned heterosexual roles.

Multiple oppressions

LGBT People of Color often face the task of facing oppression in at least two communities where they have membership. In the largely White gay and lesbian communities where they may look for potential partners, they may face racism and ethnocentrism. In their respective ethnic communities, they face homophobia as well as a salient belief that homosexuality is "a White thing" and that a gay or lesbian of color is trying to pass as White. Coming out as gay, lesbian, or bisexual can be especially difficult because it may mean taking on yet another dimension of social identity in which one is oppressed. The significant roles of the family and kinship systems in many minority cultures make the process of coming out fraught with issues of shame and guilt. Many may choose to remain closeted in their ethnic community rather than risk being ostracized. On the other hand, there may be cultural traditions within the ethnic community that allow for a different self-reference for the LGBT Person of Color. As mentioned earlier, in traditional Native American communities, gender roles and sexuality were not limited to dualistic categories, and often allowed for multiple variations in gender and sexuality roles (Tafoya, 1997). Among African American communities, homophobia may be particularly strong because, as Smith (1982) mentioned, given the lack of other forms of privilege, heterosexual privilege is often the only one that members of this community can draw upon. Moreover, the Black church plays a significant social and political role in the community and has demonstrated public opposition to homosexuality. However, Afrocentric spiritual belief systems emphasize harmony and collectivism and may lead to unspoken tolerance of same-gender relationships (Fukuyama & Ferguson, 2000). There is also a secretive phenomenon termed the *down-low,* where African American men may have sex with other men but do not consider themselves gay or bisexual. This first came to attention as the rate of HIV transmission among African American women who had only had heterosexual sex skyrocketed (King, 2004). In a similar vein, in Latino cultures, the ideal of virile manliness may suggest that men are expected to be highly sexual, even with other men, without being stigmatized as long as they assume the active sexual role. The ideal of *marianismo* for women suggests purity, self-sacrifice, submission, and lack of interesting sex. For a Latina to be sexually active with another woman would violate both sexual orientation as well as gender role expectations (Fukuyama & Ferguson, 2000). The predominant religious influence of Catholicism with its active condemnation of same-gender sexual behavior may also make it difficult for Latino LGB persons to come out in their communities.

Among Asian Americans, the family unit is highly valued, with feelings of duty and obligation to the family highlighted. Leong (1996) points out that in traditional communities, heterosexual contact was restricted but intimate same-gender friendships were accepted. Lesbian or gay relationships may not be recognized as such or not taken seriously as threatening, leading to high levels of heterosexism but low levels of homophobia. In addition, the dominant gender images of Asians as **asexual** effeminate men and exotic females may be played out in the gay community. *Rice queen* refers to White men who prefer submissive Asian partners, and many of the images underline these themes of dominance toward Asians in both heterosexual and LGB relationships (Fukuyama & Ferguson, 2000).

Due to the smaller number of LGBT Persons of Color, there is a greater likelihood that they will be engaged in interracial and intercultural relationships. Such relationships will bring their own challenges of dealing with cultural differences in the context of a gay or lesbian relationship. A White partner who is unfamiliar with racism may be oblivious to, surprised at, or overreact to external oppression. Internalized as well as external racism may be sources of conflict for the couple (Barret & Logan, 2002).

Psychosocial challenges

Other issues that specifically impact lesbians include the challenge of maintaining sexual intimacy given gender socialization for women that restricts expression of sexual interest. A high prevalence of both partners having a history of being sexually abused also makes maintaining intimacy difficult, as each struggles with recovery issues. There appear to be high rates of substance abuse present for lesbian and bisexual women. This may be both for the self-medicating and anesthetizing properties as a way of coping with social stigmatization, as well as the tendency of the gay community to socialize in bars or clubs where alcohol is common. Finally, an often unrecognized incidence of domestic violence can occur between women partners, which is a source of shame for the survivor, and due to the insensitivity and lack of understanding by service providers can serve as a barrier for women in gaining access to supportive services (Barret & Logan, 2002).

Gay men face their own challenges. Gay men who come out as adults may experience a delayed adolescence as they go through experiences that seem age inappropriate in the amount of energy that is focused on sexual pursuits (Barret & Logan, 2002). Shame and loss of privilege are even more salient for gay men as they face losing a masculine gender identity that is tied up with being heterosexual. Developing and maintaining intimacy are challenging due to learned dysfunctional relationship styles, which include a reliance on one-night stands; inhibiting shyness; seeking the most desirable partner; being only attracted to younger, attractive men; or selecting partners through peer pressure on what an appropriate partner should appear to be (Scasta, 1998).

Particular issues that carry enormous implications for gay and bisexual men are the issues of safe sex and the prevention of HIV transmission. In the late 1980s and early 1990s, a concentrated effort was made to educate the gay community on the risks of casual sex, which resulted in a reduction in the rates of infection. However, in recent years there appears to be an upward trend again as younger gay men enter the community and engage in unsafe sexual activity (Barret & Logan, 2002). Gay men who are also HIV positive have to deal with a number of issues such as dealing with the health care realities of HIV treatment, as well as shame, anger, and grief over the loss of health and the intimation of mortality (Kauth, Hartwig, & Kalichman, 2000).

Bisexuality offers its own challenges as well, distinct from those faced by gay and lesbian sexual minority identities. Based on the idea that sexuality can be fluid, bisexual sexual identity may not be consistent and may contradict across the life span. Klein (1993) offered categories of bisexuality based on these fluid constructions: (a) *transitional bisexuality*, referring to individuals who are in the coming-out phase as either gay, lesbian, or heterosexual; (b) *historical bisexuality*, referring to individuals who currently identify as gay, lesbian, or heterosexual but have had past experiences with the same or other gender, so that one's sexual orientation is not necessarily defined by the gender of one's current partner; (c) *sequential bisexuality*, referring to individuals who have relationships with members of both genders but at different periods of time; and (d) *concurrent bisexuality*, referencing individuals who simultaneously have relationships with both men and women.

Although there are countless examples of discrimination and prejudice against gay, lesbian, and transgender persons, there may be variations in what group is more acceptable or tolerated. In other words, individuals who represent these various groups may be accepted in society differentially.

REFLECTION QUESTIONS 8.3

- What might it mean, as you consider who you are attracted to, if such attraction was illegal? How might it change your self-image, thoughts, feelings, and behavior?
- To what extent do you value a person's sexual orientation as a sign of his or her worth?
- Have you ever stood up for someone being harassed or oppressed on the basis of sexual orientation? If not, why not? Has anyone ever stood up for you in this way?

- How does your understanding of sexual orientation and sexual identity affect your work with clients who are of a different orientation than you? Similar to you?
- What role does sexual orientation play in your approach to counseling?
- How does your understanding of sexual orientation create strengths for you in counseling? Limitations or blind spots for you?

REFLECTION EXERCISE **8.1**

Awareness of and Tolerance for Different Sexualities

To help you heighten your awareness about this complex issue, consider ranking the following sexualities, with 1 being the most tolerated and 10 being the least tolerated in contemporary Western society. Now, envision these persons as being of another ethnicity than your own, perhaps Native American, Asian American, or African American. Does your ranking change?

Bisexual female	_____	_____
Bisexual male	_____	_____
Gay male	_____	_____
Transgender male	_____	_____
Transgender female	_____	_____
Lesbian	_____	_____
Heterosexual male	_____	_____
Heterosexual female	_____	_____
Intersex male	_____	_____
Intersex female	_____	_____

In counseling sexual minority youth, one of the primary goals must be to empower these clients to develop a positive self-identity. The 1995 Massachusetts Youth Risk Behavior Survey data found that gay, lesbian, bisexual, and questioning youth are more than three times as likely as other students to report a suicide attempt, and it is estimated that of all adolescent suicides, almost 30% are related to sexual orientation (Barret & Logan, 2002). As Jill has become increasingly aware, society is plagued with prejudice, and she receives few positive messages about gays, lesbians, or bisexuals.

Home is not a place of comfort and safety, and appears likely to become another place of rejection. Parents, even if they would eventually accept sexual minority children, assume that their children are heterosexual and often perpetuate and further stereotypes. Given the family climate, it became impossible for Jill to share her confusion with any of her family members.

CASE STUDY **8.1**

The Case of Jill

Jill is a 14-year-old German American girl who comes in to see her school counselor, April Washington, who is African American. She begins by confiding that she feels really alone and doesn't think she has any good friends. As she gets comfortable with April, she discloses, "I guess I'll just say it—I'm different. I mean very different from all my friends and from the other kids in school. I don't even know if I can tell you, because I don't know what you'll think of me." April gently prompted her to continue, assuring her that she might feel better if she could unburden herself, and reminding her about confidentiality. Jill shared her conflict.

She talked how television shows are about some guy and girl kissing, and how she liked to watch the television show *Ellen*, but couldn't admit it in front of her family, who would make negative remarks about it. Her father told her once that "homosexuals were going

to burn in hell because they were sinners." Meanwhile, in school, she would notice how the children would harass other children who were different, beating up boys who were considered sissies and calling them names. Last week, Jill had gone to a party and met a girl who she kissed. Jill was shocked by what she had done and confused because she had enjoyed the kiss. She began to cry uncontrollably as she asked April what was to become of her.

Case Discussion
Thinking About This Case
1. Based on your understanding of identity development, where would you place Jill in the process?
2. As the school counselor, what are the constellations of your concerns as you hear Jill's story?
3. How might April help Jill to explore her issues?

Pilkington and D'Augelli (1995) state that a third of gay youth have been verbally abused and up to 10% have been physically attacked by family members due to their sexual orientation.

Although school is the environment that adolescents use to develop peer relationships and learn socialization, for LGBT youth it is often a space of harassment, alienation, and sometimes physical abuse. A 1999 national survey of sexual minority youth found that 69% reported having experienced some type of verbal, physical, and sexual harassment and/or assault while at school (Gay Lesbian Straight Education Network, 1999). Even more troubling was that of the 90% who reported that they had heard bigoted comments or name-calling, 30% reported hearing them from school faculty and staff. School becomes no place to refute negative portrayals of LGB persons.

In working with Jill, it is important for April to explore her own internalized oppressive stereotypes. She may feel that Jill is too young to be having such thoughts, though she may regularly counsel other teens who have had heterosexual sex. She may agree with Jill's family and hold similar religious views of condemning LGBT persons as sinners. It is April's responsibility to educate herself by attending workshops and conferences, reading relevant literature, and familiarizing herself with the coming-out process. After all, Jill has only enough information to confuse herself. Given the institutional pressures, it is important that April make her office a safe zone where students know they have an ally, through using "safe space" rainbow triangles and ally signs, having literature on referral organizations and support organizations prominently available, and using inclusive language. Another role that

April can take on is to educate her colleagues (i.e., school personnel) in the school, developing and facilitating training programs on the effects of homophobia, the experiences of youth and sexual identity, and the environmental effects of harassment that is unchecked by adults.

In allowing Jill to explore her sexuality, it is important that April not assume that her confusion automatically signifies that she is lesbian. Adolescence is a time of exploration, and same-gender sexual behavior does not necessarily cement sexual orientation. On the other hand, it is important that April have available information on local and community gay-affirmative youth organizations, support services, and gay-positive websites, books, and other materials. Given the lack of safety that Jill experiences, it is crucial that April ensure and respect confidentiality. Many school counselors are afraid of broaching or pursuing issues of sexual orientation due to feared parental retribution or disapproval by the administration (Barret & Logan, 2002). However, the client's rights to privacy and confidentiality are very much protected, and there have been no successful legal actions against school counselors who have provided affirmative counseling to such youth.

Jill appears to be in the first stage, identity confusion (Cass, 1979). As of now, her process is primarily one of exploring her feelings about herself and her understandings of LGB issues. If, further down the line, Jill is positive that she is lesbian and wishes to come out to her family, the counselor would have to work carefully to encourage her, support her, as well as help her to predict and deal with possible consequences of disclosure. It would be important that April process with Jill the possible repercussions prior to any disclosure so that Jill is fully prepared. Although April understands that Jill needs her family's support and acceptance, Jill may need to be prepared to deal with a gamut of reactions including shock, denial, anger, sadness, and rejection. April may need to step in to provide the family with accurate and positive information, give them referrals to support organizations such as Parents and Friends of Lesbians and Gays (PFLAG), encourage conflict resolution, and challenge verbal and physical abuse.

OPENING THE DIALOGUE ON SEXUAL ORIENTATION AND SEXUAL IDENTITY

With all of the topics discussed in this chapter, you are now challenged to think through how you would utilize this information in sessions with any number of clients from a variety of cultural backgrounds and worldviews. Questions for reflection offered to you throughout this chapter also serve as excellent process questions for opening the dialogue with clients on issues of sexual orientation, sexual identity, and experiences with heterosexism and homophobia. Some of these questions are listed here to assist you in terms of opening the dialogue with your clients:

- Who are you in terms of sexual orientation and sexual identity? How important is this in your personal and cultural identity, and what impact do these dimensions have on how you view the world and live your life?
- How do you know your own sexual orientation?

- At what point in your life did you become aware of your sexual orientation and sexual identity?
- What role did your family, peers, and the larger society play in your decision making about your sexual identity?
- Has your understanding of your own sexual identity changed over time, and if so, how? If not, why not?
- Do you recall a period of exploration and coming to a decision, or was your sexual orientation something you took for granted?
- How did your sexual definition of yourself develop, and who were some significant people in your life who helped to shape this definition?
- How has your view of sexual orientation and sexual identity been reinforced or challenged during your life?
- What does your culture say about sexual orientation and sexual identity?
- What do your family and community say about sexual orientation and sexual identity in terms of both beliefs and practice?
- How do issues of power and privilege influence your views of sexual orientation and sexual identity and your concept of heterosexism?
- How has your view of sexual orientation and sexual identity affected the way you define yourself now and at previous points in your life?
- How will your view of sexual orientation and sexual identity continue to affect the way you define yourself and the way others see you or treat you?
- How has your view of sexual orientation and sexual identity affected the way you interact with others who are similar to you versus different from you at different points in your life?
- Who are some people of your own sexual orientation and sexual identity who you look up to and why?
- How might the difference or similarity in sexual orientation and sexual identity between you (client) and I (counselor) affect your experience in the process of counseling as well as the relationship between us?
- When and how did you first become aware of heterosexism? What was your initial reaction, and how did that reaction change over time?
- What have your experiences with heterosexism been, and in what ways have those experiences shaped who you are as a person as well as the issues you are dealing with now?
- What efforts have you made to work toward positive social change with regard to the heterosexism that exists in your own life at the individual, group, and societal levels, and what other kinds of efforts would you like to make?
- To what extent do you value a person's sexual orientation as a sign of his or her worth?
- Have you ever stood up for someone being harassed or oppressed on the basis of sexual orientation? If not, why not? Has anyone ever stood up for you in this way?
- How do sexual orientation and sexual identity play into the issues you are bringing to counseling, and how can we address this in a way that is most helpful to you?

CONCLUSION AND IMPLICATIONS

In your role as a helper, it is particularly important for you to know about these various kinds of sexual orientations and how they affect your clients' psychological development. In addition, it is important to recognize the differences among the various sexualities, and know how individuals who represent these groups have been treated. In Thailand, for example, a transgender male desiring to be a woman (*kathoey*) is more accepted in Thai society than a gay male (Jackson, 1999). Indeed, there are cultural and ethnic differences in levels of tolerance and acceptance. Furthermore, when working with clients, it is important to address issues of sexuality regardless of the specific sexual orientation of the client. Gay, lesbian, and bisexual clients are estimated to seek counseling at 2–4 times greater rates than heterosexual clients, but also report far more negative interactions with mental health professionals (Perez, DeBord, & Bieschke, 2000). Innovative treatment approaches are being developed for transgender individuals (e.g., Chavez-Korell, 2006); however, few graduate training programs provide specific training in sexual minority issues, leaving personal experience and stereotypes as the major sources of knowledge about this population.

Given that sexual orientation is a fluid and constructed social category, the role of a counselor is to affirm and acknowledge the issues raised by peoples' sense of themselves as fixed or as changing (Broido, 2000). It is essential to validate the experience of those who find their sexual orientation to be a central part of their identity, and the conflicts this may often raise as they seek to maintain balance with other aspects of their lives and social networks. The ongoing discrimination and stigmatization in society of those who identify as lesbian, gay, bisexual, or transgender make it even more imperative that counseling offer a safe space to explore these concerns. The same challenge that LGBT persons face in developing and maintaining an identity in the face of conflicting forces confronts counselors who work with LGBT clients.

In this chapter's case study, some important issues that face youth are addressed. Adolescence is a difficult journey for most, and although LGBT youth struggle with the same developmental issues as their heterosexual peers, their challenges are compounded by hostile forces in the school, society, and home.

In this chapter, our aim was to present a broad perspective on sexual orientation as one aspect of all our identities, no matter where we placed ourselves on the continuum. We discussed and defined various important terms, and provided a historical context of oppression, discrimination, and harassment experienced by LGBT persons. The complexity associated with sexual orientation identity development was presented, and a variety of models were described.

Counselors need to become familiar with the cultures and environments in which their clients live, and be able to be open and supportive in working with the full range of clients. For those who are heterosexual, being an ally to LGBT individuals fulfills a significant and powerful role. Washington and Evans (1991) declare that when a supporter is not a member of the oppressed population and is a member of the dominant group, the impact of advocacy and support can often be more powerful. To be an effective ally requires that individuals recognize their heterosexual privilege. Such privileges often include legal marriage, joint income tax returns, adopting children, and being able to participate in health insurance and make health decisions for one's partner. Educating oneself about issues will be helpful, as will having a good understanding and comfort with your own sexual orientation and the process of identity development. Fears that can discourage allies include the pervasive idea that involvement in such an issue implies that the ally must also be gay, lesbian, or bisexual, an assumption that may be held by both heterosexuals and sexual minorities. The benefits of being an ally are working toward justice and equality for all persons, having opportunities to learn and interact with an additional 10% of the population, making a difference in the lives of others who may only have experienced negativity and hostility, and being more comfortable and flexible in your own identity.

GLOSSARY

Asexual: One who does not have, for a variety of reasons, sexual responses to either sex.

Bi-gender: Some gender variants in which people reject the choices of male–female and man–woman and feel that their gender encompasses "both" genders. Within some American Indians cultures, expressing both genders is referred to as *two-spirited*. Within contemporary urban life, bi-gendered people often refer to themselves as *gender queers, gender benders, third sex*, and *gender perverts* as terms of pride.

Bisexual: One who has sexual responses to either sex.

Celibacy: Describes the lifestyle of someone who chooses not to act upon sexual responses.

Coming out: The process of revealing, to self and others, one's sexual orientation.

Cross-dresser: Going beyond the older and more pathological term *transvestite*, this describes someone who prefers to wear clothing of the other sex for a variety of reasons, including eroticism and recreation. Cross-dressing is not necessarily linked to being attracted to members of one's own gender.

Female-to-male transsexuals (FtM or FTM): Female-born people who live as men. This includes a broad range of experience from those who identify as "male" or "men" and those who identify as transsexual, *transmen, female men*, or FTM as their gender identity. FtMs are often contrasted with *biomen*, or biologically born men.

Gay: Male sexual responses predominantly to one's own sex.

Heterosexism: The belief that heterosexuality is the only legitimate form of sexuality, together with institutional policies and practices that privilege heterosexuality and discriminate openly or subtly against gays, lesbians, and bisexuals. Heterosexism leads to homophobia.

Heterosexual: Sexual responses predominantly to the other sex.

Homophobia: An irrational fear and hatred of anyone perceived to be, or associated with, gays or lesbians.

Homosexual: A term used to label individuals who are attracted to someone of the same gender. This term was popularized in the 19th century and is currently used less and less due to its derogatory nature and negative stereotypes.

Lesbian: Female sexual responses predominantly to one's own sex.

Male-to-female transsexuals (MtF or MTF): Male-born people who live as women. This includes a broad range of experience including those who identify as "female" or "women" and those who identify as transsexual women. Some words used to refer to transsexual women are *Tgirls* and *new women* as compared to *GG's*, or genetic women.

Straight: A term used to describe someone who is attracted to the opposite sex.

Transgender: One who identifies with both male and female roles or as a member of an alternative gender. Often identified as a sexual orientation issue, transgenderism is more a gender identity issue.

Transsexual: A more medical term than *transgender*, the term *transsexual* describes someone who has a long-standing desire to live as the sex other than his or her biological sex. Sex reassignment is a complex process that includes therapy, electrolysis, hormonal therapy, and living in the new gender role for a prescribed period of time based on the Harry Benjamin standards.

REFERENCES

American Psychiatric Association. (1972). *Diagnostic and Statistical Manual of Psychiatric Disorders* (2nd ed.). Washington, DC: Author.

American Psychiatric Association. (1987). *Diagnostic and Statistical Manual of Psychiatric Disorders* (3rd ed. Revised). Washington, DC: Author.

American Psychiatric Association. (1994). *Diagnostic and Statistical Manual of Psychiatric Disorders* (4th ed.). Washington, DC: Author.

American Psychological Association. (1991). Avoiding heterosexist bias in language. *American Psychologist, 46*, 937–974.

Barret, B., & Logan, C. (2002). *Counseling gay men and lesbians: A practice primer*. Pacific Grove, CA: Brooks/Cole.

Bohan, J. S. (1996). *Psychology and sexual orientation: Coming to terms*. New York: Routledge.

Brammer, R. (2004). *Diversity in counseling*. Belmont, CA: Brooks/Cole-Thompson.

Broido, E. (2000). Constructing identity: The nature and meaning of lesbian, gay, and bisexual identities. In R. M. Perez, K. A. DeBord, & K. J. Bieschke (Eds.), *Handbook of counseling and psychotherapy with lesbian, gay, and bisexual clients* (pp. 13–33). Washington, DC: American Psychological Association.

Bullough, V. (2002). Transgenderism and the concept of gender. *The International Journal of Transgenderism, 4*(3). Retrieved from http://www.symposion.com/ijt/gilbert/bullough.htm

Cass, V. C. (1979). Homosexual identity formation: A theoretical model. *Journal of Homosexuality*, 4(30), 219–235.

Chavez-Korell, S. (2006). Affirmative psychotherapy and counseling with transgender clients. In K. Bieschke, R. Perez, & K. A. DeBord (Eds.). *Handbook of counseling and psychotherapy with lesbians, gay, bisexual, and transgender clients*. Washington, DC: American Psychological Association.

Cross, W. (1995). The psychology of Nigresence: Revising the Cross Model. In J. G. Ponterotto, J. M. Casas, L. A. Suzuki, L. A., & C. M. Alexander (Eds.), *Handbook of multicultural counseling* (pp. 93–122). Thousand Oaks, CA: Sage.

D'Emilio, J. (1983). *Sexual politics, sexual communities: The making of a homosexual minority in the United States, 1940–1970*. Chicago: University of Chicago Press.

Denny, D. (1997). Transgender: Some historical, cross-cultural, and contemporary models and methods of coping and treatment. In B. Bullough, V. L. Bullough, & J. Elias (Eds.), *Gender blending* (pp. 33–47). Amherst, NY: Prometheus.

Freud, S. (1905). Three essays in the theory of sexuality. In J. Strachey (Ed.), *The standard edition of the complete works of Sigmund Freud* (Vol. 7). London: Hogarth Press.

Fukuyama, M. A., & Ferguson, A. D. (2000). Lesbian, gay, and bisexual People of Color: Understanding cultural complexity and managing multiple oppressions. In R. M. Perez, K. A. DeBord, & K. J. Bieschke (Eds.), *Handbook of counseling and psychotherapy with lesbian, gay, and bisexual clients* (pp. 81–105). Washington, DC: American Psychological Association.

Gay Lesbian, Straight Education Network (1999). *National school climate survey*. Retrieved November 1, 2010, from http://www.glsen.org/binary-data/GLSEN_ATTACHMENTS/file/2-1.pdf

Herzer, M. (1985). Kertbeny and the nameless love. *Journal of Homosexuality*, 12, 1–26.

Hird, M. (2003). A typical gender identity conference? Some disturbing reports from the therapeutic front lines. *Feminism & Psychology*, 13, 181–199.

Hunter, S., & Hickerson, J. C. (2003). *Affirmative practice: Understanding and working with lesbian, gay, bisexual, and transgender persons*. Baltimore: NASW Press.

Isay, R. A. (1989). *Being homosexual: Gay men and their development*. New York: Avon.

Jackson, P. (1999). Tolerant but unaccepting: The myth of the Thai "gay paradise." In P. A. Jackson & N. M. Cook (Eds.), *Genders & sexualities in modern Thailand* (pp. 226–242). Chiang Mai, Thailand: Silkworm.

Kantor, M. (2009). *Homophobia: The state of sexual bigotry today*. Westport, CT: Praeger.

Katz, J. N. (2003). The invention of heterosexuality. In P. S. Rothenberg (Ed.), *Race, class, and gender in the United States* (6th ed., pp. 69–80). New York: Worth.

Kauth, M. R., Hartwig, M. J., & Kalichman, S. C. (2000). Health behavior relevant to psychotherapy with lesbian, gay, and bisexual clients. In R. M. Perez, K. A. DeBord, & K. J. Bieschke (Eds.), *Handbook of counseling and psychotherapy with lesbian, gay, and bisexual clients* (pp. 435–456). Washington, DC: American Psychological Association.

Kessler, S., & McKenna, W. (2000). Who put the "trans" in transgender: Gender theory and everyday life. *The International Journal of Transgenderism*, 4(3). Retrieved from http://www.symposion.com/ijt/gilbert/kessler.htm

King, J. L. (2004). *On the down low: A journey into the lives of "straight" Black men who sleep with men*. New York: Broadway Press.

Klein, F. (1993). *The bisexual option*. New York: Harrington Park.

Leong, R. (1996). *Asian American sexualities: Dimensions of the gay and lesbian experience*. New York: Routledge.

McCarn, S. R., & Fassinger, R. E. (1996). Revisioning sexual minority identity formation: A new model of lesbian identity and its implications for counseling and research. *The Counseling Psychologist*, 24(3), 508–534.

Money, J. (1998). Homosexuality: Bipotentiality, terminology, and history. In E. J. Haeberle & R. Gindorf (Eds.), *Bisexualities: The ideology and practice of sexual contact with both men and women* (pp. 118–128). New York: Continuum.

Paul, J. P. (1985). Bisexuality: reassessing our paradigms of sexuality. *Journal of Homosexuality. Special Issue: Bisexualities: Theory and research*, 11(1–2), 21–34.

Perez, R. M., deBord, K. A., & Bieschke, K. J. (2000). The challenge of awareness, knowledge, and action. In R. M. Perez, K. A. DeBord, & K. A. Bieschke (Eds.). *Handbook of Counseling and Psychotherapy with Lesbian, Gay, and*

Bisexual clients (pp 3–8).Washington, DC: American Psychological Association.

Pilkington, N., & D'Augelli, A. R. (1995). Victimization of lesbian, gay and bisexual youth in community settings. *Journal of Community Psychology,* *23,* 33–56.

Rector, F. (1981). *The Nazi extermination of homosexuals.* New York: Stein & Day.

Reynolds, A. L., & Hanjorgiris, W. F. (2000). Coming out: Lesbian, gay, and bisexual identity development. In R. M. Perez, K. A. DeBord, & K. J. Bieschke (Eds.), *Handbook of counseling and psychotherapy with lesbian, gay, and bisexual clients* (pp. 35–55). Washington, DC: American Psychological Association.

Rust, P. C. (1996). Sexual identity and bisexual identities: The struggle for self description in a changing sexual landscape. In B. Beemyn & M. Eliason (Eds.), *Queer studies: A lesbian, gay, bisexual, and transgender anthology* (pp. 64–86). New York: New York University Press.

Scasta, D. (1998). Moving from coming out to intimacy. *Journal of Gay and Lesbian Psychotherapy,* *2*(4), 99–111.

Smith, B. (1982). Racism and women's studies. In G. T. Hull, P. B. Scott, & B. Smith (Eds.), *But some of us are brave* (pp. 157–175). Old Westbury, NY: Feminist Press.

Sophie, J. (1985). A critical examination of stage theories of lesbian identity development. *Journal of Homosexuality,* *12*(2), 39–51.

Stern, K. (2009). *Queers in history: the comprehensive encyclopedia of historical gays, lesbians and bisexuals, and transgenders.* Dallas, TX: BenBella Books.

Stoller, R. (1968). *Sex and gender: Vol 1. The development of masculinity and femininity.* New York: Jason Aronson.

Swann, S. K. & Anastas, J. W. (2009). Dimensions of lesbian identity during adolescence and young adulthood. In W. Meezan and J. I. Martin (Eds.), *Handbook of research with lesbian, gay, bisexual, and transgender populations* (pp. 143–161). NY: Routledge.

Tafoya, T. N. (1997). Native gay and lesbian issues: The two-spirited. In B. Greene (Ed.), *Ethnic and cultural diversity among lesbians and gay men* (pp. 1–10). Thousand Oaks, CA: Sage.

Troiden, R. R. (1989). The formation of homosexual identities. *Journal of Homosexuality,* *17*(1–2), 43–73.

Turner, W. J. (1995). Homosexuality, type 1: An Xq28 phenomenon. *Archives of Sexual Behavior,* *24*(2), 109–134.

Van Sant, G. (Prod.), Jinks, D., & Cohen, B. (Dirs.). (2008). *Milk* [Motion picture]. Universal City, CA: Universal Pictures. (Available from Universal Pictures, 100 Universal Plaza, Universal City, CA 91608)

Washington, J., & Evans, N. J. (1991). Becoming an ally. In N. J. Evans & V. A. Wall (Eds.), *Beyond tolerance: Gays, lesbians, and bisexuals on campus* (pp. 195–204). Alexandria, VA: American College Personnel Association.

Weinberg, M. S., Williams, C. J., & Pryor, D. W. (1994). *Dual attractions: Understanding bisexuality.* New York: Oxford University Press.

White, J. W., Bondurant, B., & Travis, C. B. (2000). Social constructions of sexuality: Unpacking hidden meaning. In C. B. Travis & J. W. White (Eds.), *Sexuality, society, and feminism* (pp. 11–33). Washington, DC: American Psychological Association.

World Professional Association for Transgender Health. (2001). *Standards of care for gender identity disorders* (6th version). Retrieved from http://www.wpath.org/publications_standards.cfm

Worthington, R. L., Savoy, H. B., Dillon, F. R., & Vernaglia, E. R. (2002). Heterosexual identity development: A multidimensional model of individual and social identity. *The Counseling Psychologist,* *30,* 496–531.

CHAPTER 9

Social Class

Class is more than just the amount of money you have; it's also the presence of economic security. For the working class and the poor, working and eating are matters of survival, not taste. However, while one's class status can be defined in important ways in terms of monetary income, class is also a whole lot more—specifically, class is also culture. As a result of the class you are born into and raised in, class is your understanding of the world and where you fit it; it's composed of ideas, behaviors, attitudes, values, and language; class is how you think, feel, act, look, dress and talk, move walk; class is what stores you shop at, restaurants you eat in; class is the schools you attend, the education you attain; class is the very jobs you will work at throughout your adult life. Class even determines when we marry and become mothers. Working-class women become mothers long before middle-class women receive their bachelor's degree. We experience class at every level of our lives; class is who our friends are, where we live and work[,] even what kind of car we drive, if we own one, and what kind of healthcare we receive, if any. Have I left anything out?

From D. Langston "Tired of Playing Monopoly?" in M. L. Andersen and P. H. Collins (Eds.) *Race, Class, and Gender: An Anthology*. Copyright © 1992 by Wadsworth. Reprinted with permission.

This statement is a clear example of how *class* is a phenomenon that is omnipresent, influencing many of our human experiences. Although its impact is broad, the class construct has not received adequate attention in the psychological literature

(Liu, Ali, et al., 2004). Why has this been the case considering the differences in income levels of people living in the United States?

In 2007, approximately 37.3 million (12.5%) of the nation's population lived in poverty, up from 31.6 million (11.3%) in 2000 (U.S. Census Bureau, 2004, 2008). In addition, about 13.3 million (18%) of the nation's children under the age of 18 were considered poor by government standards. The rate of poverty for single women with families was 4.1 million (28.3%) compared to 696,000 (13.1%) for male-headed families (U.S. Census Bureau, 2008). Surely these disparities result in a hierarchical class structure that affects the kind of experiences people have, as conveyed in Langston's (1992) powerful statement.

People of color, particularly, African Americans/Blacks and Latinos, are more likely than Whites to live in poverty. In 2007, the rate of poverty was nearly 25% for African Americans and about 22% for Latinos compared to approximately 8% for Whites. For Asian Americans and Pacific Islanders, the poverty rate was approximately 10%. Equally disturbing, in 2003 single African American or Black women and Latinas heading families had poverty rates of over 35% (National Poverty Center, 2003).

The class construct, often referred to as **social class**,[1] has been widely studied within the field of sociology, advancing our understanding of differences among classes, including such aspects as social mobility and class consciousness. Drawing from the work of sociologists, Argyle (1994) points out that there are class differences in such aspects as leisure activities, social relationships, religious beliefs, and child-rearing practices. However, the field of psychology has lagged in examining the relationship between social class and mental health and well-being.

In this chapter, we define and explore social class and socioeconomic status as phenomena that lead to classism or the prejudicial attitudes and beliefs we have about people in a hierarchical class structure. We examine how social class shapes our worldview and affects physical and mental health. In addition, the intersections of social class, race, ethnicity, and gender are described.

REFLECTION QUESTIONS 9.1

- What does it mean in our society to be wealthy? Poor?
- How do you define success? How is success defined in your family? In your culture? In larger society?

SOCIAL CLASS AND SOCIOECONOMIC STATUS

In a review of the literature on using social class in counseling psychology, Liu, Ali, et al. (2004) defined *social class* as the prestige, power, economic resources, education, income, and position one holds in an economic

---

[1] Based on our review of the psychological literature, we found that the terms *social class* and *class* are used interchangeably.

hierarchy in society—that is, a low-, middle-, and upper-class structure—and the social class position of friends and peer groups. As can be gleaned by this definition, there are many parts to what constitutes social class, and it is essential to examine poverty and inequality as contextual factors that are linked to a class structure (Liu & Ali, 2008).

Quite often, the term *social class* has been used interchangeably with **socioeconomic status** (SES); however, they are conceptually different. As indicated above, *social class* refers to one's position in an economic hierarchy based on income level, education level, and occupation. One of the key ideas in understanding social class is that individuals are aware of the power and prestige given to a particular group of people belonging to a specific class. In contrast, SES is based on quantifiable measures of income, occupation, and education that stratify people in our society (Pope & Arthur, 2009). However, unlike social class, SES does not include belonging to a particular group such as the "middle-class" or "upper-class" group. When referring to SES, individuals can occupy a particular place in a social class hierarchy and can move into a higher status by using a variety of resources at their disposal that are often referred to as human, material, and social capital (Liu, 2001).

A variety of social class systems have been created to group individuals.[2] Typically, these systems are also based on objective indices of income, education, and occupation. For example, Thompson and Hickey (2005) describe a five-class model:

- Extreme wealth is described as the "upper class," consisting of individuals with significant economic and political power, prestige, and prominence. Types of occupations include those of government officials, CEOs, and prominent business leaders and typically earn six-figure salaries.
- "Upper middle class" are those who have professional jobs and advanced degrees and earn a substantial income. The types of occupations include lawyers, corporate executives, professors, and physicians.
- "Lower middle class" are those who have skilled jobs that more often than not require education beyond high school. Typical jobs include school personnel such as teachers, guidance counselors, those in sales, and mid-level supervisors.
- "Working class" consists of individuals in service jobs (e.g., blue and white collar) that normally pay minimum wage and are considered less secure occupations.
- The "lower" class consists of the unemployed, and part-time workers barely making minimum wage.

Some simply use the terms *poor*, *working*, and *affluent* or *wealthy*, whereas others use the terms *upper*, *middle*, and *lower*. Regardless of the

---

[2] Social class structures vary across societies and countries. Our intent is to describe social class structures in the United States. The source of Thompson and Hickey's (2005) social class model appears in Wikipedia ®, *Social class*. Retrieved May 29, 2009, from http://en.wikipedia.org/wiki/Social_class

terms used, there is a clear hierarchical structure. However, a major criticism of using these classification systems to group people is that they do not take into consideration the variability within each group, nor do they account for an individual's subjective perception of social class—where the individual places her or himself—which could be different from the externally created classification system (Liu, 2006). Furthermore, within the context of social class, differential treatment and inequality are often manifested. As Pope and Arthur (2009) noted, "[I]ndividuals encounter privilege or adversity based on their class membership" (p. 55).

REFLECTION QUESTIONS 9.2

- What is your perception of what makes up a person's social class?
- How does your upbringing or culture play into your definition of social class?
- What is your social class? Has it changed, and if so, why?
- What have been some of your experiences with people from different social classes? What made those experiences either positive or negative?

Social Class and Poverty

Women, particularly single women with children, and ethnic groups are the most vulnerable to poverty. As we stated earlier, the rate of poverty among these groups is considerably high. The poor are not just those who are unemployed but also the working poor. The poor live in urban and rural settings, and many do not have health insurance. For those who do have health coverage such as Medicaid, they often receive differential treatment compared to those who have employment-based insurance (Lott & Bullock, 2001). Poverty exists because of the unequal distribution of resources. Based on U.S. Census data in 2007 (U.S. Census Bureau, 2008), for example, women earned less than men (78 cents for every dollar earned by men, approximately), 18% of all children (18 years and younger) were federally classified as poor, and more than two-thirds of children live in households where at least one parent works. As stated earlier, the poverty rates for African Americans, Latinos, and Native Americans continued to hover between 22% and 25%, compared to the rate for population as a whole, which is about 8%. In terms of health care, about 10% of the population does not have health insurance; Latinos, African Americans, and Native Americans have the highest rates of being uninsured (32%, 20%, and 32%, respectively). The uninsured rate among Asian Americans actually rose from about 16% in 2006 to approximately 17% in 2007 (U.S. Census Bureau, 2008).

These statistics are powerful indicators of the inequities in this country that influence our beliefs and attitudes about class privilege and power differences. Stereotypes about the poor are pervasive and reinforced by the media. Their negative portrayal in popular television is ubiquitous. For example, the poor are more likely to appear in so-called real-life TV talk shows (Lott & Bullock, 2001, p. 231) that often center on conflict between family members, spouses, boyfriends, and so on; infidelity; and teen pregnancies (e.g., *The Jerry Springer Show*). Even more distressing is that many of these episodes show physical aggression on the air. African American and Latino men are overrepresented on TV shows about drug-related crimes in which they are portrayed as coming from low-income backgrounds. In contrast, the images of the middle class are often Whites who play the role of the young professionals with authority and power (Bullock, Wyche, & Williams, 2001). The lack of diversity in the media as well as the portrayal of ethnic minorities as poor, uneducated, and criminals fuel the negative stereotypes that already exist. How many times have you heard someone say, "There just aren't enough roles for an African American or Latino actor"? Why would such a question be asked?

Health and Social Class

"The rich may have more money, members of higher classes may have bigger houses and cars, but do they feel any better for it? Do they have better health, mental health, happiness or self-esteem?" (Argyle, 1994, p. 260). Argyle argued that, indeed, there are class differences in health, and the most important indicators of this difference involve people's lifestyle, the environment in which they live, and access to and use of medical care. With respect to mental health, he informs us that the working class and the poor are the most vulnerable to stress, have a lower sense of control over their environments, and use fewer coping strategies that are focused on problem solving (Gallo & Matthews, 2003).

It is widely acknowledged that SES and social class are related to a variety of health outcomes. For example, numerous studies have consistently shown that the higher the SES, the lower the mortality and morbidity rates (e.g., Backlund, Sorlie, & Johnson, 1996), pointing to health disparities between classes. In an attempt to explain this phenomenon, researchers have found that specific psychological risk factors, such as depression (Lorant et al., 2003), and substance abuse (Diala, Muntaner, & Walrath, 2004) are related to lower SES. Likewise, Hudson (2005) found that the incidents of hospitalization and reported mental illness were highest among low- and middle-income groups, and concludes that economic conditions such as poverty and unemployment are contributing factors.

There is mounting evidence that the inequality associated with access to recreational facilities is related to lower SES, which leads to poorer health outcomes. Specifically, individuals of lower SES, including ethnic minorities, are less likely to have access to recreational facilities, thereby decreasing physical activity and increasing the risk of being obese or overweight compared to individuals with higher SES (Gordon, Nelson, Page, & Popkin, 2006).

The notion that subjective social status or standing may be a stronger predictor of health and psychological well-being than objective indices, such as occupation, education, and income is gaining more attention. For instance, factors such as level of stress, negative affective, pessimism, and body fat have been linked to subjective social class (Adler, Epel, Castellazzo, & Ickovics, 2000).

REFLECTION EXERCISE **9.1**

Assessing Your Subjective Social Class

One of the ways to assess subjective social class is illustrated in this exercise.

The Ladder:

"Think of this ladder [below] as representing where people stand in society. At the top of the ladder are the people who are best off—those who have the most money, most educated and the best jobs. At the bottom of the ladder are the people who are the worst off—who have the least money, least education and the worst jobs or no job." (Adler et al., 2000, p. 587)

The higher you are on this ladder, the closer you are to people at the very top; and the lower you are, the closer you are to the bottom. Where would you put yourself on the ladder? Please place an 'X' on the rung where you think you stand.

=

_____

_____

_____

Source: From N. E. Adler, E. S. Epel, G. Castellazzo, and J. R. Ickovics (2000) "Relationship of Subjective and Objective Status with Psychological and Physiological Functioning: Preliminary Data in Healthy White Women." *Health Psychology*, 19, pp. 586–592.

Using the ladder as a representation of perceived social class, Singh-Manoux, Adler, and Marmot (2003) found that there was a significantly higher prevalence of illness (i.e., angina, diabetes, and respiratory illness) among individuals who placed themselves at the lower end of the ladder compared to those who placed themselves at the higher end. These research findings, as well as the approach to examining subjective social class, have important implications for counseling practice. First, they provide additional information about potential stressors in the client's life that may be contributing to psychological and physical illness. For instance, does the client experience stress because of poor living conditions or unemployment? Second, they offer an opportunity to identify the external barriers that may be related to the client's social class. For example, does the client have access to quality health care?

Classism

Whereas SES appears to allow for social mobility, social class is perceived as more permanent and often a target for prejudice and discrimination known as **classism**. Essentially, classism can be conceived as prejudicial attitudes and behaviors toward people who belong to a particular class. Its divisive force has created dichotomous groups, such as the "oppressed and the oppressor, the powerful and the powerless or the have and have nots" (Sandu & Aspy, 1997, p. 24). In many respects, class distinction has been about creating a system that keeps power and wealth in the hands of a few and the systemic oppression of groups who do not have economic power, social influence, and privilege (Harley, Jolivette, McCormick, & Tice, 2002; Smith, 2008; Smith, Foley, & Chaney, 2008). Classism affects educational attainment, the range of career and employment opportunities, and overall quality of life (Robinson, 1993).

Classism is also manifested in where people live. For example, the poor live in rural and urban settings, and the middle and wealthy live in suburbs. Another way of viewing these geographic differences is that they are segregated communities, not by race but by class. This notion is clearly exemplified by Moon and Rollison (1998) when describing the "trailer park": It is considered the place where the poor Whites live. The derogatory term *White trash* has been associated with people who live in such areas, and yet the middle class who live in trailers refer to their place of residence as a "mobile-home community" (p. 125).

From a somewhat different angle, Liu et al. (2004b; Liu, 2006) argued that classism is a complex phenomenon in that it can occur not only between higher-class and lower-class individuals but also across individuals in the same social class. For instance, classist attitudes, beliefs, and behaviors can occur by the upper class toward those perceived to be in the lower class, by the lower class toward those perceived to be in higher social classes, and among individuals who perceive themselves to be in the same class (Liu, 2006).

Equally importantly, classism can be internalized and manifested by feelings and emotional states that lead to depression. Russell (1996) provides valuable insight into the manifestations of **internalized classism** based on clinical practice. For example, from a developmental perspective, children may be motivated to separate from the family (i.e., distancing) much earlier than normal because of their desire to escape from an impoverished environment. According to Russell, this desire to psychologically separate from the family may bring about feelings of grief and shame.

The experience of being poor often triggers feelings of guilt and shame that become internalized. For example, parents may be inadvertently blamed for not getting the proper medical care for a sick child, causing them to feel shame. Children may feel anger and resentment toward parents because they do not have the same material possessions as their peers. Moreover, it is not uncommon for individuals who have moved upwardly from a lower social class to feel like they don't belong. Once again, feelings of guilt may surface in situations where the individual tries to act differently in order to fit in.

 REFLECTION QUESTIONS 9.3

- To what extent do you value prestige, power, economic resources, education, income, or status as a sign of someone's worth?
- Have you ever stood up for someone being harassed or oppressed on the basis of social class? If not, why not? Has anyone ever stood up for you in this way?

CASE STUDY **9.1**

The Case of John

John was a 40-year-old Caucasian male who entered counseling on the advice of a good friend. He was heavily drinking, and it began to affect his performance at work. Born and raised in a small rural town in the Midwest, John was the first and only one of four children in his family to go to college and obtain a master's degree in business administration (MBA). His parents could not afford to contribute to his college education, so John worked part-time while he went to school. Because he worked to pay for his education, he often took courses on a part-time basis; thus, it took nearly 11 years to complete requirements for both the undergraduate degree and MBA. Soon after graduation, John obtained an entry-level position in a prestigious company. He excelled in his job, moving up the company ladder, and finally became a manager of one of the largest divisions of the company. His salary steadily increased, allowing him to purchase a sporty car and a large house in an "upper-class" neighborhood. At 37, John married a woman who was raised in this affluent suburban community and whose parents own several restaurants and small businesses in the area. John tells the counselor that he worked very hard to "get where I'm at" and yet feels like he doesn't belong in this neighborhood. Even though he excelled in the company, John sometimes thinks he "isn't good enough." Every time he goes back to his hometown to visit his younger brother, two sisters, and parents, he feels guilty because he left his hometown to "better himself." He also disclosed that, at times, he feels ashamed of his family.

Case Discussion
Thinking About This Case
1. What are some of the factors that may be contributing to John's negative self-image?
2. What may be contributing to his heavy drinking?
3. How might you work with John in sorting out his feelings about his family?

It is conceivable that counselors make assumptions about their clients based on objective economic indicators, such as income and education. Yet, as illustrated in this case, social class has a powerful influence on shaping identity. John seems to be struggling with self-identifying as "upper class," even though he lives in such a community. Likewise, John continues to devalue himself even though he worked hard to achieve an education and has a successful career. The heavy drinking could be associated with the guilt and shame that he has toward his family, low self-esteem, and pressure to continue excelling in his career.

Classist Attitudes and Beliefs

The attitudes and beliefs about individuals in different classes also influence behavior toward them. Beliefs such as that the wealthy are well mannered, always pleasant, intelligent, and sophisticated, and that the poor are lazy, aggressive, and uneducated, will most likely influence the way one interacts with individuals who are perceived to belong to one of these groups. The mere fact that we classify people into hierarchical categories, such as *high*, *middle*, and *low* is an example of how our society values different income levels. Similarly, scholars describe the "social distancing" effect that often occurs between members of different classes as a result of the attitudes and beliefs held about people. Lott and Bullock (2001) concluded that the middle class is fairly insulated and ignorant about the issues surrounding poverty because they live, eat, shop, and engage in leisure activities in settings different from people in lower social classes.

We know little about what contributes to the perceptions we formulate about people who are members of a particular class. Surprisingly, there is

EXAMPLE **9.1**

Privileges of the Middle Class

Another way to examine middle-class attitudes and beliefs about people from lower social classes is with the notion of "White middle class privilege" as described by Liu, Pickett, and Ivey (2007). Specifically, they categorize a set of privileges of the middle class that influence attitudes and behaviors. These include the privileges associated with housing and neighborhoods, economic freedom, leisure activities, self-fulfillment, and power. Within these various categories, there are a set of corresponding beliefs. For example:

Housing and Neighborhood
- "I can be assured that I have adequate housing for myself and my family."
- "I can easily stay away from parts of my town or area where those who have less money live and have all my needs met."

Economic Liberty
- "I can buy not only what I need to have but also what I want."
- "I can be assured of three meals a day with a variety of choices and good nutrition."

Power
- "I have the resources to make choices regarding my medical care."
- "I feel able to influence schools and other institutions to treat my family fairly and give them advantages when they deserve it."
- "I feel entitled to a good education."

Self-Fulfillment
- "I feel I am what others strive to be."
- "I can look at my life and feel that it has been reasonable successful."

Leisure
- "I can leisurely engage in activities that do not supplement my income."
- "I can expect to have vacation time each year."

Source: From W. M. Liu, T. Pickett, Jr., & A. E. Ivey, "White Middle-Class Privilege: Social Class Bias and Implications for Training and Practice," *Journal of Multicultural Counseling and Development*, 35, pp. 205–206. Copyright © 2007 by the Journal of Multicultural Counseling and Development, American Counseling Association. Reprinted with permission.

little research on attitudes about the poor. In a recent study, Cozzarelli, Wilkinson, and Tagler (2001) found that participants consistently endorsed more positive characteristics to the middle class (e.g., hardworking, healthy, family oriented, happy, strong, and capable) compared to the poor (unmotivated, physically ill, depressed, alcoholic, abusive, and weak). This type of perspective also extended to endorsing more negative stereotypes about the poor as compared to the middle class. More troubling is that negative attitudes and beliefs about the poor are linked to racial and ethnic minorities because they have higher poverty rates (e.g., Wyche, 1996). The implication of these research findings is that differential attitudes, including the prevalence of stereotypes, are likely to influence beliefs about welfare and policies, such as welfare reform (Cozzarelli et al., 2001).

REFLECTION QUESTIONS 9.4

- What is your definition of the "American dream"?

Upward Mobility: The Elusive American Dream

Undeniably many African Americans, Latinos, Asian Americans, and other minorities have made economic gains in the last several decades, reaching middle-class status. More ethnic minorities own their own homes and businesses, attend college, and are earning middle-class incomes (Rodriguez, 1996). However, recent data suggest that the promise of the "American dream" is not that easy to achieve and income inequality persists. For instance, in 2007 African Americans were earning, on average, $33,916, and yet their income was $21,000 less than the average for Whites, $54,920 (U.S. Census Bureau, 2008a). Likewise, the income for Latinos was $38, 679, slightly higher than African Americans, but significantly lower than the non-Latino White population. In contrast, Asian Americans had the highest median income of $66, 103 (U.S. Census Bureau, 2008b). Unfortunately, there has been a shift in the kinds of jobs available (e.g., a dramatic loss of manufacturing jobs) that provide economic stability in the United States. Hence, ethnic minority groups continue to have low-wage service-type jobs that oftentimes have limited or no health insurance coverage (Klein, 2004). Moreover, they have been hit especially hard with the most recent recession of 2008, in which the unemployment rate for African Americans was about 11.5% and for Hispanics was nearly 9%, compared to 6% for Whites (Logan & Weller, 2009).

With respect to educational attainment, more ethnic minorities are obtaining a college education than ever before. However, there are marked differences in the financial burden they encounter upon graduation. For example, upon graduation more African Americans have fairly large loan repayments, and tend to obtain lower wage jobs than Whites. Consequently, ethnic minorities are more likely to be in considerable debt right after college, making the process of upward mobility even more challenging. In 1999–2000, 84% of African American graduates borrowed on average $2,000 more than other graduates, and although Hispanics had lower than average student loans upon graduation, their burden of debt exceeded 8% of their monthly wages (King & Bannon, 2002).

In addition to these economic challenges, it is not uncommon for many ethnic minorities to experience difficulties in being accepted into the middle class. Many ethnic minorities experience a great deal of ambivalence and guilt about "moving up the ladder" and leaving their old neighborhoods.

More troubling is that blatant forms of racism still abound once they move into these communities. Moreover, African Americans who obtain white-collar and professional positions characteristic of middle-class occupations still experience tokenism and discrimination in and out of the workplace (Cole & Omari, 2002). These experiences can create a great deal of stress as well as mixed emotions. Leanita McClain (1986), author of *The Middle-Class Burden*, illustrates this point:

> *My life abounds in incongruities. Fresh from a vacation in Paris, I may, a week later, be on the milk-run Trailways bus in deep South backcountry attending the funeral of an ancient uncle whose world stretched only 0 miles and who never learned to read. Sometimes when I wait at the bus stop with my attaché case, I meet my aunt getting off the bus with other cleaning ladies on their way to do my neighbors' floors.*
>
> *But I am not ashamed. Black progress has surpassed our greatest expectations; we never even saw much hope for it, and the achievement has taken us by surprise.*
>
> *In my heart, however, there is no safe distance from the wretched past of my ancestors or the purposeless present of some of my contemporaries; I fear such a fate can reclaim me. I am not comfortably middle class; I am uncomfortably middle class.*
>
> *I have made it, but where? Racism still dogs my people. There are still communities in which crosses are burned on the lawns of black families who have the money and grit to move in.*
>
> *What a hollow victory we have won. My sister, dressed in her designer everything, is driven to the rear door of the luxury high rise in which she lives because the cab driver, noting only her skin color, assumes she is the maid, or the nanny, or the cook, but certainly not the lady of any house at this address. (p. 13)*

SOCIAL CLASS WORLDVIEW

As stated earlier, one's lived experiences are influenced by social class. Liu et al. (Liu, Ali, et al., 2004; Liu, Soleck, et al., 2004) argued that we should broaden our understanding of this construct because focusing on demographics, such as income, education, and occupation alone will only provide superficial information that does not capture the "psychological" aspects of these factors. Accordingly, social class can be conceptualized as broader, much like the opening statement in this chapter in which Langston sees it as affecting how we think, feel, and act because it is such a central part of our daily lives. Given its broad influence, social class can include an individual's worldview. According to Liu (2001; Liu, Ali, et al., 2004; Liu, Soleck, et al., 2004), **social class worldview** is the beliefs and attitudes held by an individual in a particular economic class and the expected behaviors associated with membership in that class. One of the unique aspects of his model is the attention given to the effects of classism. This expanded conceptualization allows counselors to contextualize a client's economic circumstances, explore his or her experience with classism, and identify emotions, such as guilt and shame as illustrated in the case of John. Liu, Ali, et al. (2004) capture its importance by stating,

SCW is the intrapsychic framework (i.e., lens) through which people make sense of the economic cultural expectations and filter the demands into meaningful actions to meet expected economic goals. The worldview consists of a person's relationship to property (materialism), social class behavior (e.g., mannerisms and etiquette), lifestyle choices (e.g., vacation time), referent groups (family, peers, and a group of aspiration), and consciousness about social class. (p 10)

Liu (2001) and Liu, Soleck, et al. (2004) also offer a framework called the **social class worldview model (SCWM)** that may be useful in counseling clients. The model is illustrated in Figure 9.1 and briefly described herein.

At the center of the framework are social class saliency, consciousness, and attitudes. Social class saliency occurs in situations where there is a realization that one's position in a given class is different from those of everyone else. One example is moving into an affluent neighborhood and believing that you don't fit in. Likewise, consciousness is the awareness that one belongs to a given social class, including the awareness that there are external forces that contribute to a class structure (e.g., hierarchy, barriers, and oppression). The attitudes are the beliefs, values, feelings, and attributions one has about social class that are shaped by personal experiences, parental influence, friends, and peers. For example, an individual who grew up in an affluent upper middle-class community may believe that people who are poor are uneducated

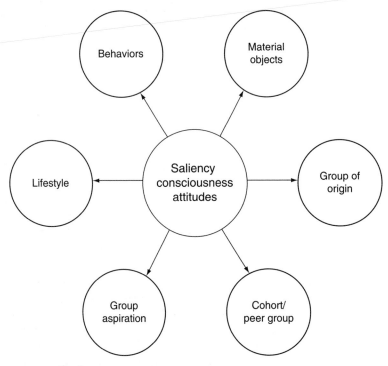

FIGURE **9.1** Social Class Worldview

and, therefore, not capable of obtaining employment that pays higher wages. Although this individual has had contact with hardworking, talented, and intelligent domestic help and/or gardeners who work in these affluent communities, their work is often devalued or simply goes unappreciated.

Social class referent groups are those people who were instrumental in the formation of the individual's worldview, and subsequently influence the way he or she behaves toward members of the same class or other social classes. Liu (2001) identifies three types of referent groups: (a) The "group of origination" consists of parents or caretakers, childhood friends, and relatives; (b) the "cohort group" represents those people who the individual associates with and feels comfortable; and (c) the "group of social class aspiration" are those people who he or she wants to be like and in emulation of whom, therefore, the individual strives to obtain a particular status. However, depending on one's circumstances and economic means, these referent groups may not function in the same way. As Liu noted, someone who comes from an affluent background may not aspire to be wealthier but may strive to maintain the wealth. In this case, the group of aspiration may not be important. Furthermore, a poor individual constantly faced with limited resources may focus on the cohort group for mere survival. In this case, the aspiration group plays a very small role.

The **relationship to material objects** is an integral aspect of the framework because it gives us a sense of their relative importance. Material possessions represent a particular lifestyle, and they are a reflection of the individual as well as a particular reference group, whether it is the original, cohort, or aspired group. Liu and colleagues also postulated that these reference groups have particular expectations about certain kinds of material objects that are valued as important. So, if the reference group highly values a particular object, so will the individual.

Social class lifestyle involves the socialization experiences within a particular class as well as how one lives. According to Liu (2001), it "represents the way people organize their [social class worldview] and economic resources to carry out a preferred pattern of action and behaviors" (p. 158). They go on to state that it derives a sense of accomplishment and satisfaction as long as it is consistent with the worldview.

Finally, **perceived class and status position** represent the individual's belief about his or her location in the socioeconomic hierarchy. This overarching aspect of the model can be conceptualized as the *subjective* sense of where one belongs based on objective indicators, such as income, education, occupation, and the other dimensions of the model. This aspect of the model is important because it focuses on the individual's internal experiences and provides valuable information about the meaning of such experiences. Ultimately, this helps to contextualize social class.

In sum, this framework makes an important contribution because it helps us to understand that social class is more than just income, education, and occupation. One of the limitations, however, is that it does not take gender, race, and ethnicity into account. As we discussed in previous chapters, gender, race, and ethnicity are central in understanding worldview and, therefore, would also have an impact on perceived class and status position. Moreover, there is an implicit assumption that certain desirable behaviors are associated with a particular class, and not with other classes. For instance, "having good table manners" and "speaking correct English" are described as middle-class behaviors. We would argue that these examples only perpetuate stereotypes. Nonetheless, they comprise a useful tool in obtaining a broader picture about an individual's worldview.

SOCIAL CLASS, RACE, ETHNICITY, AND GENDER

Based on our previous discussion, it is clear that the discourse on social class differences includes race, ethnicity, and gender. Each contributes uniquely in shaping an individual's identity; however, these dimensions also operate interdependently to influence experiences and worldview.

Gender and Social Class

Gender and class are related in a number of ways. First, women are overrepresented in low-paying and gender-segregated occupations with less status and opportunity for advancement. In 2007, the average earnings of men who worked full-time year-round was $45,113 compared to $35,102 for women (U.S. Census Bureau, 2008). Likewise, the ratio of earnings for women who were full-time workers was 78% of that for men, representing a 22% wage gap (Institute for Women's Policy Research, 2008). Thus, gender differences in the type of job and salary associated with it, and the wage disparity, dictate class position. For example, women who are overrepresented in clerical and service occupations could be classified as working class (Thompson & Hickey, 2005). Another way in which gender and class intersect is through socialization. Specifically, gender socialization experiences combined with inequality in access greatly influence career aspirations and eventually the types of jobs sought (Wright, 2001).

Although wage disparities continue to exist, there has been a steady increase in the number of women entering middle-class occupations such as marketing, sales, finance, and law. These women are earning wages that increase their ability to support a household, and many of them are postponing their childbearing years and/or having fewer children (Crompton, 2001). However, women of color continue to be concentrated in low-wage service occupations that are minimally rewarding.

Race, Ethnicity, and Social Class

Just as gender and social class are interconnected, so are race, ethnicity, and social class. One of the common features across these constructs is that they are conceptualized as power hierarchies in which the dominant group (e.g., Whites) historically has had the opportunities and access to resources that people of color have not (Constantine, 2001). As noted earlier, ethnic and racial groups are overrepresented among the low-income social class, particularly among the poor. As Smith et al. (2008) pointed out, the "gaping racial wealth divide continues to characterize the American class structure" (p. 304).

Although there is evidence that people of color are moving into middle-class ranks, the wealth gap between Whites and ethnic groups (e.g., African Americans, Asian Americans, Latinos, and Native Americans) is significant and persistent. Ethnic groups continue to face barriers that do not allow them to move up the social class ladder. Barriers, such as access to higher education directly limit employment options and opportunities. This, in turn, keeps a significant proportion of these ethnic and racial groups in the low-income social class (Armas, 2007).

CASE STUDY **9.2**

The Case of Gloria

Gloria, a 27-year-old woman of Mexican heritage who was the first generation of her family born in the United States, went to see her physician because she was having difficulty sleeping at night, was extremely tired and irritable, and had no appetite. Her physician concluded that there was no physical basis for her complaints (i.e., the tests came back negative), so he referred her to a mental health service provider. Gloria reluctantly agreed to make an appointment with a counselor at a local community-based agency that provided mental health services. She was not familiar with the counseling process and was confused about her physician's recommendation. She also thought that she just didn't have time to see a counselor. Her thinking was that working full-time, taking care of two young children, and dealing with the responsibilities of running a household took up most of her time. Gloria, who had a two-year associate's degree in accounting, got married to Jorge right after college and decided to have children right away. Jorge didn't want her to work full-time, insisting that his salary was sufficient to raise their children. Gloria also wanted to work only part-time so that she could spend more time with her children. Both Jorge and Gloria had strong family values and wanted to raise their children knowing and practicing Mexican traditions. They lived in a comfortable two-bedroom apartment in town. However, the recent divorce from her husband left Gloria with a substantial reduction in income. She had to find full-time work to pay the rent, bills, and groceries because Jorge was providing very little financial support. It was increasingly difficult to maintain the lifestyle she had before the divorce. An added expense was child care, which she didn't anticipate would be so expensive. She was working full-time as an assistant accountant, and yet was having difficulty paying the bills on time. Her new job offered limited health coverage, so when the children were taken to the pediatrician she was paying more out-of-pocket expenses. At times, she felt overwhelmed with everything but tried to keep these feelings hidden.

Case Discussion
Thinking About This Case
1. Considering Gloria's ethnic background, what cultural factors would you explore with her?
2. How would you explore her social class background, and do you think it has changed?
3. Why do you think Gloria is resistant to counseling, and what would you do to help her understand the process?

At first glance, we see that Gloria's divorce, a significant life transition, has had a major impact on her financial situation. She is clearly showing signs of distress (e.g., no appetite, difficulty sleeping, and feeling irritable and tired). Gloria's financial burden adds to her distress and sense of being overwhelmed. She doesn't understand why her physician recommended seeing a counselor, nor understands how counseling could help her. Perhaps she believes that her health insurance does not cover mental health services, and/or that counseling is for people with severe mental illness. Areas to explore with Gloria would include determining the extent to which she has immediate and extended family support and identifying cultural and traditional gender roles that are important to her. In addition, assessing for possible depression is necessary given her symptoms.

OPENING THE DIALOGUE ON SOCIAL CLASS

With all of the topics discussed in this chapter, you are now challenged to think through how you would utilize this information in session with any number of clients from a variety of cultural backgrounds and worldviews. Questions for reflection offered to you throughout this chapter also serve as excellent process questions for opening the dialogue with clients on issues of social class and experiences with classism. Some of these questions are listed here to assist you in terms of opening the dialogue with your clients:

- What does it mean in our society to be wealthy? Poor?
- How do you define success? How is success defined in your family? In your culture? In larger society?
- What is your social class? Has it changed, and if so, why?
- What have been some of your experiences with people from different social classes? What made those experiences either positive or negative?
- Who are you in terms of social class? How important is this in your personal and cultural identity, and what impact does this dimension have on how you view the world and live your life?
- How did your class-based definition of yourself develop, and who were some significant people in your life that helped to shape this definition?
- How has your view of social class been reinforced or challenged during your life?
- What does your culture say about social class?
- What do your family and community say about social class in terms of both beliefs and practice?
- How do issues of power and privilege influence your view of social class and concept of classism?
- How has your view of social class affected the way you define yourself now and at previous points in your life?
- How will your view of social class continue to affect the way you define yourself and the way others see you or treat you?
- How has your view of social class affected the way you interact with others who are similar to you versus different in age to you at different points in your life?
- Who are some people of your own social class that you look up to, and why?
- How might the difference or similarity in social class between you (client) and I (counselor) affect your experience in the process of counseling as well as the relationship between us?
- When and how did you first become aware of classism? What was your initial reaction, and how did that reaction change over time?
- What have your experiences with racism been, and in what ways have those experiences shaped who you are as a person as well as the issues you are dealing with now?
- What efforts have you made to work toward positive social change with regard to the classism that exists in your own life at the individual, group, and societal levels, and what other kinds of efforts would you like to make?

- To what extent do you value prestige, power, economic resources, education, income, or status as a sign of someone's worth?
- Have you ever stood up for someone being harassed or oppressed on the basis of social class? If not, why not? Has anyone ever stood up for you in this way?
- What is your definition of the "American dream"?
- Can you think of anyone for whom the American dream is not possible, and if so, why?
- How does social class play into the issues you are bringing to counseling, and how can we address this in a way that is most helpful to you?

CONCLUSION AND IMPLICATIONS

Counselors who are of middle- to upper-class backgrounds may not be sensitive to the life circumstances of people of lower social classes, due, in part, to their limited knowledge base and lack of self-awareness of privileges that they have by virtue of their class position. Likewise, counselors may intentionally not address classism and its impact altogether because they perceive their class status to be the same as their clients and, therefore, do not give it any importance during the counseling process. Another reason for not giving it adequate attention is that counselors may have had very little exposure to social class issues in their training programs (Constantine, 2001; Smith et al., 2008). This is compounded by the fact that many of the counseling theories, approaches, and interventions taught in training programs are based on middle-class values (Sue & Sue, 2003). Nonetheless, as counselors you are urged to consider the following:

1. Although you may be working with a client who is of the same socioeconomic and social class as you, it is important to recognize that counselors still hold a relatively privileged position.
2. Be aware that many clients of lower-social-class ranks may be more interested in working with you to meet basic needs rather than focus on psychological phenomena.
3. Understand that clients of lower classes may be unfamiliar with the counseling process; this, therefore, requires you to give special attention to explaining what it is, as well as what to expect.

4. Recognize that you may have to take on an advocacy role in helping clients of lower classes to locate needed resources (employment, food, shelter, clothing, etc.).
5. Understand that social class is intimately connected to gender, race, and ethnicity, and that they produce multiple identities, and you need to consider how they are related in conceptualizing your client's presenting problems.
6. Acknowledge that there are societal barriers that prevent your clients from reaching desired goals.

This chapter began with a discussion of the complex nature of social class, and the impact of poverty, especially among women with children and ethnic-racial groups, on overall health and well-being. Understanding the manifestations of classism, including classist attitudes and beliefs, as important contributors to inequalities in educational attainment, wages, housing, and employment was explored in this chapter. The social class worldview model by Liu et al. (2001, 2004a; 2004b) offers a broader lens from which to explore an individual's experiences with classism, including lifestyle and perceptions about his or her location in a socioeconomic hierarchy. Understanding how race, gender, ethnicity, and social class intersect helps counselors to better understand not only their clients' experiences but also their impact on health and well-being.

GLOSSARY

Classism: Prejudicial attitudes and behaviors toward other people who are members of a particular class.

Internalized classism: The acceptance of classism by individuals in a given social class. It can be manifested by feeling inferior to those in higher social classes, or superior to those lower on the class spectrum. Individuals internalize prejudicial attitudes and behaviors toward people in a given social class.

Social class: An individual's position in an economic hierarchy based on income, education, and occupation. Social class is membership in a particular group (e.g., middle class, working class, or upper class). Social class structures vary across societies and countries.

Social class worldview: The beliefs, attitudes, and behaviors of an individual in a particular social class.

Social class worldview model (SCW): A framework developed by Liu (2001) and Liu et al. (2004b that consists of the individual's relationship to property, social class behaviors, lifestyle, referent groups, and awareness of social class. The model consists of the following:

- *Social class referent groups:* Key people in an individual's life who help to shape the person's worldview such as friends, family members, and aspirational peers
- *Relationship to material objects:* Material possessions that represent a certain social class
- *Social class lifestyle:* Specific actions and behaviors tied to economic resources
- *Perceived class and status position:* A subjective sense of one's location within a particular socioeconomic hierarchy

Socioeconomic status: Based on quantifiable measures of income, occupation, and education that stratify people in our society. SES does not include belonging to a particular group such as the "middle-class" or "upper-class" group.

REFERENCES

Adler, N. E., Epel, E. S., Castellazzo, G., & Ickovics, J. R. (2000). Relationship of subjective and objective status with psychological and physiological functioning: Preliminary data in healthy White women. *Health Psychology, 19,* 586–692.

Argyle, M. (1994). *The psychology of social class.* New York: Routledge.

Armas, G. C. (2007). Wealth gap between races widens. In P. S. Rothenberg (Ed.), *Race, class, and gender in the United States* (pp. 341–344). New York: Worth.

Backlund, E., Sorlie, P. D., & Johnson, N. J. (1996). The shape of the relationship between income and mortality in the United States: Evidence from the national Longitudinal Mortality Study. *Annals of Epidemiology, 6,* 12–20.

Bullock, H. E., Wyche, K. F., & Williams, W. R. (2001). Media images of the poor. *Journal of Social Issues, 57,* 229–246.

Cole, E. R., & Omari, S. R. (2002). Race, class and the dilemmas of upward mobility for African Americans. *Journal of Social Issues, 59,* 785–802.

Constantine, M. (2001). Address racial, ethnic, gender, and social class issues in counselor training and practice. In D. Pope-Davis & H. K. Coleman (Eds.), *The intersection of race, class, and gender in multicultural counseling* (pp. 341–350). Thousand Oaks, CA: Sage.

Cozzarelli, C., Wilkinson, A. V., & Tagler, M. J. (2001). Attitudes toward the poor and attributions for poverty. *Journal of Social Issues, 57,* 207–221.

Crompton, R. (2001). The gendered restructuring of the middle classes. In J. Baxter & M. Western (Eds.), *Reconfiguration of class and gender* (pp. 39–54). Stanford, CA: Stanford University Press.

Diala, C. C., Muntaner, C., & Walrath, C. (2004). Gender, occupational, and socioeconomic correlates of alcohol and drug abuse among U.S. rural, metropolitan, and urban residents. *American Journal of Drug and Alcohol Abuse, 30,* 409–428.

Gallo, L. C., & Matthews, K. A. (2003). Understanding the association between socioeconomic status and physical health: Do negative emotions play a role? *Psychological Bulletin, 129,* 10–51.

Gordon, P., Nelson, M. C., Page, P., & Popkin, B. M. (2006). Inequality in the built environment underlies key health disparities in physical activity and obesity. *Pediatrics, 117,* 417–424. Retrieved from http://pediatrics.aappublications.org/cgi/content/full/117/2/417

Harley, D. A., Jolivette, K., McCormick, K., & Tice, K. (2002). Race, class, and gender: A constellation of positionalities with implications for counseling. *Journal of Multicultural Counseling and Development, 30,* 216–238.

Hudson, C. G. (2005). Socioeconomic status and mental illness: Tests of the social causation and selection hypothesis. *American Journal of Orthopsychiatry, 75,* 3–18.

Institute for Women's Policy Research. (2010). The gender wage gap: 2009 [Fact sheet]. Washington, DC: Author. Retrieved from http://www.iwpr.org/pdf/C350.pdf

King, T., & Bannon, E. (2002). *The burden of borrowing: A report on the rising rates of student loan debt*. State PIRG Higher Education Project. Retrieved from http://www.pirg.org/highered

Klein, A. (2004, December). A tenuous hold on the middle class. *Washington Post*, p. A01. Retrieved from http://www.washingtonpost.com/wp-dyn/articles/A8839-2004Dec17.html

Langston, D. (1992). Tired of playing monopoly? In M. L. Andersen & P. H. Collins (Eds.), *Race, class, and gender: An anthology* (pp. 110–120). Belmont, CA: Wadsworth.

Liu, W. M. (2001). Expanding our understanding of *multiculturalism*: Developing a social class world-view model. In D. Pope-Davis & H. K. Coleman (Eds.), *The intersection of race, class, and gender in multicultural counseling* (pp 127–170). Thousand Oaks, CA: Sage.

Liu, W. M. (2006). Classism is much more complex. *American Psychologist, 61*, 337.

Liu, W. M., & Ali, R. S. (2008). Social class and classism: Understanding the psychological impact of poverty and inequality. In S. D. Brown & R. W. Lent (Eds.), *Handbook of counseling psychology* (pp. 159–175), Hoboken, NJ: John Wiley.

Liu, W. M., Ali, S. R., Soleck, G., Hopps, J., Dunston, K., & Pickett, T. (2004a). Using social class in counseling psychology. *Journal of Counseling Psychology, 51*, 3–18.

Liu, W. M., Pickett, T., & Ivey, A. E. (2007). White middle-class privilege: Social class bias and implications for training and practice. *Journal of Multicultural Counseling and Development, 35*, 194–206.

Liu, W. M., Soleck, G., Hopps, J., Kwesi, D., & Pickett, T. (2004b). A new framework to understand social class in counseling: The social class model and modern classism theory. *Journal of Multicultural Counseling and Development, 32*, 95–122.

Logan, A., & Weller, C. E. (2009, January). The state of minorities: The recession issue. Center for American Progress. Retrieved from http://www.americanprogress.org/issues/2009/01/state_of_minorities.html

Lorant, V., Deliege, D., Eaton, W., Robert, A., Philippot, P., & Ansseau, M. (2003). Socioeconomic inequalities in depression: A meta-analysis. *American Journal of Epidemiology, 157*, 98–112.

Lott, B., & Bullock, H. E. (2001). Who are the poor? *Journal of Social Issues, 57*, 189–206.

McClain, L. (1986). The middle-class Black's burden. In L. McClain, *A foot in each world: Essays and articles* (Ed. C. Page, pp. 12–14). Evanston: IL: Northwestern University Press.

Moon, D. G., & Rollison, G. L. (1998). Communication of classism. In M. L. Hecht (Ed.), *Communicating prejudice* (pp. 122–135). Thousand Oaks, CA: Sage.

National Poverty Center. (2003). *Poverty in the United States: Frequently asked questions*. Retrieved from http://www.npc.umich.edu/poverty/

Pope, J. F., & Arthur, N. (2009). Socioeconomic status and class: A challenge for the practice of psychology in Canada. *Canadian Psychology, 50*, 55–65.

Robinson, T. (1993). The intersection of gender, class, race and culture: On seeing clients whole. *Journal of Multicultural Counseling and Development, 21*, 50–59.

Rodriguez, G. (1996). *The emerging Latino middle class*. Malibu, CA: Pepperdine University Institute for Public Policy and AT&T.

Russell, G. M. (1996). Internalized classism: The role of class in the development of self. *Women and Therapy, 18*, 59–71.

Sandu, D. S., & Aspy, C. B. (1997). *Counseling for prejudice prevention and reduction*. Alexandra, VA: American Counseling Association.

Singh-Manoux, A., Adler, N. E., & Marmot, M. G. (2003). Subjective social status: Its determinants and its association with measures of ill health in the Whitehall II study. *Social Science and Medicine, 56*, 1321–1333.

Smith, L. (2008). Positioning classism within counseling psychology's social justice agenda. *The Counseling Psychologist, 36*, 895–924.

Smith, L., Foley, P. H., & Chaney, M. P. (2008). Addressing classism, ableism, and heterosexism in counselor education. *Journal of Counseling & Development, 86*, 303–309.

Sue, D. W., & Sue, D. (2003). *Counseling the culturally diverse: Theory and practice* (4th ed.). New York: John Wiley.

Thompson, W. E., & Hickey, J. V. (2005). *Society in focus: An introduction to sociology*. Columbus, OH: Allyn & Bacon.

U.S. Census Bureau. (2004). *Poverty: 2003 highlights*. Current Population Survey (CPS). Retrieved from http://www.census.gov/hhes/poverty/poverty03/pov03hi.html

U.S. Census Bureau. (2008a). *Household income rises, poverty rate unchanged, number of uninsured down*. Retrieved from http://www.census.gov/

Press-Release/www/releases/archives/income_wealth/cb08-129html

U.S. Census Bureau. (2008b). *Income, poverty, and health insurance coverage in the United States: 2007*. Retrieved from http://www.census.gov/prod/2008pubs/p60-235.pdf

Wright, E. O. (2001). A conceptual menu for studying the interconnections of class and gender. In J. Baxter & M. Western (Eds.), *Reconfiguration of class and gender* (pp. 28–38). Stanford, CA: Stanford University Press.

Wyche, K. F. (1996). Conceptualizations of social class in African American women: Congruence of client and therapist definitions. In M. Hill, & E. D. Rothblum (Eds), *Classism and feminist therapy: Counting costs* (pp. 35–43). New York: Haworth Press.

CHAPTER **10**

Spirituality and Religion

*If we pass a strainer through the world's religions to lift out their
conclusions about reality and how life should be lived, those
conclusions begin to look like the winnowed wisdom of the human
race. What are the specifics of that wisdom? In the realm of ethics the
Decalogue pretty much tells the cross-cultural story. We should avoid
murder, thieving, lying, and adultery. These are minimum guidelines
but they are not nothing, as we realize if we reflect on how much
better the world would be if they were universally honored.*

*Processing from this ethical base to the kind of people we should
strive to become, we encounter the virtues, which the wisdom
traditions identify as basically three: humility, charity, and veracity.
Humility is not self-abasement. It is the capacity to regard oneself in
the company of others as one, but not more than one. Charity shifts
the shoe to the other foot; it is to regard one's neighbor as likewise
one, as fully one as oneself. As for veracity, it extends beyond the
minimum of truth-telling to sublime objectivity, the capacity to see
things exactly as they are. To conform one's life to the way things are
is to live authentically....*

*At the center of the religious life is a particular kind of joy, the
prospect of a happy ending that blossoms from necessarily painful
beginnings, the promise of human difficulties embraced and
overcome. We have only hints of this joy in our daily life. When it
arrives we do not know whether our happiness is the rarest or the*

commonest thing on earth; for in all earthly things we find it, give it, and receive it, but cannot hold on to it. When those intimations are ours it seems in no way strange to be so happy, but in retrospect we wonder how such gold of Eden could have been ours. The human opportunity, the religions tell us, is to transform our flashes of insight into abiding light.

The world at large, however, particularly the modern world, is not persuaded by this view of things; it cannot rise to the daringness of the claim. So what do we do? This is our final question. Whether religion is, for us, a good word or bad; whether (if on balance it is a good word) we side with a single religious tradition or to some degree open our arms to all: How do we comport ourselves in a pluralistic world that is riven by ideologies, some sacred, some profane?

We listen.

Source: H. Smith, *The World's Religions* (New York: HarperCollins). Copyright © 1991 by Houston Smith. Reprinted with permission.

DEFINING SPIRITUALITY AND RELIGION

Spirituality and religion are significant aspects of social identity. Similar to the experience of diversity, the terms **spirituality** and **religion** can have multiple meanings for different people. Perceptions and reactions vary, and some concepts are embraced and associated whereas others may not be. In this chapter, we seek to distinguish the two constructs, defining *spirituality* as being an overarching impulse toward a relationship with the infinite or a sense of connectedness or wholeness that goes beyond the bounds of the individual, whereas *religion* is often the social vehicle, the organizing framework and/ or institution within which a person expresses his or her spiritual identity (Faiver, Ingersoll, O'Brien, & McNally, 2001).

In many ways, spirituality is an innate human quality that can encompass many different expressions, which may or may not be translated into a recognizable religious framework. The framework, depending on the religion, can be constructed in various ways and levels of complexity. For instance, the Roman Catholic Church has a complex framework that combines many dimensions of spiritual theory and ritual, and has a complex structure that organizes and manages vast numbers of worshippers, clergy, churches, and groups that make up the body of the church. On the other hand, the Islamic religion, although it has not had the kind of worldwide impact as Christianity, is considered the second largest and fastest growing world religion (Wikipedia, n.d.-a).

A related set of concepts that may be useful in the discussion of spirituality and religions are esoteric and exoteric expression. The **exoteric** is the external, public form of a spiritual impulse, often expressed through religion that may involve adhering to a creed, following specific rituals of worship, and professing a set of stated beliefs. This frame is much affected and shaped by the cultural constructs that are present. The **esoteric** is the inner, subjective experience of the spiritual impulse, sometimes considered the quality of faith or enlightenment; it is experiential, affective, and not necessarily framed within any particular belief system.

It is important to recognize that spirituality is not necessarily a belief in the Divine. As Canda (1988) defines it, *spirituality* can be perceived as the whole process of human life and development as it is associated with a person's search for a sense of meaning, self-fulfillment, and building satisfying relationships with others. This process can be about God, Humanity, a Higher Power, or any combination of these (Kilpatrick, 1999). The constructs of spirituality and religion can be related or unrelated, and may play out in a variety of ways. For instance, a person may be a member of a church, attend services regularly, and follow the religious practices, but feel no spiritual beliefs. On the other hand, another person may care deeply about the meaning of life, engage in spiritual practices, such as meditations, practice compassion toward others, but not be affiliated with a religion. Alternatively, a person may attend synagogue regularly, be faithful to the Torah, keep kosher, and find both inspiration in these activities and support in the institution, being both religious and spiritual simultaneously.

Spiritual and religious identities are significant to counseling for a number of reasons. First, some forms of spiritual and religious beliefs and practices are present in most human cultures, signifying their importance. Second, healers who have existed in every culture have various religious persuasions

REFLECTION EXERCISE **10.1**

Spiritual Biography

As you read this chapter, we recommend engaging in the following exercises:

1. Write a spiritual autobiography: Start with the earliest memories you have of religion and/or spirituality in your home or family life, and move through childhood, adolescence, and into adulthood. Reflect on where you are with religion and spirituality at this time in your life.
2. Answer these difficult questions to which spiritual and religious belief systems often provide guidance. For instance:

    *   How do you understand the nature of human beings? Are humans good, bad, or neutral?
    *   How do you explain death, and what happens to people after they die?
    *   Do people have free will, or are their destinies fated?
    *   Why do bad things happen to good people?

TABLE **10.1**
Spirituality Competencies

Culture and worldview	1. The professional counselor can describe the similarities and differences between spirituality and religion, including the basic beliefs of various spiritual systems, major world religions, agnosticism, and atheism.
	2. The professional counselor recognizes that the client's beliefs (or absence of beliefs) about spirituality and/or religion are central to his or her worldview and can influence psychosocial functioning.
Counselor self-awareness	3. The professional counselor actively explores his or her own attitudes, beliefs, and values about spirituality and/or religion.
	4. The professional counselor continuously evaluates the influence of his or her own spiritual and/or religious beliefs and values on the client and the counseling process.
	5. The professional counselor can identify the limits of his or her understanding of the client's spiritual and/or religious perspective and is acquainted with religious and spiritual resources, including leaders, who can be avenues for consultation and to whom the counselor can refer.
Human and spiritual development	6. The professional counselor can describe and apply various models of spiritual and/or religious development and their relationship to human development.
Communication	7. The professional counselor responds to client communications about spirituality and/or religion with acceptance and sensitivity.
	8. The professional counselor uses spiritual and/or religious concepts that are consistent with the client's spiritual and/or religious perspectives and that are acceptable to the client.
	9. The professional counselor can recognize spiritual and/or religious themes in client communication and is able to address these with the client when they are therapeutically relevant.
Assessment	10. During the intake and assessment processes, the professional counselor strives to understand a client's spiritual and/or religious perspective by gathering information from the client and/or other sources.
Diagnosis and treatment	11. When making a diagnosis, the professional counselor recognizes that the client's spiritual and/or religious perspectives can (a) enhance well-being, (b) contribute to client problems, and/or (c) exacerbate symptoms.
	12. The professional counselor sets goals, with the client, that are consistent with the client's spiritual and/or religious perspectives.
	13. The professional counselor is able to (a) modify therapeutic techniques to include a client's spiritual and/or religious perspectives, and (b) utilize spiritual and/or religious practices as techniques when appropriate and acceptable to a client's viewpoint.
	14. The professional counselor can therapeutically apply theory and current research supporting the inclusion of a client's spiritual and/or religious perspectives and practices.

Source: Adapted from the Association of Spiritual, Ethical, and Religious Values in Counseling (2009). Spiritual Competencies. Retrieved from http://www.aservic.org/competencies.html

and engage in the care of people's souls (Kurtz, 1999). Third, it is quite common for people who are in crisis to seek religion or spirituality for comfort and help (Armstrong, 1999 in Faiver et al., 2001). A counselor who does not acknowledge or inquire about religious or spiritual beliefs may be doing a disservice to his or her clients. In terms of multicultural considerations, the cultural frames that shape spirituality need to be understood in order to understand a client's worldview (Fukuyama & Sevig, 1999). Finally, questions and concerns about responsibility, mortality, and loneliness are existential considerations, often present in counseling. Much of the richest work can occur in honoring and exploring clients' spiritual beliefs.

Counselors need to be sensitive in helping clients address the spiritual dimensions of their lives. In 1995, the Association for Spiritual, Ethical, Religious and Value Issues in Counseling (ASERVIC), a division of the American Counseling Association, formulated nine counselor competencies regarding the integration of religion and spirituality into counseling (Burke, 1998; Burke, Hackney, Hudson, Miranti, Watts, & Epp, 1999), which were later revised in 2009 to make a total of 14 competencies. (See Table 10.1.)

In accordance with these competencies, we encourage you to begin the process of self-examination of your own spiritual and religious belief systems, introduce models of spiritual and religious identity development, discuss some major premises of world religions, and discuss strategies and interventions through which a client's spiritual aspects can be acknowledged and incorporated into the process of counseling. Case Study 10.1 illustrates the need for counselors to become competent in these areas rather than merely well intentioned.

REFLECTION QUESTIONS 10.1

- How do you define spirituality and religion in your own life, and how are these two constructs similar or different for you?
- How comfortable are you with conversations around spirituality and/or religion? If there is discomfort for you around this topic, from where does that discomfort come?
- In what spiritual tradition, if any, were you raised, and have you deviated from that tradition at all? If so, why?
- How important is your spiritual and/or religious tradition to you, and in what ways?

Historical Background of Psychological and Religious Thought

In his theory of psychoanalysis, Sigmund Freud often critiqued religion (specifically Christianity) vigorously, believing that it was a result of wish fulfillment and fantasy, and that the rituals and liturgies were neurotic obsessions. In his view, religious doctrine created fear-induced repression that was antagonistic to objective critical thinking (Wulff, 1996).

Trained in these traditions, Carl Jung, however, significantly deviated from Freud about the role of spirituality and religion. He was interested in

CASE STUDY **10.1**

The Case of Sarah

Sarah came in to see Carla, a counselor in private practice, for assistance in handling her boyfriend Matt's pressure to attend church with him. Sarah, who is Jewish, was not interested in getting involved in Christianity, though she was not a regular attendee at the synagogue and had not observed any of the major religious days in the past few years. However, she was very much in love with Matt and was concerned that she might lose the relationship if she didn't show some appreciation of his religion. Carla had been raised Catholic but had discontinued her relationship with the church when she decided she could not support its position on birth control, abortion, and women's ordination. She empathized with Sarah's reluctance to get involved with a religion she didn't believe in. She focused on gender issues and encouraged Sarah to be assertive with Matt about her opinion of his religion. Sarah appreciated the support but still felt torn between her religious heritage and the man she hoped to marry.

Case Discussion
Thinking About This Case
1. How do you think Carla handled Sarah's issues around religion?
2. How did Carla's own history with spiritual and religious beliefs influence the way in which she worked with Sarah?
3. What might you recommend that Carla do in subsequent sessions with Sarah?

In this case, the counselor's own reaction is influencing her work with the client. Although Sarah is looking to find a balance between her faith and her relationship, her counselor has moved the issue to self-assertion. In many ways, the counselor and the client must explore the impact of their respective faiths in terms of their expectations of each other. Several questions to reflect on are as follows: 1. Are compromises possible? 2. Does Sarah feel that the pressure to attend with Matt is an ultimatum, and that she needs to agree to do this for the sake of the relationship? In further sessions, such questions could lead to other important issues that will frame the life that the couple hopes to build, including issues of possible parenting.

the ways in which one's awareness of the sacred could play a positive role in psychological adjustment. He postulated the existence of a *collective unconscious,* "the deep universal layer of the psyche" (Wulff, 1996, p. 54), as a space, shared by all human beings, that serves as a repository for universal mythic symbols. Jung created archetypes, such as the *persona,* which is the face we offer for public presentation; the **animus** and **anima,** which denote the masculine and feminine aspects of the self; and the **shadow,** which includes the dangerous, powerful, dark parts of the human experience. To become individuated or whole, people must be able to accept all the parts of themselves. The myths, rituals, stories, and images that are a part of all religious traditions have embedded in them these archetypes as ways to promote individuation (Wulff, 1996).

Erik Erickson's ego psychology also looked favorably on the role played by religion, linking it to an expression of human yearning, hope, and fear. In several places along the stages of psychosocial development he posited, religion plays an important part, whether in developing trust or in being able to move into generativity (e.g., having a sense of accomplishment and civic responsibility) (Wulff, 1996).

William James had a similar perspective as Jung, and his work on the psychology of religion focused more on spiritual expressions rather than on organized religious belief systems. He believed that the dogmatism, oppression, violence, and rigidity, in prescribing appropriate behavior, that arise in some religious organizations could be pathological distortions, but the merger of faith and reason could lead to positive psychological development. Other early significant figures in the field of psychology who appreciated and discussed the role that spiritual development could play included Abraham Maslow, who developed the mystical concept of peak experiences that allowed persons to experience a sense of wholeness and unity with the cosmos; and Erich Fromm, another humanistic psychologist who believed that humans needed a guiding framework and a place of worship to cope with the realities of existential aloneness and death. Victor Frankl, one of the founders of the existential approach in counseling, developed the concept of spiritual consciousness referring to the potential transcendence that could emerge. Frankl, through experiencing the horrors of the Holocaust, focused on the human search for meaning (Frankl, 1963).

In non-Western models of helping, religion and spirituality have often been inextricably linked with helping as opposed to separated from it (Moodley & Sutherland, 2009). For instance, in many tribal societies, the shaman was a figure who guided spiritual and emotional development. Often there is a much less rigid separation between mind, spirit, and body. For instance, Javaheri (2006) describes the use of prayer healing in Iran, where healers pray with and for their clients using adjuncts, such as prescribing herbal supplements and special diets as well as talking about the problem. Vontress (1991), in a discussion of traditional healing modalities in Africa, remarked on the holistic nature of the healing, with healers recognizing that mind and body are interactive and spirit can be assaultive to both. Healers acknowledge the interrelated physical, spiritual, and psychological dimensions within which their clients exist. In Hinduism, although Yoga is thought of primarily as a set of physical postures in the West, it is actually psychological in nature with the ultimate intent of practitioners to become more enlightened about themselves and the nature of the universe (Aranya, 1983). Case Study 10.2 illustrates an approach whereby the counselor works holistically with spiritual development to address psychological aspects of the client's presentation.

Models of Religious and Spiritual Identity Development

In this section, we offer an overview of developmental models that describe how people can grow and change in relation to their faith. Such frameworks are useful because they enable counselors to assess and understand how clients are incorporating faith into their lives, and gain some idea of the resultant influence. Categorizing religious and spiritual perspectives in these ways allows for more comparative perspectives and an understanding and acceptance of different manifestations of religion or spirituality. One important limitation of these models is that none was developed within a non-Western perspective, and although they may discuss transpersonal and ecumenical perspectives, they are grounded in a Judeo-Christian context (Frame, 2003).

CASE STUDY **10.2**

The Case of Shawn

Shawn is a 15-year-old Thai American boy who was adopted by European American parents when he was 7 and brought to the United States. He was mandated to counseling because he was convicted of a drug offense and was in an alternative school. He was also considered aggressive because though small in stature he would fight at any perceived sign of disrespect from peers. His parents refused to attend family counseling sessions. Shawn presented as apathetic and stated that he had no need of counseling. He appeared to be quite depressed. When asked about his cultural background, he declared that he didn't care about Thailand because his parents had told him that he lived in the United States now, and Thailand was not important in his new life.

Case Discussion
Questions to Think About
1. How might the counselor approach Shawn to establish a relationship despite his resistance?
2. Given Shawn's age at the time of adoption, it is probable that he has many memories and cultural affiliations with Thailand that he has not been permitted to hold on to. How might these be useful in therapy?

The counselor in this case had actually traveled to Thailand and was familiar with the country. He started by mentioning this, and Shawn, expressing interest, asked about his experience. The counselor brought in a picture book that Shawn devoured. Turning to a picture of monks meditating in a Buddhist temple, he stayed staring at the picture for a long time in silence. The counselor gently mentioned that one of the characteristics he had noticed among the Thai people was a commitment to maintain harmony and have a calm bearing. Shawn nodded mutely, then blurted out that his parents had never mentioned religion to him, and he felt he remembered Buddhism but not in any detail. When asked if he would like to learn some practices, he agreed enthusiastically with an energy markedly different from his earlier apathy. Shawn started with basic breathing exercises to facilitate calmness, and then mindfulness exercises focused on observing and monitoring his anger. At times, the counselor meditated with Shawn, and over a period of weeks, Shawn slowly changed his behavior. He also read introductory readings on Buddhism from the local library and was very struck by the notion of the Four Noble Truths. These are that life is filled with tension and suffering; desire is the source of our tension; if we cease desire, we reduce tension and suffering; and we can do this by following the eightfold path. He recast his drug use as a way of desiring escape from his feelings of alienation, and, using mindfulness and meditation, began to address that hurt. His parents were not opposed to this path and were happy with the cessation of his previous aggressive behavior, though they still refused to participate in his counseling. Finally, Shawn reported that he felt he was beginning to like himself and understand himself as Thai, and this felt much more stable for him.

Source: Adapted from Hanna, F. J., & Green, A. (2004). "Asian Shades of Spirituality: Implications for Multicultural School Counseling." *Professional School Counseling*, 7(5), pp. 326–333.

Allport's religious sentiment theory

Allport (1950) was one of the first modern psychologists to theorize about faith development. He described the development of religious sentiments in a chronological, linear, three-stage model. *Raw credulity*, Stage 1, is linked to young childhood, where children accept everything they hear from significant authority figures such as parents. In middle childhood, due to the need to feel a sense of belonging, children do not question the beliefs and values they have learned. When adults still hold these rigid, unquestioned beliefs, Allport believed that they became illogical, juvenile, and suppressive. In *satisfying ratio-nalism*, Stage 2, adolescents begin to seek an identity separate from that of their families, and begin questioning the beliefs they learned. Some youth may stay devoted to their childhood belief systems, whereas others feel alienated and still others experience a wavering faith. Stage 3, *religious maturity*, is more characteristic of adulthood in which individuals are connected to a spiritual or religious tradition, but have also approached it critically. They hold on to the beliefs that are useful and meaningful and reject those that do not meet their needs. Religion, in this phase, has a liberating rather than oppressive quality. Allport also believed that many persons never achieve religious maturity, and included are those adults who identify as agnostic or atheist.

Fowler's theory of stages of faith

Based on an empirical study of 359 individuals who were interviewed about their religion, values, and spiritual experiences over a period of a decade, Fowler (1981) developed a theory of seven stages of faith development, describing faith as a dynamic and genuine human experience, and a universal quality of meaning making. Although these stages are linked to certain ages, a person must sequentially pass through them. Therefore, although it is not possible to skip a stage, some persons may stay in stages for long periods.

The first stage is *primal faith*, which occurs in infancy during the period when infants are learning to trust their caregivers. Similar to Erickson's (1963) psychosocial stage of trust versus mistrust, babies form bonds with their nurturers while learning to differentiate themselves from others.

The next stage is *intuitive-projective faith*, which occurs in early childhood where children begin to make meaning of the world using their perceptions and feelings through images and symbols that represent both hazardous and safe characteristics of life. Some adolescents and adults can demonstrate this stage as well, but Fowler would characterize such emotional liability as dysfunctional. For instance, members of cults who ingest poison because they believe in the leader's view of the world and the afterlife may be exhibiting characteristics of this stage.

Mythic-literal faith occurs in middle childhood and is marked by the emerging cognitive ability to think logically and move away from magical thinking. Children in this stage are able to understand that persons may have different perceptions and perspectives than their own. Beliefs that are consistent with this stage include anthropomorphizing an image of the Divine, understanding the supreme being as a cosmic ruler who rewards goodness and punishes evil, and exhibiting perfectionism to be rewarded or self-abasement in expectation of punishment. Many of these beliefs are unidimensional and literal.

Synthetic-conventional faith spans from puberty into adulthood, and characteristically begins to take form in early adolescence during which adolescents are able to reflect general meaning from their experiences. Typically, during this time of adolescence, formal operational thinking (Piaget, 1972) emerges and opens the way for reliance on abstract ideas and concepts for making sense of one's world. Therefore, in this stage adolescents engage in critical reflection that often results in clashes with the previously valued authorities or perhaps a rejection of authorities, resulting in atheism.

Before *individuative-reflective faith* can emerge in young adulthood, individuals must both be willing to critically examine their belief systems and take responsibility for a self-authored worldview. In a sense, persons commit to religions through conscious choice rather than unexamined acceptance. Analyzing meanings and translating them into conceptual formulations gain clarity of faith, resulting in the exercise of responsibility and choice in regard to the spiritual communities to which a person belongs.

Conjunctive faith emerges in midlife and beyond, and many adults do not reach this stage. This is a stage, also called *paradoxical-consolidative faith*, that involves embracing and integrating the polarities in one's life. Persons may acknowledge multiple perspectives without being forced to choose in any direction. In a way, there is a reworking of the power of symbols to gain access to deeper truths. Individuals in this stage develop a commitment to justice beyond the boundaries of any one religious community, class, race, culture, or nation.

Finally, the apex of Fowler's model, *universalizing faith*, is a rare stage that only a few persons may transition into late in life. Persons are grounded in their connection to the Divine, and are committed to and aware of universal values. These individuals' lives are focused on God, but that does not make them perfect. Examples of some of those who achieved this stage may include Mother Teresa, Mahatma Gandhi, or Martin Luther King Jr.

Oser's five stages of religious judgment

Describing the term *religious judgment* as a balancing of competing values, beliefs, and views, and a struggle for faith and for developing viable explanations for the incongruence and unevenness in the world, Oser (1991) believed that religion was a continually evolving construct. As persons age, they go through stages and transformations of faith, and they connect their life experiences to an Ultimate Being in different ways through the life span. In Stage 1, persons view the Ultimate Being as all powerful, intervening in events and causing everything that happens. In Stage 2, persons still believe that the Ultimate Being is omnipotent, but that they can influence decisions through prayers, deeds, and vows that will result in being rewarded. In Stage 3, the Ultimate Being is in a transcendent realm removed from individual and secular concerns where human will is dominant. In Stage 4, persons regain a sense of the Ultimate Being as present and acting in concert with human autonomy. There may be a sense of a divine plan that gives meaning to life's situations and allows for human freedom. Similar to Fowler's final stage, Oser's Stage 5 is achieved by only a few. In this stage, persons are intensely aware of and committed to the Ultimate Being in every moment and aspect of their lives, and the universal aspects of all religions are central to their beliefs.

Genia's developmental typology of faith

Grounded in psychoanalytic theory, this five-stage model does not necessarily describe development in a linear fashion (Genia, 1995). Often people can regress to less mature stages or alternate peaks of spiritual development with long stays in certain stages. Emotional difficulties could cause persons to fail to move along the continuum as well as develop unhealthy forms of faith.

In Stage 1, *egocentric faith*, religion is rooted in fear and needed for comfort. Arising from childhood mistreatment or deprivation, persons in this stage have self-deprecating beliefs and behaviors, feel victimized by God when disappointed by life, and strive to be perfect to appease a vengeful God. In Stage 2, *dogmatic faith*, there is great fear of offending God, and a correspondingly strict adherence to religious prescriptions and rules to please. According to Genia (1995), persons in this stage often strive to please authoritarian parents and in their religious lives are drawn to groups that are intolerant of ambiguity and are centered on allegiance to religious authority.

Stage 3, *transitional faith*, is marked by a critical examination of religious beliefs, an exploration of new spiritual paths, and beginning to depend more on conscience than on dogma. Experimentation with different ideologies, changing religious affiliations, and having diverse spiritual experiences are characteristic of this stage, as is the sense of being disconnected and unbalanced as persons strive to find a meaningful spiritual orientation. Stage 4, *reconstructed faith*, occurs once persons have chosen a faith that provides purpose and fulfillment of their spiritual needs. Persons conform to religious prescriptions because they are congruent with inner convictions, and relate to God as a nurturing source of sustenance and support. They offer thanks as well as petition in their prayers and are aware of their human frailties. Although Genia (1995) considers such persons to have achieved significant religious maturity, the risk is that they may stay in this stage without further growth. The final Stage 5, *transcendent faith*, captures the rare experience of those persons who have a transcendent relationship to something greater than themselves, whose actions and lifestyle are congruent with their spiritual values, and who appreciate spiritual diversity while being committed to a faith that they have critically examined.

As you may have gathered from the models described here, current theories of spiritual development roughly correspond to and appear consistent with models of ego, cognitive, moral, and psychosocial development. Similar to the limitation of worldview discussed earlier, some other limitations are also present in these theories. For instance, many of these theories promote the idea that those in more advanced stages of the model are superior to those in earlier stages, an implicit assumption in hierarchical, linear models. Furthermore, much of the research does not address the views of diverse cultures or religions. For example, only 3% of the participants in the study by Fowler (1981) were African American, and there were no Muslim, Buddhist, or Hindu participants. In addition, it would be difficult for counselors who do not have a psychodynamic orientation to effectively use the stages of Genia's work. Nonetheless, the contribution made by such models outweighs the deficits by enabling counselors to perceive clients as engaged in a dynamic process of spiritual transformation. Case Study 10.3 may exemplify the use of developmental stages in spirituality as an intervention in counseling.

CASE STUDY **10.3**

The Case of Helen

A middle-aged, middle-class European American couple, Janet and Ralph, came in to see a family counselor because of their concern about Janet's mother, Helen. Sixty-four-year-old Helen had been living with them after her husband Jake's death 2 years prior. Janet was concerned about Helen's mental health because of what she characterized as "bizarre" ideas and behavior. Apparently, in grieving Jake's death, Helen had become increasingly involved in spiritual activities, and immersed herself in practices, such as meditation. She had also embraced a new political and social activism that both Janet and Ralph could not reconcile with their previous image of Helen. Additionally, Ralph was concerned that Helen was involving herself with all kinds of disreputable people with whom she appeared to be developing strong connections. Positive changes that they acknowledged were that Helen seemed very accepting of her physical limitations and failing health, while not being a prisoner to them.

Case Discussion

Thinking About the Case

1. How do you make sense of Janet and Ralph's concerns?
2. How might the family counselor assess Helen?

3. Would it be more productive to focus on Helen, or involve Janet and Ralph in counseling?

Given that the counselor is accustomed to working with families, it would be helpful to invite Helen to a session with Janet and Ralph to be able to hear from her directly and to understand the changes that have been occurring. This would provide the counselor with an opportunity to assess where Helen is in her spiritual journey. It would also give the counselor insight into Janet and Ralph's discomfort and unease. In such joint conversations, Helen could be asked about what has been happening in her life in the past year. As she describes the changes she has undergone in coming to terms with Jake's death, the counselor will be able to identify a theory of spiritual development and a stage that might be appropriate. It is likely that Helen is undergoing a stage where she is moving from more conventional expressions of faith to a deeper understanding. Her becoming more committed to social activism is characteristic of later stages, such as Fowler's Conjunctive Faith or even Genia's stage of Transcendent Faith. The counseling task will be to normalize conversations about faith and Helen's spiritual journey.

RELIGIOUS SYSTEMS AND SPIRITUAL BELIEFS

In Chapter 3, we discussed the construct of worldview and defined it as the unique way that an individual sees, interprets, and gives meaning to the world based on life's experiences. In terms of religious and spiritual belief systems, worldview encompasses a number of different criteria. The basic aspects of worldview include ideas and beliefs about how the universe was created. A second criterion is the notion of a Divinity, Ultimate Being, God, Goddess, or form of deity who is viewed as the source and center of all things. Beliefs regarding the origin of the world, how it was created, its destiny, as well as the origin and fate of human beings are usually present. In addition, belief systems also tend to have some instrument that mediates between the ultimate and the human that explains how we know our origins, our destinies, the path we take, and the assistance we may receive in achieving our destinies. In various cases, this instrument can be a personal revelation, or can be experiential, institutional theology, or revealed by priesthood. On a practical level, most religions have a code of what is expected of its members in terms of worship, practices, and behavior in the context of the religion as well as socially. Finally, every religion has some kind of sociological and institutional structure that allows the religion to preserve and implement its teachings and practice, develop a structure of leadership, as well as interact with the larger society. Table 10.2 shows a description of select world religions according to this schema.

One of the ways that various religions have been grouped is by their core beliefs as being monotheistic, polytheistic, or pantheistic. Specifically a **core belief** is whether the faith believes in a singular Supreme Being, a multiplicity of Divinities, or an equation of divinity with the universe such that it is considered all-encompassing and pervasive. Western religions are by and large monotheistic; Judaism, Christianity, and Islam can also be grouped as "People of the Book" because all three have a sacred text in common. Zoroastrianism, emerging from Persia, is also monotheistic. However, Wicca and other neo-Pagan traditions are considered pantheistic. Eastern religions, such as Hinduism, Buddhism, Taoism, and Shintoism tend to be polytheistic or pantheistic.

It is also important to note that within a religion, there are a number of distinct groups, sects, and practices that may deviate slightly or significantly from the major beliefs. Thus, Judaism can be orthodox, conservative, or reform. Three major divisions in Christianity are Roman Catholicism, composed of those who acknowledge the supreme authority of the pope, descended from St. Peter, in matters of faith; Eastern Orthodoxy that spreads from central and eastern Europe and is based on liturgy, tradition, and the idea that humans are to achieve divinity (Young, 2000); and Protestantism, which encompasses a diversity of denominations but is united by rejecting the authority of the pope and focusing on the authority of the Bible and the importance of individual faith. Evangelical and Fundamental Christianity are significant forces in the United States, whose members tend to be conservative both theologically and socially. Beyond following the Bible, such groups also tend to oppose homosexuality, extramarital sex, abortion, and divorce, and may expect women to take a submissive position to men (Thurston, 2000).

Most world religions are represented and practiced in the United States. In 2001, whereas the majority of the population was a denomination of Christianity (76%), other groups were also represented (4%), such as Jewish, Muslim, Buddhist, Hindu, Native American, Baha'i, Taoist, Rastafarian, Sikh, Wiccan, Druid, and Santeria (U.S. Bureau of the Census, 2003). Of the Christian denominations, the largest by far was Catholic, followed by Baptist and Methodist. It is necessary to note that there is a large minority that did not identify themselves as belonging to a religious faith (14%).

Green (1994) described the United States as a pioneer in separating church and state as a part of its foundation in the First Amendment, and enshrining a value of freedom to practice one's own religion. However, Siegel, Choldin, and Orost (1995) point out that regardless of this constitutional protection, Christianity has been closely woven into mainstream culture that has influenced the legal system. The dominance of Christianity as the majority religion of the United States has led to Christian privilege such that

TABLE **10.2**
Fundamental Features of Various Religions

Aspect	Judaism	Christianity	Islam	Hinduism	Buddhism	Shintoism	Wicca
Basic worldview	Universe is an arena for humans to live in, exercising free will, in cooperation with G-d's guidance.	A world fallen from harmony with God's will; Jesus Christ bridges the gap, and faith and love are required.	The world is for humans but under the absolute rule of God.	The universe is one even though it goes through surface changes and cycles; it is the ultimate expression of the divine.	The universe is infinite in terms of both time and space, and the universe is created and then destroyed over and over again, in a process of natural evolution.	The universe is pluralistic with many gods, and is growing and changing. There is no sharp demarcation between the divine, nature, and humanity.	The universe consists of *akasha*, a universal all-encompassing, nurturing soul of energy.
God or ultimate reality	Singular, sovereign, personal, creator represented as G-d or YHWH.	Sovereign, personal, all-good creator. God's son who is divinity in human form is Jesus.	*Allah*, who is sovereign, revealing Himself and giving specific guidance to humanity.	Brahma or the Universal Mind expresses itself like a flame taking many shapes, leading to a pantheon of local deities who depict aspects of divinity.	Dharma means ultimate truth, both about the nature of human existence and about the nature of the universe and the world. Dharma is not a being or a god who controls human existence; instead, it is an eternal principle that transcends everything else, but is also present everywhere around us.	There are many *kami* who may be deities such as Amaterasu, the Japanese sun goddess, or natural forces, guardians, exceptional people, or abstract creative forces.	Akasha is represented as a goddess and Her consort.
Origin and destiny of the world	Created by G-d, and will be led through historical unpleasant events, until the beginning of a messianic age that brings paradise.	Created by God and will be judged at the end of time and remade into a paradise.	Created by Allah and will be destroyed on the last Day of Judgment.	With no real beginning or end, the world goes through endless cycles of creation and destruction.	The world we know now is the product of an endless cycle of creation and destruction.	Created by the gods, the destiny is unknown, but historical progress has meaning.	Born out of the Goddess and will grow as her child.

TABLE **10.2**
Fundamental Features of Various Religions (Continued)

Aspect	Judaism	Christianity	Islam	Hinduism	Buddhism	Shintoism	Wicca
Origin and destiny of humans	Created individually by G-d and to be in this world. With divine help and human cooperation, the human condition can become increasingly paradisiacal.	Created individually by God, and will be resurrected and judged on the last day, and those so judged will gain eternal life.	Are created by Allah and will receive reward or punishment in the Second Creation.	Individuals have countless lifetimes determined by karma, which may include reincarnation as nonhumans, or even deities, until achieving oneness with the Universal Mind.	A person's actions have consequences in this life, but also shape destiny in subsequent lives. All people are reborn again and again, in a cycle called samsara, until they achieve spiritual enlightenment and reach nirvana. How they are reborn in the next life depends on how they behave in this life. A person's behavior and the consequences resulting from his or her behavior are called karma.	Are descended from kami, and may merge with kami or become kami depending on their deeds.	Humans are children of the Goddess and are to learn to be a part of the universe.
Revelation between the human and the ultimate	The scriptures, especially the Torah (the Hebrew Bible) and the collection of interpretations in the Talmud.	Supreme mediation by Jesus Christ, through the Bible combining the Hebrew scriptures or Old Testament, the four gospels, Acts, the letters attributed to the Apostle Paul, and Revelation. Also the tradition, authority, and teaching of the church in Catholicism and Eastern Orthodoxy.	The revelation of Mohammed, the last and greatest of the Prophets of Allah (acknowledging earlier messengers described in the Hebrew and Christian texts), is contained in the Koran.	Authorities include the Vedic scriptures, the Brahmin priesthood, the gods, and those saintly humans who have achieved a state of transcendence and can be followed as spiritual guides.	Buddha, or the Enlightened One, revealed the four Noble Truths about human existence, and developed the eightfold path. There are many teachers and persons, known as Bodhisatvas who continue to move along the path to enlightenment.	Ceremonial prayer called norito, myths, traditions, festivals, and rituals at shrines dedicated to particular kami.	Lessons from nature, tradition, and ritual; sometimes texts, such as the Book of Shadows.

Practical expectations	To honor and serve G-d by following the law of Moses, maintain the identity of the people, and promote the ethical vision of the great prophets. Jewish customs are followed in the home as well as outside.	To seek to know God, to worship him. To practice the ethic of love and service and follow the teachings of Jesus Christ.	To worship and serve God; to observe the Five Pillars: (1) *Shahadah:* there is no God but Allah, and Muhammad is his prophet; (2) *Salah:* ritual prayer performed 5 times a day; (3) *Zakat:* the sharing of wealth with the needy; (4) *Sawm:* fasting from sunrise to sunset during the Islamic month of Ramadan; and (5) *Hajj:* a pilgrimage to Mecca.	To follow *dharma,* or the right way through rituals, behavior, and righteous deeds. To seek *moksha* or liberation, and to practice meditation or devotion under the guidance of a guru.	To live a moral and ethical life. Although Buddhists do strive for spiritual enlightenment, the primary focus is on the here and now. It is imperative to treat others with respect, and to behave in a way that promotes harmony among all living things.	To remember and celebrate the gods, remain pure and sincere, preserve family and tradition, give honor to ancestral spirits and *kami,* and treat nature as sacred.	To do good, to respect the life energy of other organisms, and to revere nature and be a part of it.
Major social institutions	After the Jewish people, the basic unit is the congregation of Jews forming a synagogue or temple. The Jewish family is also a significant unit.	The Church, divided into many denominations, monastic orders, missionary works, and numerous associations.	The whole Islamic community; the local Friday Mosque community; the *Ulama* or body of teachers and preachers; Sufi orders; as well as the ideal role models of Islamic society.	The caste system; temples as places for the worship of gods, gurus or spiritual advisors, the family, and the Brahmin priesthood.	Temples, monasteries, and community centers. There are leaders in each of the branches, called *Theravada, Mahayana,* and *Vajrayana.* The Dalai Lama is considered the spiritual head of the Vajrayana branch.	Shrines that each have an *ujiko* community, Family, work, and regional ties with each shrine are important.	Communities of practicing Wiccans called *covens.*

American Christians are unaware of how much they are entitled to as a result of their faith, whereas members of other religions experience both overt and subtle discrimination. This can take the form of attacks against synagogues, mosques, and other places of worship; the targeting of non-Christian persons; or simply overlooking the religious significance of particular holy days in other religions while institutionalizing the celebration and commemoration of Christian-based holidays as universal. Historically, thousands of people were tortured and executed in America and Europe for allegedly practicing witchcraft; the most notable example in America was the Salem witch trials that occurred in the 17th century in Massachusetts. The conflation of witchcraft, a nature-based faith, with Satanism, a belief practice that grew out of opposition to Christianity and was based on the deliberate perversion of Christian beliefs, contributed to this persecution. Similarly, there is a long history of Jews being persecuted, forcibly converted, hounded, and killed for their beliefs. A religious justification for anti-Semitism was a Christian belief that Jesus was killed by the Jews; therefore giving people the right to persecute them. In the current period, much hostility has been experienced by American Muslims, who are often targeted for discrimination and specific profiling. In the aftermath of the terrorist attacks of September 11, 2001, many mosques and Islamic centers were attacked and Muslims were threatened including Indian American Sikhs who wear turbans as part of their faith.

Given the space constraints of this chapter, we offer only a brief overview of religion and its significance. In learning about religions, extensive reading is crucial. Beyond reading, we encourage students to attend services of faiths not their own to begin to get a sense of the diversity of practices and beliefs.

REFLECTION QUESTIONS 10.2

- To what extent do you value a person's religious affiliation and/or spiritual traditions as a sign of his or her worth?
- Have you ever stood up for someone being harassed or oppressed on the basis of religion or spiritual tradition? If not, why not? Has anyone ever stood up for you in this way?
- What types of clients or client problems involving spirituality or religion would be most challenging for you? Why?
- What does it mean to you to be effective in working with someone who is dealing with issues around spirituality or religion?

Cults

An issue related to religion and spirituality is that of cults. These are differentiated from religions, which interact closely with mainstream society, and from sects that continue to interact with society while breaking off from established religions. According to Woody (2009), there are conflicting definitions of the word **cult**, and he cautions us to be mindful on how we describe it. He notes that historically, the definition has had a negative connotation and groups have been labeled cults depending on their size, their perceived acceptance in society in terms of beliefs and practices, and the group leader's role and influence. Along these lines, Fielding and Llewelyn (1996) outlined specific characteristics about a cult that includes (a) a common set of beliefs that are deviant from those of mainstream culture, (b) strong cohesiveness within the group and a separation from mainstream culture, (c) a pressure to conform to group norms, and (d) perception of the leaders of the group as charismatic and divine. Furthermore, Deikmann (1990) cautioned that the focus on labeling extreme groups has diverted attention from cult dynamics that might be present in socially sanctioned groups. Such dynamics include (1) compliance with the group where members are recruited based on their vulnerability and allegiance by isolating them from other sources of support and esteem; (2) dependence on the leader where the leader is placed on a pedestal, invoking feelings of inferiority among members; and (3) devaluation of others who are outside the group (Deikmann, 1990). As you will note, this description of a cult is quite negative and can be generalized to include many new religious groups. For instance, the Church of Jesus Christ of the Latter-Day Saints (also known as the Mormons) has been called a cult (Woody, 2009). As a result of this controversy, the use of the word *cult* has been widely criticized, and many are opting to use terms such as "new religious movement, alternative religious movement, emergent religion, or marginal religious movement" (Woody, 2009, p. 220). Nonetheless, the negative views of a cult persist in contemporary society, so much so that many scholars are using a different terminology to describe religious and spiritual groups as noted here. To support this, Olson (2006) found that in a randomly selected sample of approximately 2,400 people living in Nebraska, an overwhelming 81% indicated that they would feel uncomfortable if their neighbor joined a cult, whereas the majority (63%) felt comfortable if the neighbor joined a "new religious movement." More striking was that nearly 90% of the sample endorsed feeling comfortable if their neighbor joined a "new Christian group."

Intersections of Spirituality and Religion with Ethnicity

Many cultural groups have an identified religious or spiritual orientation that pervades much of the culture (Albanese, 1992). For instance, many of the edicts in the Koran are directly related to Middle Eastern culture, and the sacred text is written in Arabic. Catholicism as practiced in Mexico has unique features and celebrations that are indigenous to the culture and that even non-Catholics may well celebrate, such as the Day of the Dead. As mentioned earlier, Christianity, in its aspects as a monotheistic religion that places human beings at the apex of creation, is woven into the dominant cultural fabric of the United States. However, it is crucial not to overgeneralize the connections between culture and religion. For example, not all Arabs are Muslims, not all Chinese are Buddhists, not all African Americans are Baptists, not all Indians are Hindus, and not all Europeans are Christians. A culture-oriented approach to spirituality and religion legitimately highlights diversity rooted in culture. At the same time, it is important to balance the group identification, both the universal aspects of spirituality common to all people across cultures, as well as the unique aspects that allow individual expression of spiritual beliefs. In this section, we provide an overview of some features that are significant to the practice of religious and spiritual traditions within select groups.

African American spirituality

Spirituality is considered an integral part of African American identity and a major part of surviving slavery and continuing struggles. Perhaps the most visible expression is in the Black church, consisting of Methodist, Pentecostal, and Baptist denominations, which provides a place of worship, prayer, catharsis, validation of life experiences, as well as fellowship, community, parental and child support, political activism, education, and refuge from discrimination (Boyd-Franklin & Lockwood, 1999). Music is also a significant medium, with many Black traditions of music being rooted in a communal expression of liberation and solidarity. Although many African Americans follow Christian traditions, Spiritism and West African–derived forms of spirituality also exist within the community. **Santeria**, a Caribbean religion that originated with the Yoruba people in what is now Nigeria, includes saint worship, feasts, festivals, rituals, offerings, and sacrifices through the worship of **orishas** that are deities and spirit manifestations (Gonzalez-Wippler, 1992). **Vodou** (sometimes called *voodoo* or *vodoun*), prevalent particularly in such places like Louisiana and Haiti, is based on an earth religion that involves the worship of ancestors and deities, and includes magic and ritual in everyday life (Falicov, 1999). In addition, **Kwanzaa** is an African American communal celebration initiated by Dr. Karenga in the late 1960s as both a way to celebrate the new year and a reminder of the history of black communities in the United States. Patterned on the African celebration of harvest, it consists of a 7-day celebration, marked by principles that serve as building blocks for the community, during which tribute is paid to the ancestors and to God while at the same time the participants pray for another benevolent year. These principles, also known as **nguzo saba**, consist of *umaja* (unity), *kujichagulia* (self-determination), *ujima* (collective work and responsibility), *ujamaa* (cooperative economics), *nia* (purpose), *kuumba* (creativity), and *imani* (faith) (Karenga, 2008). The celebration has also become an opportunity for African American communities to teach younger generations about African culture, values, symbols, and language. There are a variety of religions that are indigenous to Africa, of which some might be practiced in the United States; however, it is not our intent to provide an exhaustive description of these religions due to page limitations. We encourage the reader to seek out resources to learn more about them.

REFLECTION QUESTIONS 10.3

- What are some of the beliefs, images, or stereotypes you have held about African American spirituality?
- Where did these beliefs, images, or stereotypes come from?
- How have they changed over time, and what caused them to change for you?
- How do these beliefs, images, or stereotypes affect your work with people who practice these traditions?
- What have been some of your experiences with African American spirituality, if any?
- In what ways is African American spirituality similar to or different from your own religious or spiritual tradition?

Asian American spirituality

Similar to Latino immigrants, many Asians bring a heritage that is influenced by Eastern spiritual thought from Confucianism, Taoism, Shintoism, Buddhism, and Hinduism (Tan & Dong, 2000). Many of these religions emphasize harmony and interdependence in the natural world as well as in society. Many also emphasize the importance of the family unit, which leads to the close-knit and collectivist, as well as patriarchal and hierarchical, family structure that is common in Asian societies. Mind–body–spirit interconnectedness is another core aspect, often leading to psychosomatic experiencing of distress, rather than singularly psychological labeling of mental illness. Islam is also a factor, particularly in Asians from Indonesia and Malaysia, where a large portion are Muslim. Christianity is also common due to the efforts of missionary churches, so that Busto (1996) reported that about 60% of Asian Americans reported themselves to be a member of a Christian denomination. Quite a few young Asian Americans are often involved in evangelical and fundamental Christian groups in communities and on college campuses. It is important to keep in mind the connection between traditional values and beliefs that are present even in the context of being an adherent of a faith that may not hold such values. Thus, many Asian Americans may not seek mental health services because of a reluctance to look outside the family, as well as a value in enduring suffering and being in harmony.

REFLECTION QUESTIONS 10.4

- What are some of the beliefs, images, or stereotypes you have held about Asian American spirituality?
- Where did these beliefs, images, or stereotypes come from?
- How have they changed over time, and what caused them to change for you?
- How do these beliefs, images, or stereotypes affect your work with people who practice these traditions?
- What have been some of your experiences with Asian American spirituality, if any?
- In what ways is Asian American spirituality similar to or different from your own religious or spiritual tradition?

European American spirituality

The majority population in the United States, most European Americans have been influenced significantly by Judeo-Christian beliefs. The various ethnic groups that comprise European Americans are most visible in the arena of religion, with Irish Catholics, Scottish Presbyterians, German Lutherans, Greek Orthodox, and Eastern European Jews as examples of the bonds between ethnicity and religion. This may also lead to diverse expressions of the same religious denomination. For instance, Irish, Polish, and Italian Catholics hold a variety of expressions of the same religion, such that with the Irish the Church is primary, whereas with the Italians the family is primary with the Church being secondary, and with the Polish there is no separation between Church and family (Giordano & McGoldrick, 1996).

Regionalism too plays a role in the diverse expression of religious and spiritual beliefs. Thus Southern Baptists may be stricter and more conservative in their observance of moral codes than Baptists in the North.

Many European Americans may be less influenced by ethnic heritage in their religion, as they lose touch with specific ethnic roots and perceive themselves to be ethnically neutral or too mixed to be able to trace allegiance to any particular ethnic heritage. They may choose religious affiliation based on a variety of factors, such as the theological belief system, the religious leader, engagement with activism, closeness to home, and room for family and children in the religious community. A large minority reject religion and prefer to consider themselves atheist or agnostic, whereas others explore Eastern religions, such as Buddhism or European Pagan spiritual beliefs, such as Wicca.

REFLECTION QUESTIONS 10.5

- What are some of the beliefs, images, or stereotypes you have held about European American spirituality?
- Where did these beliefs, images, or stereotypes come from?
- How have they changed over time, and what caused them to change for you?
- How do these beliefs, images, or stereotypes affect your work with people who practice these traditions?
- What have been some of your experiences with European American spirituality, if any?
- In what ways is European American spirituality similar to or different from your own religious or spiritual tradition?

Latino/a spirituality

As mentioned earlier, although Catholicism is a major religious affiliation for many Latinos due to the colonization of Latin and South America by the Portuguese and Spanish, indigenous customs and practices are very much present. Because so many Latinos in the United States have a history of migration, such practices fortify ties with their heritage (Falicov, 1999). Many may share belief in the supernatural and have explanations for chronic problems that are based on witchcraft. *Mal puesto* (an illness or condition caused by a hex) can explain infertility or mental illness, and *brujeria* (witchcraft) can cause relationship difficulties. Folk healing is practiced by **curanderos** (folk healers) who use a variety of herbal remedies, incantations, consultations with spirits, trances, and cleansing rituals. *Curanderismo* (the use of natural remedies, such as herbs and religious rituals to cure physical and spiritual ailments) focuses on harmony between individuals, families, communities, and the environment (Foster, 1960). *Espiritistas* (spiritual healers), who have the ability to communicate with spirits and to access power for healing, are also among the indigenous healers available (Falicov, 1999). Santeria, mentioned earlier, is also prevalent among Cubans, Puerto Ricans, and others from the Caribbean. It is possible for many Latinos to embrace their Catholic beliefs as well as incorporate other spiritual and magical rituals and practices. Icons of saints, statues of the Virgin Mary, and sanctified items, such as devotional texts are often prominently displayed, and belief in miracles, proprietary rituals, such as lighting candles in church, promises, and prayers shape Latino religious life. It is also important to note the presence of many Latino Jews.

REFLECTION QUESTIONS 10.6

- What are some of the beliefs, images, or stereotypes you have held about Latino/a spirituality?
- Where did these beliefs, images, or stereotypes come from?
- How have they changed over time, and what caused them to change for you?
- How do these beliefs, images, or stereotypes affect your work with people who practice these traditions?
- What have been some of your experiences with Latino/a spirituality, if any?
- In what ways is Latino/a spirituality similar to or different from your own religious or spiritual tradition?

Native American spirituality

Native American spirituality believes that immaterial forces, such as a Supreme Being, can appear in many manifestations and have power in determining what happens in people's everyday lives and that all aspects of life are interrelated through the spiritual dimension. A person's mind, body, and emotions form an interconnected triad; whatever alters one component also influences the others. Lack of wellness within mind–body–spirit is often the result of suppressed emotions, such as anger and fear, resulting in physical and mental deterioration. Mental health concerns are said to involve a weakening of the spirit, and the goal is to identify natural or unnatural causes that have contributed to the life problem and rectify them. In various tribe affiliations, the medicine wheel is symbolic of mind–body–spirit–nature. The four compass directions in the wheel have east representing birth, future, and beginnings; south representing trust and the building of foundations; west representing strength and courage; and north representing wisdom. Health is attained by balancing the four directions (Trujillo, 2000). This represents both personal growth as well as the cycle of the seasons, emphasizing the interconnection between humans and nature.

In the tribe, the shaman is one who has a special relationship with the natural world and spirit powers, and makes use of rituals, ceremonies, and prayers to help tribal members. Some of the ceremonies across different tribes include the purification ritual in the sweat lodges, the Sun Dance, the vision quests among the people of the plains, as well as the use of peyote in some rituals to experience spiritual visions. All of these are focused on experiencing transcendence, finding the inner self, or connecting with the spirit powers (Trujillo, 2000).

Christianity has been a thorny issue among Native Americans because they experienced much oppression early on from missionaries who tried to "civilize" them by attempting to eradicate their culture and values. On the other hand, one of the manifestations of Christianity incorporated with indigenous practices has been the establishment of the Native American Church as a pan-Indian movement that is a source of strength, resilience, and pride (Hammerschlag, 1988).

 REFLECTION QUESTIONS 10.7

- What are some of the beliefs, images, or stereotypes you have held about African American spirituality?
- Where did these beliefs, images, or stereotypes come from?
- How have they changed over time, and what caused them to change for you?
- How do these beliefs, images, or stereotypes affect your work with people who practice these traditions?
- What have been some of your experiences with Native American spirituality, if any?
- In what ways is Native American spirituality similar to or different from your own religious or spiritual tradition?

CASE STUDY **10.4**

School Counselor Christine

Christine is an experienced school counselor in a wealthy private school located in a large Midwestern city. Although nonsectarian, the school has a large concentration of Anglican teachers, parents, and students. Christine is also Anglican, and participates in a prayer breakfast with many others in the school cafeteria once a week. She wears a discreet gold cross on a necklace every day. One day one of the parents, Fatima, calls Christine about Abdullah, her 14-year-old son. Christine had earlier recruited Fatima to sit on a parent advisory council that Christine convenes monthly. Fatima reports that Abdullah has become unusually withdrawn at home, reluctant to talk with either of his parents and somewhat surly. She further notes that when she approached him, he said he was "fed up" with a "Christian student" who, in the course of an argument, addressed him with a racial epithet. Christine reflects that Abdullah has been an outstanding student who seemed to get along well with his peers, and begins to plan how she might invite him to talk, only to be surprised when Fatima asks for a referral to "someone who would be able to work with

him," because she expects that Christine will be unable to work with him because he is a Muslim.

Source: "Counselors, communities, and spirituality: Ethical and multicultural considerations" (p. 321) by S. D. Lonborg & N. Bowen, 2004, *Professional School Counseling*, 7(5), 318–325. Copyright 2004 by *Professional School Counseling*. Adapted with permission.

Case Discussion
Thinking About the Case
1. Should Christine be surprised at Fatima's assumptions and stance?
2. Should Christine find a Muslim counselor referral for Abdullah, or should she encourage him to see her first?
3. How might she handle the interaction with Fatima to reassure her that Abdullah's needs will be met?
4. What interventions can Christine use to integrate Abdullah's religious beliefs as well as his experience in the school?

As mentioned in the case study, Christine has clearly communicated her spiritual beliefs to students through her participation in the prayer breakfasts and wearing of the cross. Although the school is in accordance with her religious beliefs, and there is no penalty for her activities, because in her capacity as counselor Christine serves students from other faiths, her involvement in such activities may convey unwillingness, inability, or disinterest in respecting other spiritual traditions. How can Christine communicate her respect for diverse traditions? Her recruitment of Fatima to serve on the council is one indication that she desires diverse viewpoints, but the proof will be in her ability to hear this diversity of viewpoints when expressed. For instance, if she chooses to work with Abdullah, how safe will he feel in confiding to her that he is being harassed by a group of students who all attend her prayer breakfast? If he is able to tell her, how might she handle the situation? Beyond simply addressing it as a student conflict, there may be ways in which Christine can incorporate an institutional responsibility to create a safer environment for students of minority faiths. Moreover, Christine may want to work with Abdullah herself, but if both Fatima and Abdullah choose to work with an external referral, it is necessary that Christine be well acquainted with the resources in the local community. At the very least, she should have an acquaintance with the local Muslim professionals or imams to be able to consult with them in her work.

REFLECTION EXERCISE **10.2**

Mindfulness of five things

This is a simple exercise to center yourself and connect with your environment. Practice it at any time during the day, especially anytime you find yourself getting caught up in your thoughts and feelings. The steps are as follows:

1. Pause for a moment,
2. Breathe in and out with attention to your breath for five breaths,
3. Look around, and notice five things you can see.
4. Listen carefully, and notice five things you can hear.
5. Notice five things you can feel in contact with your body (e.g., your watch against your wrist, your pants against your legs, the air upon your face, your feet upon the floor, and your back against a chair).

Notice what thoughts are passing through your mind as you do this. Notice what feelings are passing through your body. Observe those thoughts and feelings without judging them as good or bad, and without trying to change them, avoid them, or hold onto them. Simply observe them. Notice what it's like to observe those thoughts and feelings with an attitude of acceptance.

OPENING THE DIALOGUE ON SPIRITUALITY AND RELIGION

With all of the topics discussed in this chapter, you are now challenged to think through how you would utilize this information in sessions with any number of clients from a variety of cultural backgrounds and worldviews. Questions for reflection offered to you throughout this chapter also serve as excellent process questions for opening the dialogue with clients on issues of religion and spirituality. Some of these questions are listed here to assist you in terms of opening the dialogue with your clients:

- How do you understand the nature of human beings? Are humans good, bad, or neutral?
- How do you explain death and what happens to people after they die?
- Do people have free will, or are their destinies fated?
- Why do bad things happen to good people?
- What does it mean to you to be spiritual? What does it mean to be religious?
- In what spiritual tradition, if any, were you raised, and have you deviated from that tradition at all? If so, why?
- How important is your spiritual and/or religious tradition to you, and in what ways?
- Who are you in terms of spirituality and religion? How important is this in your personal and cultural identity, and what impact do these dimensions have on how you view the world and live your life?
- How did your spiritual and religious definitions of yourself develop, and who were some significant people in your life who helped to shape this definition?
- How has your view of spirituality and religion been reinforced or challenged during your life?
- What does your culture say about spirituality and religion?
- What do your family and community say about spirituality and religion in terms of both beliefs and practice?
- How do issues of power and privilege influence your view of spirituality and religion and your concept of oppression based on religious or spiritual tradition?
- How has your view of spirituality and religion affected the way you define yourself now and at previous points in your life?
- How will your view of spirituality and religion continue to affect the way you define yourself and the way others see you or treat you?
- How has your view of spirituality and religion affected the way you interact with others who are similar to you in age (versus different from you) at different points in your life?
- Who are some people of your own spirituality and religion that you look up to, and why?
- How might the difference or similarity in spirituality and religion between you (client) and I (counselor) affect your experience in the process of counseling as well as the relationship between us?

- When and how did you first become aware of religious or spiritual-based oppression? What was your initial reaction, and how did that reaction change over time?
- What have your experiences with religious or spiritual-based oppression been, and in what ways have those experiences shaped who you are as a person, as well as the issues you are dealing with now?
- What efforts have you made to work toward positive social change with regard to the religious or spiritual-based oppression that exists in your own life at the individual, group, and societal levels, and what other kinds of efforts would you like to make?
- To what extent do you value a person's religious affiliation and/or spiritual traditions as a sign of his or her worth?
- Have you ever stood up for someone being harassed or oppressed on the basis of religious or spiritual tradition? If not, why not? Has anyone ever stood up for you in this way?
- How do religion and spirituality play into the issues you are bringing to counseling, and how can we address this in a way that is most helpful to you?

CONCLUSION AND IMPLICATIONS

Obtaining information about a client's religious and spiritual background is just as important as assessing psychosocial identity, history, and functioning. The topic can be addressed directly in gathering general descriptive information about the centrality of religion and spirituality in the client's life, including specific practices and beliefs, as well as determining the extent to which they serve as a source of support.

Clients may also seek help for specific problems of a religious or spiritual nature. These include conversion to a new faith that is either forced or voluntary, where the client must complete a certain amount of grief work and adjustment to the demands of the new faith and way of life; loss or questioning of faith, which may sometimes result in ostracism from a close-knit community; faith or beliefs that may be serving as a barrier to wellness such as conditional love based on pleasing performance, constant maintenance of inner peace even in the face of trauma, or belief that real faith implies healing on demand of proper prayers. Other spiritual problems for which clients may seek assistance include mystical experiences and near death experiences that the client may have difficulty integrating into his or her life, chronic or terminal illnesses that may influence one's spiritual beliefs, as well as membership in cults or cult-like groups.

For counselors to incorporate spirituality into the counseling relationship requires some general ground rules. Fukuyama and Sevig (1999) developed three guidelines: the need for the counselor to seek clarity about his or her own spiritual and religious beliefs; to develop an in-depth understanding of the client's spiritual and religious beliefs; and, finally, to maintain ongoing participation in supervision and consultation to enhance ethical practice in using certain interventions. In terms of developing interventions, Faiver et al. (2001) advise five major prescriptions that they consider helpful: (1) affirming the client's spiritual belief system to be able to create an empathic and strong alliance, (2) using compatible vocabulary and imagery to enter the client's worldview, (3) consulting with other religious or spiritual authorities in the client's life to gain insight and deepen the power of interventions, (4) using stage models of spiritual identity development to ascertain the client's position, and (5) being cautious and careful but willing to distinguish toxic versus healthy practices and values in the client's spiritual system. This last guideline requires further exploration. On the one hand, counselors must seek to be open to clients' religious and spiritual beliefs, but these can also create conflicts. The time to intervene is when these situations conflict with legal and ethical obligations, such as when clients claim that child sexual abuse is a spiritual practice, or are being commanded to commit suicide. The 1978 mass suicide of over 900 American people living in the Jonestown settlement located in Guyana is an example of the powerful influence of a leader, Jim Jones, in ordering the residents to ingest poison. Spiritual interventions often focus on the esoteric, encouraging the client to explore the subjective meanings of experiences, such as meditating amidst nature or with close kin. Religious interventions utilize the client's exoteric religious path, such as by encouraging attendance at religious events. Similarly, interventions that are religious can be denominational or ecumenical (i.e., utilizing the theology specific to the client's religious denomination, or being more universal in nature). They may occur within the session or outside it. In other words, a client can be directed to pray for guidance in accordance with his or her religious belief system while at worship, or they may develop a prayer in the session. Bibliotherapy, through using texts meaningful to the client's belief system, is another intervention. More particularly, sacred texts such as the Bible or Koran can be used for quotations,

teaching specific concepts, or challenging irrational beliefs.

Religion and spirituality have become increasingly important in American society. A majority of Americans identify themselves with a particular religion (U.S. Bureau of the Census, 2003), and consider it a significant part of their lives. As Houston Smith (2001) states in the opening quote for this chapter, one of the primary means of staying open and attentive to the diversity of belief systems that people bring with them is to listen. In many ways, our religious and spiritual beliefs are significant because no matter what their content, they are our attempt to answer the unanswerable, to seek help to sustain, challenge, nurture, and guide us in our lives. As we strive to assist clients who struggle with problems, we cannot overlook the resources, values, and beliefs they bring that may help or hinder them in their struggles.

GLOSSARY

Anima: Carl Jung's archetype for the feminine side of the self.

Animus: Carl Jung's archetype for the male side of the self.

Brujeria: Witchcraft practiced in Spanish-speaking countries, and in some Latino communities in the United States.

Core belief: A fundamental faith-based belief.

Cult: Often used to refer to a group that has (a) a common set of beliefs different from the mainstream, (b) a specific leader who directs and guides the group, (c) strong coherence among its members, and (d) members who separate themselves from the mainstream society. The term *cult* has negative connotations.

Curanderismo: The use of natural remedies, such as herbs to cure an illness. It is practiced in Latino communities across the United States, and in Spanish-speaking countries such as Mexico.

Curandero/a: A folk healer who practices *cuanderismo*.

Espiritista: A spiritual healer who has the ability to call spirits for assistance in curing an illness or personal problem.

Esoteric expression: The inner sense of consciousness, sometimes referred to as a *spiritual state of enlightenment*.

Exoteric expression: The external or public that is expressed through organized religion and religious beliefs.

Kwanzaa: A 7-day celebration that honors African culture and history based on seven fundamental principles known as *nguzo saba*. During this time, people gather to celebrate ancestors, community, and family.

Mal puesto: An illness or abnormality caused by a hex in Latino culture.

Nguzo saba: The seven principles of African culture, which are *umaja* (unity), *kujichagulia* (self-determination), *ujima* (collective work and responsibility), ujamaa (cooperative economics), *nia* (purpose), *kuumba* (creativity), and *imani* (faith).

Orishas: An African spirit or deity that has specific roles and purposes, such as Shango, the male worrier representing power, and Oshun, the female representing fertility, beauty, and love (Wikipedia, n.d.-b).

Religion: A set of beliefs and devotion to some organized faith. It is also the social vehicle and organizational framework to express and practice specific faith-based beliefs.

Santeria: A belief system that comes from the Yoruba religion, which is a combination of African, indigenous, and Roman Catholic traditions and practices. It is practiced mostly in the Caribbean Practices include animal sacrifices, communicating with ancestors, and spirits (Orishas) such as Obatalá, Oggún, and Changó

Shadow: Carl Jung's archetype for the part of the self that is impulsive, instinctual, and viewed as the dangerous or dark side of the human experience.

Spirituality: A desire to understand human existence, the universe, and a sense of connectedness or wholeness beyond the physical; not tied to any one religion.

Vodou: The worship of deities and ancestors that includes rituals and magic. Sometimes referred to as *voodoo*.

REFERENCES

Albanese, C. L. (1992). *America: Religions and religion* (2nd ed.). Belmont, CA: Wadsworth.

Allport, G. W. (1950). *The individual and his religion.* New York: Macmillan.

Aranya, H. (1983). *Yoga philosophy of Patanjali.* Albany: State University of New York Press.

Armstrong, T.D. (1999). The impact of spirituality on the coping process of families dealing with pediatric HIV or pediatric nephritic syndrome (Doctoral dissertation, University of North Carolina at Chapel Hill, 1998). *Dissertation Abstracts International*, 59 (12-B), 6482.

Boyd-Franklin, N., & Lockwood, T. W. (1999). Spirituality and religion: Implications for psychotherapy with African American clients and families. In F. Walsh (Ed.), *Spiritual resources in family therapy* (pp. 90–103). New York: Guilford.

Burke, M. T. (1998). From the chair. *The CACREP Connection*, 2.

Burke, M. T., Hackney, H., Hudson, P., Miranti, J., Watts, G. A., & Epp. L. (1999). Spirituality, religion, and CACREP curriculum standards. *Journal of Counseling and Development*, 77, 251–258.

Busto, R. V. (1996). The gospel according to the model minority? Hazarding an interpretation of Asian American evangelical college students. *Amerasia Journal*, 22, 133–147.

Canda, E. R. (1988). Spirituality, religious diversity, and social work practice. *Social Casework*, 69, 292–298.

Deikmann, A. (1990). *The wrong way home: Uncovering the patterns of cult behavior in American society.* Boston: Beacon Press.

Faiver, C., Ingersoll, R. E., O'Brien, E., & McNally, C. (2001). *Explorations in counseling and spirituality: Philosophical, practical, and personal reflections.* Belmont, CA: Wadsworth.

Falicov, C. J. (1999). Religion and spiritual traditions in immigrant families: Therapeutic resources with Latinos. In F. Walsh (Ed.), *Spiritual resources in family therapy* (pp. 104–120). New York: Guilford.

Fielding, R. G., & Llewelyn, S. (1996). The new religions and psychotherapy: Similarities and differences. In G. Claxton (Ed.), *Beyond therapy: The impact of eastern religions on psychological theory and practice* (pp. 271–289). Dorset, UK: Prism.

Fowler, J. W. (1981). *Stages of faith.* New York: Harper & Row.

Frame, M. W. (2003). *Integrating religion and spirituality into counseling: A comprehensive approach.* Pacific Grove, CA: Brooks/Cole.

Frankl, V. E. (1963). *Man's search for meaning.* Boston: Beacon Press.

Fukuyama, M., & Sevig, T. (1999). Spiritual issues in counseling: A new course. *Counselor Education & Supervision*, 36, 224–232.

Genia, V. (1995). *Counseling and psychotherapy with religious clients: A developmental approach.* Westport, CT: Praeger.

Giordano, J., & McGoldrick, M. (1996). European families: An overview. In M. McGoldrick, J. Giordano, & J. K. Pearce (Eds.), *Ethnicity and family therapy* (2nd ed., pp. 427–441). New York: Guilford Press.

Gonzalez-Wippler, M. (1992). *The Santeria experience.* Saint Paul, MN: Llewellyn.

Green, W. S. (1994). Religion and society in America. In J. Neusner (Ed.), *World religions in America* (pp. 293–301). Louisville, KY: Westminster/John Knox Press.

Hammerschlag, C. (1988). *The dancing healers: A doctor's journey of healing with Native Americans.* New York: HarperCollins.

Hanna, F. J., & Green, A. (2004). Asian shades of spirituality: Implications for multicultural school counseling. *Professional School Counseling*, 7(5), 326–333.

Javaheri, F. (2006). Prayer healing: An experiential description of Iranian prayer healing. *Journal of Religion and Health*, 45(2), 171–182.

Karenga, M. (2008). *Kwanzaa: A celebration of family, community and culture.* Los Angeles: Sankore Press.

Kilpatrick, A. C. (1999). Ethical issues and spiritual dimensions. In A. C. Kilpatrick & T. P. Holland

(Eds.), *Working with families: An integrative model by level of need*. Boston: Allyn & Bacon.

Kurtz, E. (1999). The historical context. In W. R. Miller (Ed.). *Integrating spirituality into treatment: Resources for practitioners* (pp. 19–46).Washington, DC: American Psychological Association.

Lonborg, S. D., & Bowen, N. (2004). Counselors, communities, and spirituality: Ethical and multicultural considerations, *Professional School Counseling*, 7(5), 318–325.

Moodley, R., & Sutherland, P. (2009). Traditional and cultural healers and healing: Dual interventions in counseling and psychotherapy. *Counselling and Spirituality*, 28(1), 11–32.

Olson, P. J. (2006). The public perception of "cults" and "new religious movements." *Journal of the Scientific Study of Religion*, 45, 97–106.

Oser, F. K. (1991). The development of religious judgment. In F. K. Oser & W. G. Scarlett (Eds.), *Religious development in childhood and adolescence* (pp. 5–25). San Francisco: Jossey-Bass.

Piaget, J. (1972). *The psychology of the child*. New York, NY: Basic Books.

Siegel, R. J., Choldin, S., and Orost, J. H. (1995). Impact of three patriarchal religions on women. In J. C. Chrisler & A. H. Helmstreet (Eds.), *Variations on a theme: Diversity and the psychology of women* (pp. 107–144). Albany: State University of New York Press.

Smith, H. (1991). *The world's religions*. New York: HarperCollins.

Tan, S-Y., & Dong, N. J. (2000). Psychotherapy with members of Asian American churches and spiritual traditions. In P. S. Richards & A. E. Bergin (Eds.), *Handbook of psychotherapy and religious diversity* (pp. 421–444). Washington, DC: American Psychological Association.

Thurston, N. S. (2000). Psychotherapy with evangelical and fundamentalist Protestants. In P. S. Richards & A. E. Bergin (Eds.), *Handbook of psychotherapy and religious diversity* (pp. 131–153). Washington, DC: American Psychological Association.

Trujillo, A. (2000). Psychotherapy with Native Americans: A view into the role of religion and spirituality. In P. S. Richards & A. E. Bergin (Eds.), *Handbook of psychotherapy and religious diversity* (pp. 445–466). Washington, DC: American Psychological Association.

U.S. Bureau of the Census. (2003). Self-described religious identification of adult population: 1990 and 2001. *2003 statistical abstract of the United States.* Retrieved from http://www.census.gov/prod/2004pubs/03statab/pop.pdf

Vontress, C. E. (1991). Traditional healing in Africa: implications for cross-cultural counseling. *Journal of Counseling & Development*, 70(1), 242–249.

Wikipedia: The free encyclopedia. (n.d.-a). Islam. Retrieved from http://en.wikipedia.org/wiki/Islam

Wikipedia: The free encyclopedia. (n.d.-b). Orisha. Retrieved from http://en.wikipedia.org/wiki/Orisha

Woody, W. D. (2009). Use of *cult* in the teaching of psychology of religion and spirituality. *Psychology of religion and Spirituality*, 1, 218–232.

Wulff, D. M. (1996). The psychology of religion: An overview. In E. P. Shafranske (Ed.), *Religion and the clinical practice of psychology*. Washington, DC: American Psychological Association.

Young, T. R. (2000). Psychotherapy with Eastern Orthodox Christians. In P. S. Richards & A. E. Bergin (Eds.), *Handbook of psychotherapy and religious diversity* (pp. 89–104). Washington, DC: American Psychological Association.

CHAPTER **11**

Disability

Growing up, I wanted to dis-identify myself with the image or label of being a cripple. I wanted to be normal.... I avoided other disabled people. I refused to see myself as part of that group.... I drank excessively, consumed drugs and cigarettes, acted out my anger in violent outbursts, ended up in jails and hospitals. Finally, through some mysterious grace, I woke up and found myself in the company of an excellent therapist....

I joined a group of disabled women on the advice of my therapist. I hated the idea, but to my surprise they were marvelous, dynamic women. They shared so many of what I had always thought were my own isolated, personal experiences that I began to realize that my supposedly private hell was a social phenomenon.

Source: From J. Tollifson, "Imperfection is a Beautiful Thing: On Disability and Meditation," in K. Fries (Ed.) *Staring Back: The Disability Experience from the Inside Out* (New York: Plume)

Disability is a complex aspect of identity. Although the range and kind of disabilities are extremely varied, ranging from physical, to intellectual or psychiatric, an experience that persons with disabilities have in common is being devalued by society and often shunned. However, those who are able-bodied are only temporarily so, by chance and luck, a condition that will inevitably change with increasing age or by accident. Paradoxically, those who consider themselves able-bodied perceive a gulf between themselves and those with disabilities, even though the separating boundary is neither absolute nor clearly defined. In this chapter, we will examine some of the constructs of disability, looking at the historical development of such an identity, the sociopolitical aspects, and the experience of disability.

REFLECTION QUESTIONS 11.1

- What does it mean to have an ability or disability?
- What abilities or disabilities have you dealt with in own your life?

Notice that the Americans with Disabilities Act (1990) definition can encompass many conditions we do not generally associate with disability. By this definition, impairments can be temporary or permanent, reversible or irreversible, progressive or regressive, or serious or minor (Bickenbach, 1993). Many persons may believe that they are not disabled, but even if all one ever had was a broken arm or leg, a bad sprain, or a serious illness, that constitutes a temporary experience of disability. Beyond such temporary experiences, it is also necessary to acknowledge that impairment itself does not need to be as significant as being paraplegic, but can be an invisible condition such as Asperger's syndrome, or a socially insignificant condition such as having double-jointed fingers (Stone, 1995).

EXAMPLE **11.1**
ADA 1990

The Americans with Disabilities Act (1990) defines a person with a disability in three ways: (A) an individual who has a physical or mental impairment that substantially limits one or more of the major life activities of such individual; (B) A record of such impairment; or (C) Being regarded as having such impairment. *Physical or mental impairment* means: (1) Any physiological disorder or condition, cosmetic disfigurements, or anatomical loss affecting one or more of the following body systems: neurological, musculoskeletal, special sense organs, respiratory (including speech organs), cardiovascular, reproductive, digestive, genitourinary, hemic and lymphatic, skin, and endocrine; or (2) Any mental or psychological disorder, such as mental retardation, organic brain syndrome, emotional or mental illness, and specific learning disabilities. *Major life activities* means functions, such as caring for oneself, performing manual tasks, walking, seeing, hearing, speaking, breathing, learning, and working. *Substantially limits* means: (i) Inability to perform a major life activity that the average person in the general population can perform; or (ii) Significantly restricted as to the condition, manner, or duration under which an individual can perform a particular major life activity as compared to the condition, manner, or duration under which the average person in the general population can perform that same major life activity.

Note: Americans with Disabilities Act (1990) Section 1630.2.

REFLECTION EXERCISE **11.1**

Disability Awareness

- Go through your neighborhood and survey cars parked over drive-ways, unleashed dogs, sidewalks and curb cuts, color contrast on stairs (people with low vision need this), branches that can hit a blind person, and audible cues (such as horns honking).
- Look at the entrance to your favorite cafe or bookstore. Is it flat? Is there a small step? Are there lots of steps? What would need to be altered to make it accessible? Sometimes there's a loading ramp in back a disabled person can use. What do you think about having to enter that way?
- Go to a local clothing shop in the mall. Notice how much space there is between racks of clothes. What would this be like for someone who is blind or who has a mobility disability?

OVERVIEW OF DISABILITY

All human beings face limitations on their abilities. Given time to think about it, many of us can remember being in situations where we could not perform an activity because of boundaries our bodies could not cross. Whether it is being unable to reach a can on the highest shelf, unable to lift a suitcase due to its weight, missing a bus because of not being able to move fast enough, or taking the wrong turn because the sign was too small to read, our bodies told us in those instances that we had met a limit. However, Stone (1995) argued that most of us tend not to focus on such awareness of inability, which enables us to treat people with disabilities as "other," fundamentally different from ourselves in kind as opposed to degree. She pinpointed several aspects of dominant culture for this, particularly focusing on what she terms as "the myth of bodily perfection" (p. 413). In Western traditions, there is a consistent theme about the desirability and possibility of achieving perfect bodies. Christian beliefs that distinguish between the spirit and the body, regarding the body as essentially a temple for the spirit, result in the body being viewed as a reflection of morality and purity. So, disease or dysfunction in the body is evidence of spiritual and moral imperfection. The inability to manage disease or to be cured, as well as the inability to be normative, is then failure of the person (Livneh, 1982). In some other cultures, there may be causal explanations given for disability, so that a child with a disability is perceived as a sign of divine punishment of the parents, whereas in other cultures, disability is understood as infectious so that a pregnant woman, for instance, is discouraged from seeing or hearing or touching someone with a disability for fear of passing it on to her child (Groce, 2005).

Together with such prevailing values, the late 20th-century belief in technology and medicine as all-powerful led to the notion that all bodily failures were potentially fixable. In the 1950s, when many children lost the ability to walk due to the polio epidemic, they were subjected to numerous agonizing operations designed to allow them to walk again. This occurred repeatedly, even though the operations required long periods of painful recovery yet rarely achieved the desired result. To accept that one's child would not walk again and focus on making necessary adjustments was seen as defeatist and harshly judged. Normalization at any cost was perceived as better than having a disability (Kaufert & Kaufert, 1984).

These deeply rooted beliefs about health, attractiveness, productivity, competence, and the value of human life create an environment where those with physical, mental, cognitive, or sensory disabilities are treated with discrimination. **Ableism** is the manifestation of oppression against individuals with physical, mental, or developmental disabilities that is characterized by the belief that these individuals need to be repaired or cannot serve as full members of society (Castafieda & Peters, 2000). Because having a disability has been viewed as a deficiency rather than an aspect of difference, disability has only recently been recognized as a multicultural concern by practitioners (Smith, Foley, & Chaney, 2008).

The distorted and negative images of disability present in the dominant culture serve to discourage most people from acknowledging and accepting the wide range and number of disabilities present. So, a man who has a "bad back" that prevents him from doing heavy lifting does not see himself as impaired, nor does the woman who considers herself in excellent health but no longer drives because she suffers from sudden fainting spells. When persons with disabilities are objectified, it is easy to pretend one has nothing

---

EXAMPLE **11.2**
Disability in the Margins

My Blackness has been an integral part of my identity repertoire as I have negotiated the sometimes troublesome terrain of higher education. It influences the alliances I cultivate, the hypotheses I probe and the strategies I employ to simply stay sane in the face of disconnection from a mainstream academic culture. But my Blackness is not always my predominant identity. Many times throughout my studies my disability has ascended and my Blackness has been rendered subsidiary. Thus, even during my attendance at predominantly Black institutions—supposed safe spaces that can act as refuges from the torrent of otherness that can pelt Blacks at majority White institutions—otherness continued to rain down upon me. In short, as a disabled Black man, my disability can leave me drenched in otherness in a manner that my Blackness does not. Thus, for me, the dearth of discussions on ableism that students with disabilities can face during matriculation makes some diversity panels less diverse than their names might imply.

Source: Excerpted from A. Rahman Ford (2009) "It's Not Just About Racism, but Ableism: When Talking About Diversity, the Ableism that Students with Disabilities Face Should Be Part of the Conversation." *Diverse Issues in Higher Education*, 26(4), 16.

in common with such people and ignore the commonality we share as universally living in imperfect and limited bodies. *Passing*, a term first used in the context of People of Color who were sufficiently light-skinned to appear to be White, is also applicable here. Hillyer (1993) pointed out that passing as normal rather than disabled enhances the possibility of being accepted as an individual, as well as the ability to connect with those who would shun a person if he or she were seen as belonging to such a devalued group.

Disability is perceived as a condition to be avoided, and those who are visibly disabled find that their disability is not merely a salient part of their identity but also the exclusive means by which they become identified. Thus, someone in a wheelchair is not expected to climb a flight of stairs, but is often assumed to not be able to do anything else either. Being defined by this difference is a sign of oppression, particularly when the difference is seen as pathological. The use of a wheelchair by Franklin D. Roosevelt, one of the great American presidents and the man credited with leading the United States out of the Great Depression, was hidden from the public, because his use of the device would be seen as a sign of weakness (Blotzer & Ruth, 1995). In today's era of saturation media coverage, he would probably not even be elected. Even recently, having a 10-foot statue of him in a wheelchair at the FDR memorial in Washington, DC, was controversial.

The condition of disability is perceived as absolute; one either is or isn't. In actuality, some disabilities fluctuate across the continuum of visible and invisible. These fluctuations may be based on a change in the degree of disability, circumstances, or environment (Peters, 1993). An individual may have a psychiatric disorder such as schizophrenia, which may go into remission, leading to a change in the degree of disability. In some cases, the circumstances influence the visibility of the disability, so a person who is mobility impaired and employed as a receptionist behind a large desk may have a less visible disability versus this same person in a gym. Finally, the environment can also shape the perception of visibility, such that an adolescent with a learning disability working at a fast-food restaurant might have the disability invisible in such a context (Peters, 1993).

REFLECTION QUESTIONS 11.2

- To what extent do you define yourself around your abilities or disabilities?
- Are there any abilities you have that you think you've taken for granted at any point in your life?

Historical Context

Throughout history, there have been people with disabilities who have made their mark through their achievements and accomplishments. Often, the disability is overlooked or made invisible in the context of accomplishment, leaving the notion of disability as equated with impairment and inability. For instance, the *Rig Veda*, written in Sanskrit between 3500 and 1800 B.C., recounts the story of a warrior, Queen Vishpala, who lost her leg in battle, was fitted with an iron prosthesis, and returned to battle. In 218 B.C., Marcus Sergius, the Roman general who fought against Carthage, sustained many injuries and an amputation of his right hand, which was then fitted with an iron hand to hold his shield so he could return to battle. Beyond people such as Helen Keller, who was an activist and visionary for the rights of people who were blind and visually impaired, there are also other figures. Harriet Tubman, who spent her life fighting for civil rights and rescuing slaves, had epilepsy; as mentioned earlier, Roosevelt who was president of the United States for four terms, had polio; Frida Kahlo, world famous for her paintings, also contracted polio in childhood; and Wilma Mankiller, a principal chief of the Cherokee Nation, had muscular dystrophy.

In disability history, much has changed in the ways in which disability has been defined and people with disabilities have come to define themselves. Three different constructs of disability have existed across history (McColl & Bickenbach, 1998). The earliest is the *moral construct*, whereby disability is perceived as divine intervention or retribution. Disability is seen to be caused by a failing in the moral fiber of the individual, resulting in a manifestation of character flaws, a punishment by God, or a curse by the Devil. This sort of thinking can be seen in the debates of the 1990s where some who acquired HIV as a result of blood transfusions were seen as "innocent victims" of the disease whereas gay men who contracted it through sexual intercourse were thought to be punished for their "sinful lifestyle." In the 1800s, the *medical model* arose, which saw disability as something to be cured, an abnormality or pathology that could be fixed so that individuals could return to "normalcy." Many elements of the medical model of conceptualization are flourishing today, with emphasis on curing people to allow them to live normal lives. Finally, the *social model* began to gain acceptance in the 1960s, focusing on the cultural context in which attitudes about disability are shaped. Recognizing disability as a social identity, there is the acknowledgment that many of the barriers faced by persons with disabilities come from society rather than from internal limitations. For instance, when a person with a mobility impairment cannot go to the local movie theater because there are no ramps for her wheelchair, the limitation is one created by the lack of accommodation rather than by her use of a wheelchair.

Through the ages, persons with disabilities have struggled for change in the ways they are perceived and treated. In 1500, Girolamo Cardano was the first physician to recognize that being deaf was not the same as an inability to reason. Bonifacio published a treatise on sign language in 1616, and the first oral school for the deaf was established in 1755 in Germany. In 1790, Philippe Pinel in Paris had people with mental illness unshackled (Disability Social History Project, 2005).

The early 1900s saw both activism and discrimination. In 1935, a group in New York City called the League for the Physically Handicapped formed to protest discrimination by the Works Progress Administration (WPA). The 300-odd members of the league, mostly disabled by polio and cerebral palsy, had been turned down for WPA jobs. Members of the league protested through sit-ins and eventually generated a couple of thousand jobs nationwide.

At the same time, Dr. Alexis Carrel, a Nobel Prize winner, published his book *Man the Unknown*, where he suggested the removal of the mentally ill and the criminal by small euthanasia institutions equipped with suitable gases. This idea was taken up by the Nazi government, and a euthanasia program was instituted in 1939 to order the "mercy killing" of those who were sick and disabled. It is estimated that more than 100,000 people were killed by this program. The 1970s saw the rise of disability activism though the independent living program, and women with disabilities began organizing. In 1990, the Americans with Disabilities Act was signed into law (Disability Social History Project, 2005).

It is important to note that the consideration of disability as a unified concept is not universal (Groce, 2005), and in many cultures there may be no single word describing disability. In some cultures, disabilities are grouped by specific types of impairments, for instance placing those who are blind in separate categories from those who are deaf. The idea of disability as a category that encompasses people with a range of physical, emotional, intellectual, or sensory impairments is relatively recent.

Overview of the Americans with Disabilities Act (ADA)

As mentioned earlier, the ADA defined *disability* as meeting one of three conditions. Essentially, this law prohibited discrimination on the basis of disability in employment, state and local government, public accommodations, commercial facilities, transportation, and telecommunications. It also applies to the U.S. Congress.

Title I of the ADA covers employment and requires employers to provide qualified individuals with disabilities an equal opportunity to benefit from the full range of employment-related opportunities available to others. For example, it prohibits discrimination in recruitment, hiring, promotions, training, pay, social activities, and other privileges of employment. It restricts questions that can be asked about an applicant's disability before a job offer is made, and it requires that employers make reasonable accommodation to the known physical or mental limitations of otherwise qualified individuals with disabilities, unless it results in undue hardship.

Title II focuses on state and local governments and requires them to give people with disabilities an equal opportunity to benefit from all of their programs, services, and activities, such as public education, transportation, recreation, health care, social services, courts, or voting. When constructing new buildings or altering buildings, specific architectural standards must be followed; however, undue financial and administrative burdens are not required as long as reasonable modifications are made to policies and practices to avoid discrimination.

Title III covers public accommodations of those businesses and nonprofit service providers, such as restaurants, day care centers, funeral homes, homeless shelters, or fitness clubs and requires them to comply to prohibit exclusion, segregation, and unequal treatment. Title IV addresses telephone and television access for persons with hearing and speech disabilities.

In addition to the ADA, there is a structure of legal protections available such as the 1984 Voting Accessibility for the Elderly and Handicapped Act that required polling places across the United States to be physically accessible to persons with disabilities for federal elections. Similarly, the 1993 National Voter Registration Act strove to increase the historically low registration rates of marginalized communities by requiring all state-funded programs providing services to persons with disabilities to provide applicants with voter registration forms, as well as assistance in completing and transmitting the completed forms. The Individuals with Disabilities Education Act requires all public schools to make available to all eligible children with disabilities a free appropriate public education in the least restrictive environment appropriate to their individual needs (U.S. Department of Justice, 1992).

DISABILITY CULTURE

Beyond laws and legislation, a growing movement in the disability community has focused on developing a collective identity as a group. Although disability does not fit a strictly anthropological definition of culture, Bryan (1999) argues that people with disabilities do share common experiences, such as being perceived as damaged, or being considered extraordinary if one were to be successful. Unlike more normatively cultural groups such as ethnic groups, people with disabilities have historically been isolated and segregated not only from the mainstream society but also from each other. People with psychiatric disabilities were kept in institutions, and children with intellectual disabilities were removed from their families and placed in large institutions. People with disabilities often lived in poverty, given lack of access to employment and education, appropriate transportation, and housing. For those with physical disabilities, the lack of attendant care often made survival the focal point of existence. Environmental and communication barriers isolated persons with visual impairments and deafness. However, since the 1960s, social and political activism, the increased availability of adaptive technology, and attendant care have facilitated the communication of persons with disabilities to develop a more collective identity, drawn together by the commonalities of experience they share. This has changed much, from social perceptions to internalized perceptions of persons with disabilities. Swain and Cameron (1999) describe the process as "coming out as disabled" (p. 76) through rejecting the negative labels of normalcy, developing a positive recognition of impairment, and redefining disability as a valid social identity.

Although disability culture has provided a new context and perspective on the experience of disability, challenging the dominant sociocultural constructions of such an identity, this is still an evolving field. Disability studies comprises an interdisciplinary field drawing from social, historical, political, and economic sources to examine and articulate the construction of disabilities, and how people with disabilities are stigmatized (Kielhofner, 2005). There is much variety in even the terminology used and found acceptable. For instance, although *disabled* is acceptable as a label descriptor for many, others prefer *physically challenged*. In the United States, people-first language is preferred, whereby it is preferable to put the person before the condition, as

CASE STUDY **11.1**

Case of Peter

An automobile accident left Peter, a European American man in his early 30s, with paraplegia. It was devastating to him. He had been an enthusiastic athlete and saw no way he would participate in sports again. He told his wife to divorce him and find a "whole" man. He found it humiliating to be seen in public in his wheelchair. His disability was understood by him in the context of all the messages he had received about his role as an able-bodied man. He described himself as freakish and expressed suicidal thoughts of "being better off dead than half a man."

In an earlier period, Peter would have stayed isolated in his disability and surrounded by persons who shared his construction of his disability as terrible. More recently, however, he met with others with spinal cord injuries (SCI), who had all gone through the shock he had undergone: They had lost the ability to walk, lost volitional control over their bladders, and experienced the assumptions of the nondisabled people around them. Peter began to participate in a SCI subculture. When he referred to himself as a "T-12 para," everyone in his newfound group understood him to mean that he had a spinal cord injury at the 12th thoracic level. When people talked about a *TAB*, all knew the reference was to a "temporarily able-bodied" person. In a sign of solidarity about their shared experience, they might refer to each other as *gimp* or *crip*, using hate words from the dominant culture much as other marginalized groups might amongst themselves—an insider language not permitted to nondisabled outsiders.

Gradually over time, Peter adapted to his new life, and his disability lost its negative meaning. He began to participate again in sports, with wheelchair basketball, adapted track and field, and waterskiing, and felt a vital part of the new community and culture of which he was a member.

Case Discussion
Thinking About This Case
1. If Peter came to you for assistance immediately after acquiring his disability, how would you characterize him? What would you see as the main presenting problem?
2. If Peter came to you much later, presenting with depression, must his emotional state be connected with his disability?

As you read the case above, it becomes clear that Peter has undergone significant, meaningful changes in terms of both how he deals with his disability and earlier sense of loss, and how his own disability identity has shifted through his identification as a member of the SCI subculture. It would be interesting to explore with Peter how he sees himself now, how things have changed for him over time, and what kind of active role he played in that change. As a function of better understanding his cultural identity now, his sense of strengths and renewed purpose, and his sense of his own life, it could be important to explore with Peter what happened with his marriage and what part that has played in who and how he is now.

---

in *people with disabilities*, as opposed to identifying persons by their condition, as in *disabled people* or *the disabled*. However, in some activist circles, identifying themselves as disabled first is a way of signifying proud membership in the collective identity of disability (Gill, 2001). Although this may seem confusing, it is a normal aspect of any marginalized group's process of developing a sense of identity. Marginalized groups have historically been objectified and defined by others, and the process of empowerment involves developing acceptable language to self-identify. Inevitably, given the diversity amongst any collection of individuals who share one common group status, this is a dynamic process because social norms as well as oppressive conditions shift and change.

In *The Body Silent* (1987), author Robert Murphy describes his personal journey as he becomes degeneratively paralyzed by an inoperable spinal cord tumor. He writes the book virtually quadriplegic, hitting the keys of his computer with the eraser end of a pencil held in place by a 'universal cuff' wrapped around his palm. His riveting though uncomfortable narrative details the experience of profound physical alteration, its impact on his relationship with significant others, such as his wife on whom he becomes increasingly dependent, an unflinching exploration of the self, and a study of the social construction of disability as he is perceived as increasingly "other" by society.

FACTORS IMPACTING THE DISABILITY EXPERIENCE

In the context of the helping profession, our concern is to understand the sociopolitical and cultural milieux in which disability is constructed, as well as to understand the ways in which individual persons interact with these social constructions and are influenced. In this section, based on the important work of Vash and Crewe (2004), we discuss some of the general delineating factors that may influence how individuals experience and perceive their disabled status. Three major aspects are the disability, the person, and the environment, with each aspect having complex facets.

The Disability

The nature of the disability that a person has is a profound impact on the experience of the disability. The *time of onset* of the disability, whether present from birth or acquired later in life, is influential. For instance, speaking intelligibly is more difficult for those who became deaf before language acquisition. Furthermore, for acquired disabilities, one's developmental stage of life also shapes one's reactions. Being born with a disability or acquiring one in childhood may mean being subjected to isolation, overprotection or rejection from caretakers, and separation in family life, play, or education. On the other hand, a person who becomes disabled later in life may experience greater loss of well-established life activities, or no longer have resiliency. A study by Krause and Crewe (1991) suggested that in terms of spinal cord injuries, there was more effective adjustment to the disability by those who acquired it as young adults as opposed to later in life.

The *type of onset* of disability can also impact reactions, because it influences the kind of blame or responsibility attached to the disabling outcome. It is difficult to predict how a prolonged and progressive onset as opposed to a sudden one, or a self-generated versus other-produced injury, will affect an individual's reactions. For some, feeling some responsibility for their disability may lead to a greater sense of control, rather than feeling at the mercy of a random chance or malice. For others, the issues that influence adjustment may include opportunities to express anger or feel that adequate punishment has been handed out to the perpetrator.

Although persons with disabilities have commonalities of experience, the kinds of *functions impaired* generate different reactions because of the different adjustments required. Many nondisabled people, when asked the disability they would fear most, identify blindness (Vash & Crewe, 2004). However, people who are blind are less apt to think that it is the worst disability.

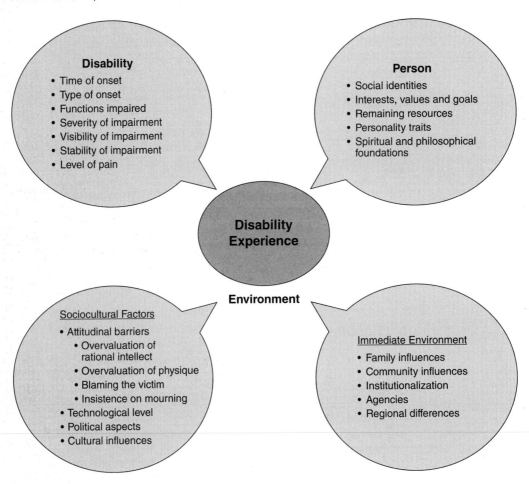

FIGURE **11.1** Factors Impacting Disability Experience

Source: Adapted from Vash, C. L., & Crewe, N. M. (2004). *Psychology of Disability, 2nd ed. Springer Series on Rehabilitation.* (New York: Springer)

The fear of blindness has generated far more wide-ranging adaptive and protective legislation than for any other disability. On the other hand, many deaf persons pride themselves on being part of Deaf Culture, and maintain that they simply communicate differently rather than have a disability. The characteristics of the person who is disabled tie in with the impact of impaired functions, so that for someone who is solaced most by the auditory stimuli of music, a mobility impairment might be perceived as less devastating than deafness.

The *severity of the disability* also shapes situational experiences. A woman with total paralysis may experience the fears of being totally dependent on others for survival, whereas the young man with a traumatic brain injury that has affected speech may experience the humiliation of seeing an interested attractive stranger turning away on hearing his words. Huebner and Thomas (1995) suggested that the greatest difficulties in adjustment may lie with those who are on either ends of the continuum of severity of disability. Associated with this issue is the *visibility of disability*, discussed earlier. In some ways, although visible disabilities generate the issues of physical appearance and cultural judgment of attractiveness, invisible disabilities can be interpersonally difficult as well because of misleading appearances of normality. For instance, the burly man who cannot lift heavy weights due to his back must always explain his inability and fear being disbelieved and judged as lazy. The *stability of the disability* is also a factor. For instance, a progressive disability with a downward course leading to death means that the individual has to adjust not only to the disability but also to an active disease process, fluctuating conditions, or issues of remission or relapse.

Finally, the degree and presence of *pain* are cardinal factors. When pain occurs, whether chronically through a progressive condition such as arthritis or in a stabilized condition such as amputation, it affects behavior, demeanor, attitude, and experience. As well as the challenges of coping with pain, because of its invisibility, one may also experience questioning by others of its validity or reality.

The Person

The characteristics of the person who is disabled are important determinants of the experience. *Issues of social identity* are key because the person's other status in society will shape how his or her disability status is perceived. Gender is one of the most important variables in shaping differential reactions and responses. Although men, who have a strong gender role expectation of being active, independent breadwinners, may be more devastated by a disability that counters such role expectations than a woman, a more stringent sociocultural demand is placed on women's aesthetic appearance that can be demoralizing to a woman with a disability who cannot meet the demands of physical perfection. In addition, identity aspects, such as socioeconomic status are crucial because so many adaptive devices can be acquired, as well as stressors ameliorated, through one's economic resources, social status, and ability to knowledgeably navigate the bureaucracy of care.

The racism associated with being a Person of Color can also impact the quality of services as well as access to services. Overall, there appears to be a higher rate of disabilities among members of racial and ethnic minority groups and among women than men (U.S. Census, 2000). Approximately 26.4% of the African American population has some type of disability, whereas Native Americans rose to 27%, as compared to 18.3% for non-Hispanic Whites. Such a high rate may be explained by other factors including the high rate of the African American population that works in semiskilled and unskilled labor, resulting in a higher likelihood of disabling injuries. There are relatively larger numbers of African Americans in the working class, leading to living conditions that pose greater hazards, such as chemical and toxic pollution, exacerbated by poor lighting, heat, and ventilation, and limited access to adequate health care (Bryan, 1999). In a similar vein, socioeconomic and cultural factors contribute to the proportionately huge increase in HIV infection among Latinos.

The *kinds of interests* a person has will also affect responses to a whole range of disabilities. For instance, it is ironic that persons who get spinal cord injuries were often extremely active and risky before their injury, and are, therefore, less prepared for a sedentary life. The range of interests is also important, because people whose interests span a wide diversity of physical, intellectual, passive, and active modes are more likely to be able to sustain a variety of interests than someone who has been singularly focused.

The *remaining resources* a person has following disability strongly influence coping. If a person develops a visual impairment but has resources, such as social poise, leadership skills, high energy, emotional stability, and/or strong career motivations, it is more likely that the person will be able to effectively build a secure and satisfying life. Such *personality attributes* of flexibility or adaptability will enhance coping.

Finally, one's *spiritual belief systems and life philosophy* create a foundation from which disability is understood and responded to. Understanding disability as punishment for sin, versus understanding it as an opportunity for spiritual development or, alternatively, as a chance occurrence in a random universe, will also lead to different responses to the disability. Ososkie and Schultz (2003) suggest that the existential issues of freedom, isolation, anxiety, meaning, and mortality are salient ones in experiencing life with a disability. For instance, due to other people's existential anxiety about disability, the person with a disability must confront isolation. Alternatively, there may be a sense of having lost freedom due to enforced physical dependency.

The Environment

One of the key ways of understanding the impact of the environment on disability experience is of delineating the difference between being disabled and being handicapped. Although being disabled is defined in terms of individual functioning, handicap refers to the restrictions and obstacles faced by a person with a disability in an ableist society. Therefore, whereas *disability* is the condition of the individual, *handicap* is the condition of the social context. The handicapping experienced by people with disabilities comes from two interrelated sources primarily: (a) the parts of the physical environment constructed by humans and (b) social customs, values, and expectations. For instance, a young man with paraplegia is handicapped when invited to dinner in a house that can only be reached thorough a flight of stairs, as well as by the social assumption carried through in architecture that stairs are the best way to go up a level even though ramps can serve both mobility-impaired and non-mobility-impaired people. These handicapping conditions impact all aspects of life depending on the disability, such as issues of housing, transportation, recreation, shopping, employment opportunity, work access, and job site. The discussion of environmental influences can be divided into two categories: the sociocultural context and the immediate environment.

Sociocultural Context

In the earlier section of this chapter, we explored the social aspect of devaluation of disability, from the extreme of the Nazi genocide of people with disabilities to the subtle and everyday segregation, avoidance, discomfort, or pity directed toward persons with disabilities. **Attitudinal barriers** are ways in which people with disabilities are grouped, categorized, labeled, or rejected by temporarily able-bodied persons. An example is the predisposition to stereotype by overgeneralizing about what persons with disabilities are like, what they are capable of, how they can be helped, or the conditions in which they should live. For instance, there is widespread feeling that persons with mental retardation should not be allowed to be sexually active, and even stronger feeling that they should not be allowed to reproduce. Institutions that house such persons often create exclusionary practices, ostensibly based on protecting the residents from harm, by restricting free movement and relationship.

In addition to the attitudinal barriers described above that are generated through societal constructions of disability, cultural aspects also impact disability experience. For instance, because of the dominant European American cultural emphasis on valuing independence, individualism, and the importance of a productive work ethic, the American rehabilitation system reflects these values. Therefore, families are discouraged from doing things for persons with disabilities that they might do for themselves; importance is placed on functional independence in daily activities of eating, sleeping, bathing, and dressing; and it is perceived as important that persons have some kind of productive employment, even if it is not meaningful, engaging, or in alignment with the person's talents. In other cultural groups, however, it may be seen as disrespectful to allow a grandparent to struggle to dress or eat without offering assistance. Yet, the available rehabilitation services and philosophy rarely take the culture of origin into account.

Technological level

The technological aids available to get around the functional limitations of disability shape the experience of disability greatly. Aids, such as powered lifts, text communication over telephonic lines, voice-to-text computer programs, electronic magnifiers, and motorized wheelchairs all impact the quality-of-life experience as well as extend the access and opportunity available for independent living. Environments where these aids are undeveloped, poorly funded, or unavailable for sociopolitical reasons magnify the handicapping conditions.

Political aspects

Independent of technological development, but related in how such development is used and made available, political philosophy and practice diverge and change over time. Protective legislation and antidiscriminatory laws are examples of political practices. A philosophy of directing resources toward assistance for independent living as opposed to seeing disability as a private economic and caretaking burden on the family is another example.

Immediate Environment

Those obstacles or resources present in the person's daily environment are profoundly important. Although the larger sociocultural aspects influence persons with disabilities in the same place and historical context similarly, the immediate environmental influences allow diversity in the experience of one individual versus another.

TABLE **11.1**
Attitudinal Barriers

Overvaluation of rational intellect	A high value is placed on logical, deductive, linear thinking since the 17th century brought in the Age of Reason. Concurrently, intuition or right-brain thinking has been devalued. Many persons labeled "mentally retarded" may be limited in their linear thinking but are often gifted in terms of nonlinear processing ability (Vash & Crewe, 2004). So, a young woman who is intellectually challenged but has a gift of being able to pierce through the communication obstacles that generate misunderstandings is rarely rewarded by society with a position that explicitly uses such talents.
Overvaluation of physique	Not only are physical beauty and prowess highly regarded by majority society but also the range of what society defines as attractive is often narrow. Therefore, in today's society, attractiveness is defined by tall, muscular, rugged men, whereas women should have minimal body fat, large breasts, and no character lines to deface delicate, regular facial features. Youthfulness and athleticism are also prized, with aging being considered particularly detrimental for women and physical prowess particularly emphasized for men. People with disabilities rarely fit within these narrow categories, and often feel unable to enter the relationship arena because of their automatic disqualification.
Undervaluation of spirituality	A materialistic society handicaps differently than one that is more spiritually oriented. The notion of community responsibility for all members diminishes in a materialistic society to a more individualistic work ethic, where human worth is defined by the production of goods and services rather than by spiritual essence and humanity. Disability negatively impacts the materialistic assessment of worth of an individual especially when coupled with the idea that persons with disability cannot be useful members of society.
Blaming the victim	The idea of randomness is difficult for humans to fully accept because it implies that we are not always in control of our fate. Sometimes known as the *just world hypothesis*, we like to believe that the universe is generally fair, and bad things only happen to bad people. To defend oneself from this consciousness of vulnerability, assigning responsibility for misfortune to the victim is reassuring. Then, if one does not do what that other did, the misfortune cannot happen to oneself. If we cannot assign logical blame, as in "Well, skydiving is a risky business" or "You should always look before crossing the road," we may even develop psychodynamic explanations of self-destructiveness. Then we can make explanations of arthritis being caused by buried hostility, cervical cancer by self-hatred, or asthma as psychosomatic.
Insistence on mourning	Those attributes possessed by the temporarily able-bodied seem precious, and give rise to an inclination to assume that loss of any such attribute must lead to mourning. Not mourning such loss might imply not finding attributes of strength, flexibility, attractiveness, power, or wealth intrinsically critical to being happy, which in turn might threaten the meaning of our own pursuits of such attributes. So disability is inevitably equated with tragedy. For instance, when a deaf person values his immersion in the deaf community and refuses to use adaptations to normalize him in hearing society, that may be perceived as reactive and dysfunctional coping—after all, how could someone *prefer* to be deaf?

Family

Family structure and dynamics, such as parental acceptance, sibling support, spousal engagement, and marital strength are significant, as are the related variables, such as the family's social status and power in the community.

Community

The size and location of the community within which a person with a disability finds him or herself can impact the available range of services and paraphernalia. Although a more sophisticated and larger community may offer more, it may also lack the human support present in a smaller town. Many rehabilitation service models are designed specifically for large urban areas with a host of medical, educational, psychosocial, and vocational resources. Communities also make a difference in their response to inclusion issues in the schools, commitment to eliminate mobility barriers, and support of volunteer services and organizations.

Institutionalization

People with disabilities may vary in their experience of institutions, whether short recovery stays in hospitals during treatment, ongoing chronic visits for rehabilitation or physical therapy, or institutional residence for a greater part of their life. For institutions to function, they appear to require residents to give up personal power and agency, often through a network of rules that convenience the administration and management of the institution but would be considered intolerable to noninstitutionalized citizens. For instance, in many nursing homes, residents have rigid rules of mealtime, recreation and socializing with others, and bedtime. Although teenagers in this society rebel over restrictive curfews, the systematic deprivation of privacy and power in these residences is taken for granted. Although these policies may be accepted, it may be psychologically damaging in the long term. A prime example is the influx of persons with mental illness who were deinstitutionalized from large state-run psychiatric hospitals in the late 1970s onward, who ended up homeless rather than integrated into the community as intended.

Agencies

Other than institutions, people with disabilities must often interact, usually on an ongoing basis, with bureaucracies who provide vital services. Navigating the "red tape" of such agencies is challenging, and can be potent sources of frustration, disempowerment, and exhausting drains on resources and energies. Those persons who have mastered social skills have an advantage, but it is a heavy demand to be assertive as well as diplomatic in dealing with persons who have positions that allow them to control the quality and direction of people's lives. For instance, when one person in a couple is a recipient of Supplemental Security Income benefits, they may have to remain unmarried to avoid a loss of income because agencies are reluctant to pay spouses for providing attendant care. Thus, they may live as recipient and provider rather than legalize their union. Because it is common for persons with disabilities to rely on services and funds from agencies to be able to live in the community, failure to receive services may mean institutionalization or being trapped in poverty. Success in being determined eligible for disability benefits can make a significant difference to quality of life.

Regional differences

Finally, based on the region there may be much variation in funding, political practice, state and local government legislation, and services available. In

CASE STUDY **11.2**

Keisha's Day

Keisha, a 47-year-old African American single woman, has rheumatoid arthritis. She lives alone, and it takes her about 2 hours in the morning to get up, bathe, toilet, dress, and eat breakfast each morning. She found a device that would reduce the 15 minutes it used to take her to button her blouse down to 3 minutes.

Her apartment is accessible, allowing her to live independently. She had to search for a longtime, finding all too often when she arrived to look them over that the apartments had just been rented. She went into debt while she was searching to pay a personal care attendant to help her.

Keisha goes to work using public transportation because she cannot drive. Although the buses are accessible, she cannot get to the bus stop on snowy winter days. There is a dial-a-ride service available and this is a great help, but it does not allow for spontaneous flexibility. Mornings when she is delayed, she can call her brother who lives close by and who will drive her to work. Although he is always supportive, she does not want to overburden him.

Her workplace has been made accessible by a ramp at a side entrance, which usually suffices for her. However, she sometimes finds that those clearing snow from the sidewalks and parking lot have dumped a pile of snow at the foot of the ramp. There is no electric door opener because the company has said it is too expensive to install at this point. She does not have access to an accessible women's restroom in the part of the building where she works, and has been given permission to use the spacious executive restroom close by the president's office. She does feel somewhat embarrassed going in there. She does love her work, not so much for its content but because her rehabilitation counselor got a special engineer to design a desk for her with everything within reach to operate independently.

In the evening, once a week, her cousin comes by to take her grocery shopping. Ironically, she found herself unable to enter the closest supermarket because of a barrier designed to prevent the theft of shopping carts. Although she has complained, there has been no action taken as yet. For recreation, she often turns to her personal computer, which has several adaptive devices for her use. Before her arthritis became too severe, she used to love to dance. Recently, a dance club close by has been renovated to be accessible, and she will take over a set of mobility-impaired friends on some weekends to "show them how we dance." Although it created a stir when they first went, now the other patrons and staff seem to have become used to them, and she is greeted with smiles.

Keisha is optimistic and usually cheerful. Although there are many obstacles in her pursuit of living independently, working, and enjoying leisure time, she feels that there is much improvement. After all, just a couple of decades ago, she would probably have been institutionalized given the extent of her disability. In fact, she feels that the frustrations themselves are a sign of progress as they are transitional blocks that occur as the process is figured out.

Case Discussion
Thinking About This Case
1. What are some things that stand out to you as being most significant in terms of who Keisha is as a person and what she struggles with on a daily basis?
2. What other kinds of things would it be important for you to know about Keisha to be most effective as a helper working with her?

When considering this case, the number of daily barriers that Keisha has to overcome in order to function independently throughout the day seems significant. It would be interesting to know how Keisha deals mentally and emotionally as well as physically with the sense of frustration, anger, or embarrassment she might feel regarding the barriers she faces daily, some of which are alleviated through accommodations, some of which are not. It is also important to note that helpful outlets for Keisha are her time with the personal computer and involvement in dance, which seem to give her a sense of fulfillment, but it would be important to understand these from her point of view as well as other possible fulfilling outlets. In addition, keeping a sense of perspective seems important to Keisha and would be worth exploring more.

addition, whereas some regions are more welcoming, accessible, and committed to independent living, there are also differences based on aspects, such as geography, climate, and building style. In mountainous states, persons may have to deal with the impact of high altitudes, whereas in northern states, having to cope with snow can take its toll.

DISABILITY IDENTITY

There is no widely accepted model of identity development in terms of disability as there has been developed for other marginalized groups, such as racial identity development theories. Specific disabilities have generated models, such as the Nash and Nash (1981) model of adaptations to deafness. In their model, *acculturation* is based on learning American Sign Language and immersing oneself in Deaf culture; *membership* involves integration into the deaf community as a means of neutralizing stigma; *advocating* is a stance of actively rejecting the stigmatizing majority views; *passing* is about achieving normative status by pretending to hear through lipreading and speech production; and, finally, *retreating* describes a marginalized position of both failing to integrate into majority society and rejecting the deaf community. One can notice in this model the commonalities with other minority identity models of various adaptation paths of consciousness, accommodation, rejection, and alienation that arise due to the particular aspect of having a group identity that is stigmatized in majority sociocultural constructions.

REFLECTION QUESTIONS 11.3

- To what extent do you value a person's abilities as a sign of his or her worth?
- Have you ever stood up for someone being harassed or oppressed on the basis of disability? If not, why not? Has anyone ever stood up for you in this way?

EXAMPLE **11.3**
Disability Identity

I sat for the first time in my life in a room filled with other disabled people. I remember how nervous I felt.... I'd always gone to "regular" schools; I'd been mainstreamed before there was a word for it. I had moved through the world as a normal person with a limp, and no thank you, I didn't need any help, I could manage just fine. And, no, I was nothing like "them." I wasn't whiny, or needy or self-pitying.

Source: Excerpted from Anne Finger (1990), *Past due: A Story of Disability, Pregnancy and Birth.* (Seattle: WA: Seal Press)

Darling (1979, 2003) developed a typology of orientations toward disability that she updated over the last 2 decades based of the changing environment and the shift from a primarily medical model to a social model in understanding disability. Originally based on a study of parents of children with disabilities, the typology focused on ways in which these parents responded. In the earlier typology, Darling (1979) used sociological theories to postulate four modes of adaptation, based on integration in mainstream society versus integration in a disability subculture. This typology was updated and expanded to provide seven modes of adaptation, and the integration aspect was widened to separate out aspects of access and acceptance (Darling, 2003). The typology is a useful way of understanding the complexity and variation among people with disabilities and their experiences and, therefore, we share it with you in some detail.

The *cultural majority* refers to acceptance or access based on majority cultural values about attractiveness, achievement, appearance, and ability. *Disability subculture* references alternative norms and values about ability and achievement based on social and political activism. Access and acceptance are separated because a given individual may have access in one area of majority culture but reject majority norms and values to identify with the subculture.

Each of the modes depicts a different type of orientation and balancing act between these two cultural value sets. *Normalization* describes those who accept the majority society values and achieve lifestyles similar to those of able-bodied individuals, welcoming technology that allows them to function more like "normal" people, for example hidden cochlear implants for those

TABLE **11.2**
A Typology of Disability Orientations

	Integration			
	Norms or goals of cultural majority		Norms or goals of disability subculture	
Modes of Adaptation	Access	Acceptance	Access	Acceptance
Normalization	+	+	+/−	−
Crusadership	−	+	+	−
Affirmation	+/−	−	+	+
Situational identification	+	+	+	+
Resignation	−	+	−	−
Apathy	+/−	−	+/−	−
Isolated affirmation	−	−	−	+

Source: Adapted from Darling, R. B. (2003), "Toward a Model of Changing Disability Identities: A Proposed Typology and Research Agenda." Disability & Society, 18(7), pp. 881–895.
Note: +having access or acceptance, − not having access or acceptance, and +/− may or may not have access.

who are hard of hearing. They may reject stigmatizing objects that would mark them visibly as disabled. This does not mean that all individuals who define themselves through normalization have accepted the stigmatized image of disability and are escaping from it by passing. Watson (2002) argues that disability is not necessarily a salient part of one's identity, and it can be managed in one's own terms of reference.

Crusadership describes those who accept the norms of the majority but do not have access to such a lifestyle. They become involved in self-advocacy and larger social movements to promote the achievement of normalization. An example of such a typology would be Christopher Reeve, the late actor who was paralyzed after an equestrian accident and became prominent as a campaigner for research into a cure for spinal injuries. In *affirmation*, however, although persons identify with the disability culture in order to achieve goals, their identification is not temporary. They tend to view disability as their salient identity and conceptualize it in positive terms rather than seek to normalize. An example of a person in this typology might be actress Marlee Matlin, who is deaf, and whose deafness is a part of the characters she plays in movies and television, though not exclusively so. *Situational identification* is a variable type to identify those who maintain multiple identities, shifting based on environment or circumstance. Thus, a person may choose normalization values when interacting in the majority culture while demonstrating affirmation when in the company of disabled peers. This type may reflect ambivalence and may eventually change to one of the more settled types of normalization or affirmation, because it is difficult to maintain the balancing act of trying to live in two different worlds.

Resignation describes the condition of those individuals who may desire but are unable to achieve normalization while not having access to disability subculture. Living in isolated areas, in poverty, or without access to a computer would mean greater exposure to majority culture values and correspondingly fewer opportunities to learn about affirmation. *Apathy* describes those who may be completely uninformed, such as persons with significant mental illness or learning disabilities, and who are unaware of the norms of both the majority and the disability subculture, though they may have access to opportunities for normalization. Finally, *isolated affirmation* describes those rare individuals who arrive at an affirmation orientation without access to disability subculture. Early leaders of the movement advocated such an identity long before it was common. Today, although there may be individuals who arrive at such an identity by themselves, they would tend to join the collective disability subculture upon becoming aware of it.

Looking at the process of disability identity development, Gill (1997) developed a theory of four types of integration reflecting the incorporation of both group and individual identities in the context of coming to terms with a minority identity status. The first, "coming to feel we belong," focused on integrating into society after the process of being alienated and marginalized from it due to the disability. The second, "coming home," described the process of integrating with the disability community; the third, "coming together," was based on internal processes of integrating one's commonality as well as difference; and the fourth, "coming out," concentrated on the interpersonal integration of self-presentation with self-concept.

In a critique of the social model, Reeve (2002) suggested that the construction of disability as being caused by externally imposed limitations and restrictions fails to acknowledge the role of illness and impairment as well as cultural dimensions on the experience of disability. She posited psychoemotional dimensions of disability that impact not only the external lives of people with disabilities but also what they internally believe and feel about themselves. An example might be a young woman who is physically disfigured, feeling ashamed when being stared at on the street. Here she has internalized the marginalization that she experiences and feels bad about herself rather than perceiving the stares as originating from the onlooker's attitudes and experiences. She may well take her resultant lack of self-esteem further by believing that she is not a sexual being anymore and has no right to participate in the society to seek relationships.

EXAMPLE **11.4**
Deaf Culture

Deafness, by federal definition, is classified as a disability. Thus, people who are part of the group commonly referred to as the deaf and hard of hearing have the right to accommodations under the Americans with Disabilities Act (ADA) as well as the Rehabilitation Act of 1973 and other pertinent laws. The term **deaf** refers to individuals with severe to profound hearing loss. The use of the lowercase *D* reflects a physical, audiological, or pathological view of such a person. **Hard of hearing** refers to individuals who typically experience hearing loss from a physical or audiological perspective. However, within this group are significant portion who consider themselves Deaf, with the capital *D* signifying a cultural identity. Those members of the Deaf community typically do not consider themselves as having a disability as much as a different human experience. The characteristics of this group fall more in line with those of other cultural or linguistic minority groups. Practitioners must integrate knowledge of Deaf culture into their policies, practices, and attitudes in order to provide culturally affirmative services.

Deaf communities are composed mostly, but not exclusively, of deaf individuals and typically include individuals who communicate via **signed languages**, individuals who attended schools for the deaf, **children of deaf parents, Children of deaf adult** and sign language interpreters. In the United States, American Sign Language is typically favored over English-like signing, and cochlear implants are rejected as are oralist methods of teaching children to speak or lip-read with limited use of signing (Ladd, 2003).

CASE STUDY **11.3**

Case of Esteban

An able-bodied man in his mid-20s, Esteban came to counseling for mixed anxiety-depressive disorder, along with a long history of abusing various substances. Though he was sober at the time of counseling, he was vulnerable to relapses of cocaine and methamphetamine abuse. He had a history of an abusive father and an early loss of his mother to cancer. Initial counseling focused on maintaining drug abstinence as well the depression and anxiety. He found and held a job, and received a promotion. Well into counseling, a crisis arose when Esteban discovered that he had Hodgkin's disease. His primary reaction was that now, after turning his life around for the better, he was being punished for his years of drug abuse and would die young like his mother. He felt overwhelmed, isolated, and unable to process much of what the doctors had told him, much less take charge of a plan for treatment. The counselor immediately called and found national support and information organizations and asked for two copies of their literature. The counselor read upon the material and learned that there were three stages of the disease, and the prognosis varied according to stage. At the next session, the counselor informed Esteban that she had received written information about the disease and handed him a packet of information, without either telling him what she had learned or pushing him to read the materials. In a later session, Esteban asked if she had read the materials, and she answered affirmatively without going into details. He wanted to discuss his stage of Hodgkin's but didn't want to have to explain it, and he was quite relieved that he did not have to.

As he came to terms with the reality of his diagnosis, it became clear that he would need considerable work accommodations for weeks of chemotherapy and radiation. Esteban was terrified that he would be fired and lose his medical insurance and have to find new work just when he was feeling the worst. At this juncture, the counselor developed familiarity with disability laws, realizing that because his employer had over 50 employees, the company was responsible for complying with the ADA. However an employer is not responsible for proving any reasonable accommodation until an employee requests it because only a disclosure of disability triggers the law. The counselor educated Esteban on key concepts such as "essential functions of the job," "reasonable accommodations," and "otherwise qualified

individual." Like many persons, Esteban was unaware that he was considered a person with a disability and, therefore, had some protections. The counselor had to be sensitive to give Esteban some important information while not giving legal advice. She encouraged him to use the basic information as a starting point to learning more on his own. She also role-played with Esteban ways to tell his supervisor about his condition. Ultimately, the company did try to fire Esteban, but by then he was well prepared with specific information that got the company to reconsider. Through this process, the counselor supported and encouraged Esteban.

Note: Adapted from Rhonda Olkin. 1999. *What psychotherapists should know about disability* (pp. 151–153). New York: Guilford Press.

Case Discussion
Thinking About This Case
1. What are some ways in which the counselor here took initiative in educating herself on disability issues that helped facilitate the therapeutic relationship? As you can see, a counselor may not be well-, versed in disability issues, but may need to gain such expertise to serve clients effectively.
2. As you read about Esteban, how would you trace his disability identity over the process of counseling? How might his identity affect the therapeutic work done?

As you read the case above, it is clear that Esteban has multiple issues that influence and affect what he is going through, and how he deals with what seems to be his primary concern now of coping with Hodgkin's disease. The counselor in the case scenario seems to take initiative for educating herself in order to best serve her client from a more informed point of view. In the case description, it seems important to note that Esteban's primary reaction was that "now, after turning his life around for the better, he was being punished for his years of drug abuse and would die young like his mother." It would seem critical to explore this reaction further in the context of cultural, religious, and spiritual beliefs perhaps, as well to explore Esteban's past processes of overcoming what could have been impossible barriers and how those previously learned skills for survival could come in handy now in dealing with this new challenge.

Source: Adapted from Rhonda Olkin (1999), *What Psychotherapists Should Know about Disability* (New York: Guilford Press)

OPENING THE DIALOGUE ON ABILITY AND DISABILITY

With all of the topics discussed in this chapter, you are now challenged to think through how you would utilize this information in sessions with any number of clients from a variety of cultural backgrounds and worldviews. Questions for reflection offered to you throughout this chapter also serve as excellent process questions for opening the dialogue with clients on issues of disability and experiences with ableism. Some of these questions are listed here to assist you in terms of opening the dialogue with your clients:

- What does it mean to you to have an ability or disability?
- To what extent do you define yourself around your abilities or disabilities? How important is this in your personal and cultural identity, and what impact does this dimension have on how you view the world and live your life?
- Are there any abilities you have that you think you've taken for granted at any point in your life?
- How did your definition of yourself based on ability or disability develop, and who were some significant people in your life that helped to shape this definition?
- How has your view of ability or disability been reinforced or challenged during your life?
- What does your culture say about ability or disability?
- What does your family and community say about ability or disability in terms of both beliefs and practice?
- How do issues of power and privilege influence your view of ability or disability and concept of ableism?
- How has your view of ability or disability affected the way you define yourself now and at previous points in your life?
- How will your view of ability or disability continue to affect the way you define yourself and the way others see you or treat you?
- How has your view of ability or disability affected the way you interact with others who are similar to you in age (versus different from you) at different points in your life?
- Who are some people of your own ability or disability that you look up to, and why?
- How might the difference or similarity in ability or disability between you (client) and I (counselor) affect your experience in the process of counseling as well as the relationship between us?
- When and how did you first become aware of ableism? What was your initial reaction, and how did that reaction change over time?
- What have your experiences with ableism been, and in what ways have those experiences shaped who you are as a person, as well as the issues you are dealing with now?
- What efforts have you made to work toward positive social change with regard to the ableism that exists in your own life at the individual, group, and societal levels, and what other kinds of efforts would you like to make?

- To what extent do you value a person's abilities as a sign of his or her worth?
- Have you ever stood up for someone being harassed or oppressed on the basis of disability? If not, why not? Has anyone ever stood up for you in this way?
- How does ability or disability play into the issues you are bringing to counseling, and how can we address this in a way that is most helpful to you?

COUNSELOR PREPARATION

One of the important aspects of counselor readiness and competence in working with clients with disabilities is to obtain good supervision and consultation—preferably from a professional who has had experience with these issues.

In thinking through some of the aspects that will impact working with clients with disabilities, go through the list of 10 etiquette rules of working with such clients (Table 11.3).

Evaluation and Assessment

It is important in medical and vocational rehabilitation programs, as well as counseling, to obtain a multidimensional understanding of the individual with disabilities to not only set goals but also determine the services necessary to attain such goals, as well as measure progress toward the goals. Interviewing, psychometric testing, and functional assessments are three methods used, often in some combination to maximize the advantages of each approach. Although interviewing is a standard approach in counseling, working with people with disabilities often involves the extensive use of testing. For instance, neuropsychological testing is often carried out to determine the extent of functional impairments and their implications for persons with brain injuries. However, tests such as the Minnesota Multiphasic Personality Inventory, Beck Depression Inventory, or Hamilton Anxiety Scale are also

REFLECTION EXERCISE **11.2**

Acquiring a Disability

Take a moment to consider and respond to the following questions:

- What is the most challenging disability you could acquire or have? What about this particular disability is so bad? How do you imagine your life with such a disability? How would you cope?
- What would be the easiest disability for you? What about this disability seems less daunting? What would be different about your life with this disability?
- How can you put aside your own considerations and beliefs about such disabilities if you are working with a client who has either of the disabilities (both the most difficult and the easiest) you have identified above?

TABLE **11.3**
10 General Rules of Etiquette with Clients with disabilities

1. Don't stare.

2. Don't tell clients with disabilities about all the other persons with disabilities you know.

3. Don't assume the person needs your help, and don't help without asking.

4. Be clear about who is the client, and don't get confused into addressing the personal assistant, interpreter, family member, or anyone else who may accompany the client into counseling.

5. Don't be afraid to say you don't understand either the words themselves or their meaning.

6. Don't worry about word choices that seem counter to the disability (such as using "Do you see what I mean?" with someone who has a visual impairment), but be careful about words that carry emotional power (such as "crippled").

7. Don't touch someone's assistive device (wheelchair, voice computer, prosthetic, crutches, etc.) without permission.

8. Nonverbal cues are often altered by disability, so you need to learn to understand the interaction among specific disabilities, and be careful of how you interpret body language.

9. Think about the temperature in your therapeutic space in terms of client sensitivity to heat or cold, and have accommodations available.

10. Don't take these rules too seriously because they are guidelines, not absolutes.

Source: Adapted from Rhonda Olkin (1999), *What Psychotherapists Should Know about Disability* (New York: Guilford Press).

used frequently (Vash & Crewe, 2004). A criticism of the use of such tests is that they have rarely been validated on individuals with physical disabilities, and they are usually oriented to determining pathology rather than identifying persons caught up in abnormal situations.

Functional assessments typically made in rehabilitation include assessing a range of daily living skills, such as the ability to bathe, groom, or eat independently (Chan, Berven, and Thomas, 2004). In vocational rehabilitation, capabilities in several areas are assessed. The Functional Assessment Inventory (Neath, Bellini, & Bolton, 1997) examines six factors: (a) adaptive behavior such as judgment, interaction with coworkers, social support, and work habits; (b) cognition, including leaning ability, memory, and form perception; (c) physical capacity, which assesses aspects of endurance, mobility, and motor speed; (d) motor functioning, which focuses on hand and upper-extremity functioning; (e) communication such as speech, hearing, and language functioning; and (f) vocational qualifications, such as skills, work history, special working conditions, and acceptability to employers.

In addition to functional assessments, it is possible to use the three prevailing models of disability to assess the client's perspective. Olkin (1999) assesses the client's model of disability to a set of questions that address differing aspects of the client's experience with the disability (see Table 11.4).

Therapeutic Issues

The evaluative process can itself have therapeutic effects as clients describe their history, situation, and problems; learn through the assessments about their

capacities and limitations; and begin to see future possibilities. Although rehabilitation counselors are specifically trained to work with persons with disabilities,
other counseling professionals may well have clients who have disabilities. Such
clients may come to meet educational and career needs, receive personal
counseling or case management, or receive marriage, family, or child counseling.
It is important that counselors do not turn such clients away, particularly if the
counseling is unrelated or only remotely related to the disability.

For persons who acquire a disability, emotional support is needed in the
recovery process to cope with the concurrent shock, fear, anger, and loss.
Those born with a disability may require similar support in the process of

TABLE **11.4**
Assessing the Client's Model of Disability

Model	Questions to Ask the Client
Moral model	Do you feel shame or embarrassment about your disability?
	Do you feel you bring dishonor to your family?
	Do you try to hide and minimize your disability as much as possible?
	Do you try to make as few demands on others as possible because it is "your problem" and hence your responsibility?
	Do you try to make your disability inconspicuous?
	Do you think your disability is a test of faith or a way to prove your faith?
	Do you think your disability is a punishment for your or your family's failings?
Medical model	Compared to FDR's time, do you think that life for people with disabilities has improved tremendously?
	Do you try to make as few demands on others as possible because you believe you should be able to find a way to do it yourself?
	Do you dress in ways that maximize your positive features and minimize the visibility of your disability?
	Do you believe that the major goals of research should be to prevent disabilities and find cures for those who already have disabilities?
	Do you think people with disabilities do best when they are fully integrated into the non-disabled community?
Minority model	Do you identify yourself as part of a minority group of persons with disabilities?
	Do you feel kinship and belonging with other persons with disabilities?
	Do you think not enough is being done to ensure rights of persons with disabilities?
	When policies and legislation are new, do you evaluate them in terms of their effects on persons with disabilities?
	Do you think the major goals of research should be to improve the lives of persons with disabilities by changing policies, procedures, funding, and laws?
	Do you think persons with disabilities do best when they are free to associate in both the disabled and nondisabled communities as bicultural people?

Source: Adapted from Rhonda Olkin (1999), *What Psychotherapists Should Know about Disability* (New York: Guilford Press).

realizing the handicapping and disadvantages they face from society. At this stage in recovery, the major therapeutic task is of assuring the individual of his or her human worth and the possibility of an optimistic future, while acknowledging and legitimizing the anger and grief. According to Vash and Crewe (2004), in the adjustment process for persons with a full range of disabilities, three significant areas of loss include the (a) loss of emotional discharge mechanisms, (b) loss of pleasure or reward sources, and (c) loss of physical and economic independence. The disjunction between the former interests, activities, and recreations of an able-bodied life and the currently experienced limitations may lead to a loss of self-esteem or life purpose. A concern is that such loss of meaningfulness, if not dealt with, can lead to dysfunctional ways of self-numbing such as substance abuse. Along with the emotional support, encourage the client to investigate and develop new ways of discharging tension, find sources of gratification, as well as explore, confront, and reorient belief systems. Some such beliefs include equating the resultant dependency with total loss of independence, as well as believing that the disruption and confusion following the disability will always be present.

Another aspect of the adjustment process where counseling can be actively helpful is assisting in interpersonal skills training. As mentioned earlier, because of the automatic discomfort and stereotyping by able-bodied individuals as well as the ongoing negotiating required to access services and sustain quality of life, persons with disabilities benefit from assertiveness training, as well as from developing interpersonal flexibility and social presentation.

Beyond the adjustment process itself, other issues may bring clients with disabilities into counseling. Some common issues include depression, anxiety, substance abuse, as well as physical and sexual trauma. In a study of persons with spinal cord injury, Krause, Kemp, and Coker (2000) found that almost half reported some form of depression. Although disability can bring about many losses, disability itself cannot explain depression because there are many persons with disabilities who are not depressed. It would be important for counselors to not focus so exclusively on the client's disability as a source of the depression that other life issues as well as biochemical and neuropsychological originators are overlooked. In terms of substance abuse, there is evidence that the incidence is higher among people with disabilities than in the general population. This could be because substances were contributors to the onset of the disability in the first place, are being used as a way to defend against loneliness and isolation, or are used to self-medicate against pain or because the person has become addicted to prescribed opiates.

Using a logotherapy approach, Ososkie and Schultz (2003) emphasize the importance of finding meaning in a dynamic process, based on a thorough exploration of the question "What do I do with my life with a disability?" It is vital that the focus of this phenomenological process is attached to the individual's life with a disability and not to the disability by itself. Otherwise, the person becomes subsumed by the disability and loses all the other aspects of identity and humanity.

Chan, Cardoso, and Chronister (2009) discuss therapeutic principles helpful in working with clients with disabilities. These include the awareness that persons with disabilities have complex inner lives and the need to work with the patient's subjective experience from a social constructionist and disability rights perspective. It is important to counter the pathologizing of disability as loss, by focusing on strengths and being flexible in considering unusual solutions as adaptive and reasonable. For instance, whining and non-cooperation as strategies have often allowed persons with disabilities to literally survive recommended medical interventions and toxic caregiving. Being creative and resisting the pressure to be too goal-oriented allow room for flexible solutions for unprecedented issues. Furthermore, counselors may need to accept more responsibility for acting outside traditional counseling as advocates, while explicitly addressing issues of locus of control and self-determination.

CONCLUSION AND IMPLICATIONS

Counselors must explore and confront their own phenomenology when assisting clients with disabilities. Otherwise, the counselor may be a barrier rather than a facilitator in the client's exploration of meaning. Meaning imposed by others is not helpful, and can be harmful to the client's own search and resolution of these concerns.

One's own discomforts with aspects of disability must be acknowledged and processed, in supervision or consultation. In addition, the counselor's experiences and meaning given to loss, and to expressions of anger and grieving, also need to be explored and understood. The counselor must be careful not to take on a caretaker role with the client, meeting one's own needs of helpfulness at the expense of the client. It is also imperative that the counselor's own discomfort with dependency or loss not cause him or her to push a search for solutions before the grieving process is resolved.

Although disabilities may be distressing or uncomfortable for some temporarily able-bodied readers, working with the issue of disability will be inevitable for practitioners. Disabilities may be historically part of the client's context or acquired in the course of counseling. To be able to serve clients effectively, disability-affirmative therapy (Olkin, 2009) requires that practitioners take responsibility for understanding the models of disability, become aware of the difference between disability and defect, value disability culture, and assess disability identity sensitively.

GLOSSARY

Ableism: A pervasive system of discrimination and exclusion that oppresses people who have mental, emotional, and physical disabilities based on beliefs about health, beauty, and productivity, leading to an environment that is often hostile to those whose physical, mental, cognitive, and sensory abilities are considered nonnormative.

Attitudinal barriers: Stereotyped beliefs or prejudices regarding people with disabilities that result in categorizing, blaming, limiting, or discriminating environments.

Child of deaf adult: A Child Of Deaf Adult is a person who was raised by a Deaf parent or guardian. Many CODAs identify with Deaf and hearing cultures.

Disability: Describes, with respect to an individual, a physical or mental impairment that substantially limits one or more of the major life activities, a record of such impairment, or being regarded as having such an impairment.

Handicap: A disadvantage for a person with a disability that occurs when they encounter cultural, physical, or social barriers that prevent their access to the various systems of society that are available to other citizens. Thus, handicap is the loss or limitation of opportunities to take part in the life of the community on an equal level with others.

Sign language: A sign language is a language which, instead of acoustically conveyed sound patterns, uses visually transmitted sign patterns to convey meaning—simultaneously combining hand shapes, orientation and movement of the hands, arms or body, and facial expressions to fluidly express a speaker's.

REFERENCES

Americans with Disabilities Act of 1990, Public Law 101-336, 42 U.S.C. 12111, 12112.

Bickenbach, J. E. (1993). *Physical disability and social policy.* Toronto: University of Toronto Press.

Blotzer, M. A., & Ruth, R. (1995). *Sometimes you just want to feel like a human being: Case studies of empowering psychotherapy with people with disabilities.* Baltimore: Paul H. Brooks

Bryan, W. V. (1999). *Multicultural aspects of disabilities: A guide to understanding and assisting minorities in the rehabilitation process.* Springfield, IL: Charles C Thomas.

Castafieda, R., & Peters, M. L. (2000). Ableism. In M. Adams, W. J. Blumenfeld, R. Castafieda, H. W. Hackman, M. L. Peters, & X. Zuniga (Eds.), *Readings for diversity and social justice* (pp. 319–323). New York: Routledge.

Chan, F., Berven, N. L., & Thomas, K. R. (Eds.). (2004). *Counseling theories and techniques for rehabilitation health professionals* (Springer Series on Rehabilitation). New York: Springer.

Chan, F., Cardoso, E., & Chronister, J. A. (2009). *Understanding psychosocial adjustment to chronic illness and disability: A handbook for evidence-based practitioners in rehabilitation.* New York: Springer Press.

Darling, R. B. (1979). *Families against society: A study of reactions to children with birth defects.* Beverly Hills, CA: Sage.

Darling, R. B. (2003). Toward a model of changing disability identities: A proposed typology and research agenda. *Disability & Society,* 18(7), 881–895.

Disability Social History Project. (2005). Retrieved from http://www.disabilityhistory.org/dshp.html

Finger, A. (1990). *Past due: A story of disability, pregnancy and birth.* Seattle: WA: Seal Press.

Ford, A. R. (2009). It's not just about racism, but ableism: When talking about diversity, the ableism that students with disabilities face should be part of the conversation. *Diverse Issues in Higher Education,* 26(4), 16.

Gill, C. J. (1997). Four types of integration in disability identity development. *Journal of Vocational Rehabilitation,* 9, 39–46.

Gill, C. J. (2001). Divided understandings: The social experience of disability. In G. L. Albrecht, K. D. Seelman, et al. (Eds.), *Handbook of disability studies* (pp. 351–372). Thousand Oaks, CA: Sage.

Groce, N. (2005). Immigrants, disability and rehabilitation. J. H. Stone (Ed.), *Culture and disability: Providing culturally competent services* (Multicultural Aspects of Counseling Series 21). Thousand Oaks, CA: Sage.

Hillyer, B. (1993). *Feminism and disability.* Norman: University of Oklahoma Press.

Huebner, R. A., & Thomas, K. R. (1995). The relationship between attachment, psychopathology, and childhood disability. *Rehabilitation Psychology,* 40(2), 111–124.

Kaufert, P. L., & Kaufert, J. M. (1984). Methodological and conceptual issues in measuring the long-term impact of disability: The experience of poliomyelitis patients in Manitoba. *Social Science and Medicine,* 19, 609–618.

Kielhofner, G. (2005). Rethinking disability and what to do about it: Disability studies and its implications for occupational therapy, *American Journal of Occupational Therapy,* 59(5), 487–497.

Krause, J. S., & Crewe, N. M. (1991). Chronologic time, time since injury, and time of measurement: Effect on adjustment after spinal cord injury. *Archives of Physical Medicine & Rehabilitation,* 72 (2), 91–100.

Krause, J. S., Kemp, B. J., & Coker, J. L. (2000). Depression after spinal cord injury: Relation to gender, ethnicity, aging, and socioeconomic indicators. *Archives of Physical Medicine and Rehabilitation,* 81, 1099–1109.

Ladd, P. (2003). *Understanding deaf culture: In search of deafhood*. Toronto: Multilingual Matters.

Livneh, H. (1982). On the origins of negative attitudes toward people with disabilities. *Rehabilitation Literature*, 43(11), 338–347.

McColl, M. A., & Bickenbach, J. E. (1998). Introduction. In M. A. McColl & J. E. Bickenbach (Eds.), *Introduction to disability*. London: Saunders.

Murphy, R. (1987). *The body silent*. New York: Henry Holt.

Nash, J. E., & Nash, A. (1981). *Deafness in society*. New York: Lexington, Heath.

Neath, J., Bellini, J., & Bolton, B. (1997). Dimensions of the Functional Assessment Inventory for five disability groups. *Rehabilitation Psychology*, 42(3), 183–207.

Olkin, R. (1999). *What psychotherapists should know about disability*. New York: Guilford Press.

Olkin, R. (2009). Disability-affirmative therapy. In I. Marini & M. Stebnecki (Eds.), *The professional counselor's desk reference* (pp.355–369). New York: Springer.

Ososkie, J. N., & Schultz, J. C. (2003). Disability acceptance theories and logotherapy. *International Forum for Logotherapy*, 26, 21–26.

Peters, S. (1993). Having a disability "sometimes." *Canadian Woman Studies*, 13, 26–27.

Reeve, D. (2002). Negotiating psycho-emotional dimensions of disability and their influence on identity constructions. *Disability & Society*, 17(5), 493–508.

Smith, L., Foley, P. F., & Chaney, M. P. (2008). Addressing classism, ableism, and heterosexism in counselor education, *Journal of Counseling and Development*, 86(3), 303–310.

Stone, S. D. (1995). The myth of bodily perfection. *Disability and Society*, 10(4), 413–424.

Swain, J., & Cameron, C. (1999). Unless otherwise stated: Discourses of labeling and identity in coming out. In M. Corker & S. French (Eds.), *Disability discourse* (pp. 74–83). Buckingham, UK: Open University Press.

Tollifson, J. (1997). Imperfection is a beautiful thing: On disability and meditation. In K. Fries (Ed.), *Staring back: The disability experience from the inside out* (pp. 106–111). New York: Plume.

Vash, C. L., & Crewe, N. M. (2004). *Psychology of disability* (2nd ed., Springer Series on Rehabilitation). New York: Springer.

U.S. Census Bureau. (2000). Disability Status 2000. Retrieved from http://www.census.gov/prod/2003pubs/c2kbr-17.pdf

U.S. Department of Justice. (1992). A guide to disability rights laws. Retrieved from http://www.ada.gov/cguide.htm

Watson, N. (2002). Well, I know this is going to sound very strange to you, but I don't see myself as a disabled person: Identity and disability. *Disability & Society*, 17, 509–527.

CHAPTER 12

Multicultural Counseling Competence

What sets worlds in motion is the interplay of differences, their attractions and repulsions. Life is plurality, death is uniformity. By suppressing differences and peculiarities, by eliminating different civilizations and cultures, progress weakens life and favors death. The ideal of a single civilization for everyone, implicit in the cult of progress and technique, impoverishes and mutilates us. Every view of the world that becomes extinct, every culture that disappears, diminishes a possibility of life.

Octavio Paz (*The Labyrinth of Solitude*, 1978)

In this chapter, we come to the end of this part of the journey. Recall when we started, we used the metaphor of a train journey. Given the lifelong nature of the process of developing and refining multicultural competence, it would be both wrong and arrogant to imply that we have arrived at a final destination. This text and other experiences you have are but stops along the way. However, after the content knowledge you have gathered on various aspects of identity such as culture, race, gender, sexual orientation, class, religion, disability, and age, you may well feel somewhat paralyzed with how to use this knowledge in practice. In this chapter, we will provide an overview of the need for cultural competence, moving beyond awareness to enter the domains of knowledge and skills. Ethical and professional issues of practice will be important to consider. We will introduce you to concepts of social justice and advocacy as part of the tools and demands made of a culturally competent practitioner. We will also cover some models of practice that add effectiveness.

REFLECTION QUESTIONS 12.1

- Given your own identities of race, culture, class, gender, sexual orientation, disability status, age, and spiritual affiliation, what kinds of clients do you think it would be challenging to work with? Are there certain issues that clients might present that would be trickier than others?
- As in the question above, considering your identities, what kinds of clients do you think might find it difficult or challenging to work with you? Why?
- Can you prepare yourself to counsel any and every client, or do you think there are limitations on your ability to stretch yourself? How might you justify or explain these limitations?

THE IMPORTANCE OF MULTICULTURAL COUNSELING COMPETENCE

Multicultural competence is the ability to work effectively and sensitively within various cultural contexts. Multicultural counseling competencies, then, can be defined as a set of practices that enable people to work effectively and sensitively, honoring and respecting the cultural worldviews and behaviors in the context of persons receiving services (President's New Freedom Commission for Mental Health, 2003). One of the most crucial skills for a culturally competent practitioner is the ability to engage a culturally different client's reality in an accepting and genuine manner. Practitioners who give equal value to others' worldview are more able to engage clients in ways that put them at ease quickly and successfully. People of marginalized social groups are adept at reading subtle cues that carry messages of disapproval, discomfort, judgment, or lack of acceptance because of one's race, culture, or ethnicity. A description of a worker as "she's all right" by a client of color in reference to a cross-cultural interaction is usually a response to an accurate reading of the worker's skill at entering a dissimilar cultural milieu. Acquiring such a fundamentally important skill can take place only through consistent practice motivated by an authentic goal to be real with others.

Prevailing practice principles are clear about the importance of developing rapport and trust with clients. Cultural differences, by their very existence, complicate the bridging of what often appear as gulfs. An inferior knowledge base, coupled with a skewed view of our multicultural reality, doom the best efforts to connect with clients in productive work. In clinical practice, for example, it is futile to expect people of color, given their oppressive experience with the dominant White society, to immediately trust the intentions of White practitioners or to honestly disclose vulnerabilities. Closing this cultural gap is the professional responsibility of the culturally competent practitioner.

EXAMPLE **12.1**
Guidelines for Culturally Competent Practice

1. *Assess the person's and family's needs with an emphasis on culturally respectful behavior.*
2. *Identify culturally related strengths and supports, including personal, interpersonal, and environmental supports.*
3. *Clarify what part of the problem is primarily environmental (i.e., external to the client) and what part is cognitive (internal), with attention to cultural influences.*
4. *For environmentally based problems, focus on helping the client to make changes that minimize stressors, increase personal strengths and supports, and build skills for interacting more effectively with the social and physical environment.*
5. *Validate clients' self-reported experiences of oppression.*
6. *Emphasize collaboration over confrontation with attention to client–therapist differences.*
7. *With cognitive restructuring, question the helpfulness (rather than the validity) of the thought or belief.*
8. *Do not challenge core cultural beliefs.*
9. *Use the client's list of culturally related strengths and supports to develop a list of helpful cognitions to replace the unhelpful ones.*
10. *Develop weekly homework assignments with an emphasis on cultural congruence and client direction.*

Questions for Reflection

1. Go through each guideline, and develop a rationale for why it may be important in cultural competence.
2. Generate examples of client counselor interactions for each guideline.

For example: In guideline 2, *Personal strengths* include pride in one's culture and identity; religious faith or spirituality; musical and artistic appreciation and abilities, such as weaving, beading, and sewing; bilingual and multilingual skills; culturally related knowledge and practical living skills, such as fishing, hunting, farming, and the use of medicinal plants; and culture-specific beliefs that help one cope with prejudice and discrimination. *Interpersonal supports* include extended families, traditional celebrations and rituals that involve an entire religious culture, storytelling activities that pass on the history of the group, involvement in political or social action groups, and having a child who is successful in school as a source of pride for the family. *Environmental supports* include space for prayer and meditation; available food, cooking, and eating of preferred foods; and access to nature for gardening, fishing, hunting, and farming.

Source: From Hays, P. A., "Integrating Evidence-Based Practice, Cognitive-Behavior Therapy, and Multicultural Therapy: Ten Steps for Culturally Competent Practice." *Professional Psychology, Research and Practice*, 40(4), pp. 354–360. Copyright © 2009 by the American Psychological Association. Reprinted by permission.

MODELS OF CULTURAL COMPETENCE

Three examples of models of cultural competence that are presented in the literature are (a) Pedersen's conceptual framework for developing cultural and cross-cultural competence, (b) Hogan-Garcia's model for cultural diversity competence, and (c) Hays's ADDRESSING model.

Pedersen's Framework for Developing Cultural and Cross-Cultural Competence

Paul Pedersen published a groundbreaking article in 1991 arguing that culture is central to all counseling and provided impetus for a culture-centered approach to counseling that set the stage for emphasis on culturally based competencies (Pedersen, 1991). Subsequently, Pedersen developed his *conceptual framework for developing cultural and cross-cultural competence model* (2003), which is comprised of the domains of awareness, knowledge, and skills. Pedersen (2003, p. 193) describes the individual stages as follows: The first stage, awareness, provides the basis for accurate opinions, attitudes, and assumptions. At the second stage, knowledge provides the documentation and factual information necessary to move beyond awareness toward effective and appropriate change in multicultural settings. The third stage, skill, provides the ability to build on awareness and apply knowledge toward effective change in multicultural settings.

Hogan-Garcia Model for Cultural Diversity Competence

Hogan-Garcia (2007) offers another model for cultural diversity competence that is focused on systemic change: "The broad objective of this training model is to work on a person-to-person basis to provide an interpersonal foundation for change while refashioning our hierarchical social structures into more collaborative, synergistic collectives" (p. 4). The training consists of the development of four skills. The first skill is the development of an understanding of the four levels of culture: (a) personal, (b) ethnic or cultural group, (c) U.S. mainstream and national (i.e., one's identity related to systemic level of culture based on home country and nationality), and (d) organizational (i.e., the systemic, structured interpersonal group or groups within which one functions). Second, an understanding of the six barriers to effective communication must be achieved. The six barriers are (a) nonverbal communication; (b) verbal communication; (c) preconceptions, stereotypes, and discrimination; (d) judgments; (e) stress; and (f) norms, policies, procedures, and programs unfriendly to cultural diversity. Next, culturally centered communication skills must be developed.

Hays's ADDRESSING Framework

Hays's (2008) ADDRESSING framework enables therapists to better recognize and understand cultural influences as a multidimensional combination of Age, Developmental and acquired Disabilities, Religion, Ethnicity, Socioeconomic status, Sexual orientation, Indigenous heritage, National origin, and Gender. The model can be used in three ways that are useful for examining biases and developing increased understanding of the specific aspects of culture that clients identify as being of utmost importance. First, the counselors can use the model to evaluate their own biases and explore areas where they may lack experience.

TABLE **12.1**
ADDRESSING Framework

The ADDRESSING Framework: Summary of Cultural Influences and Related Minority Groups	
Cultural influence	Minority group
Age or generational	Children and elders
Developmental disabilities	People with developmental disabilities
Disabilities acquired later in life	People with disabilities acquired later in life
Religion and spiritual orientation	Religious minority cultures
Ethnic and racial identity	Ethnic and racial minority cultures
Socioeconomic status	People of lower status by class, education, occupation, income, or rural or urban habitat
Sexual orientation	Gay, lesbian, and bisexual people
Indigenous heritage	Indigenous, Aboriginal, and Native people
National origin	Refugees, immigrants, sojourners, and international students
Gender	Women and transgendered people

Source: From Hays, P. A. *Addressing Cultural Complexities in Practice: Assessment, Diagnosis, and Therapy*, 2nd ed. Copyright © 2009 by the American Psychologcal Association. Reprinted by permission.

It can also be used to increase awareness of the "-isms" affecting people of color as a means to gain increased understanding of the connections between racism, sexism, and other forms of oppression. Last, by examining a particular ethnic group through the lens of the model, the tendency to make generalizations or hold inaccurate biases may be decreased.

THE THREE DIMENSIONS OF MULTICULTURAL COUNSELING COMPETENCE

As stated earlier, multicultural counseling competence has been articulated as falling into three dimensions: awareness, knowledge, and skills (Arredondo et al., 1996). Each area is, of course, inextricably linked with the other two. It is impossible to have a real therapeutic relationship without being knowledgeable about the other person and aware of how each of you shape the relationship, and it is simultaneously unfeasible to be completely aware of one's own assumptions and biases without having sustained contact with others and learning from the dissimilarities (Smith, Richards, & Granley, 2004). In this next section, we will examine each of these dimensions from a practical perspective.

REFLECTION QUESTIONS 12.2

- What does multicultural competence mean for you in practice?
- What aspects of your work with clients do you think show multicultural competence?
- Is there any difference in your mind between competence and effectiveness? If so, what?

Awareness

Counselors at all levels of expertise and training must strive toward self-awareness regarding all the various aspects of social identity and how their views are carried into the counseling relationship. Self-awareness, as a crucial dimension of culturally competent practice, appears to be an important component for counselors in anticipation of serving culturally diverse populations (Balkin, Schlosser, & Levitt, 2009). However, self-awareness is a complicated circular process of reflection and action and critical examination. In a groundbreaking essay, the poet Audre Lorde (1984) warned that the "Master's Tools Will Never Dismantle the Master's House." Too often, because of our socialization in hierarchical and dominant social structures, even when we do work for change we may go about it in ways that are themselves oppressive. Members of marginalized groups do not need a "white knight" to leap in and rescue them; in fact, such rescue serves only to reinforce their subordinate and disempowered status. When a counselor starts advocating for a client in ways such that the counselor's words and actions take precedence over those of the client, the counselor may end up being unpleasantly surprised when the client resists in both subtle and overt ways. The unreflective counselor then becomes bitter, complaining about the lack of appreciation or inherent flaws in the client. Gainor (2005) advocates consistently and critically examining the underlying values and assumptions of who is being served and whose agenda is directing and being promoted by the work. Counselors who stipulate appreciation may want to think about why they require gratitude for their efforts.

Another aspect is that embracing an agenda of justice and sensitivity does not remove the possibility that we may simultaneously resist systemic change. Even when desired and well intentioned, change can be met with covert and overt resistance. Many students, while in the process of developing cultural sensitivity and awareness, experience pressure from significant close people in their lives to regress and punishment when they do not. When they stop laughing at the racist jokes, they will be accused of having lost their sense of humor and becoming politically correct. Change, after all, is threatening to a whole carefully balanced system of privileges. When any one person in a dominant group takes a principled stand and starts refusing to be advantaged, it makes the invisible privilege uncomfortably visible to all.

Change provokes loss, because when we change we delve into unfamiliar territory where we no longer know the rules, however, oppressive they may be. Change makes us lose our sense of competency in our confusion (Evans, 1996). As advocated in Johnson's best-selling book *Who Moved My Cheese?* (1998), we can facilitate change when we identify our responses to change, attending to the attitudes and beliefs that both assist and impede change.

Finally, as persons become increasingly reflective, they may experience themselves as being hyperaware, unbearably sensitized to the constant microaggressions they notice around them. However, just as persons in marginalized groups can and do survive and even flourish under these assaults, the hyperawareness will eventually become bearable, particularly when it is possible to examine them, have a knowledge context in which to explain them, and develop ways to respond effectively.

REFLECTION QUESTIONS 12.3

- Have you ever felt the need to rescue a client? How did you handle it?
- What is the difference in your mind between rescuing a client and advocating or empowering him or her?
- What are some instances in which you've empowered a client or any person in your life? What did you do with them that worked well?
- What are examples of micro-aggressions that you or others close to you have dealt with? How did you deal with them?

Knowledge

Often practitioners in training are overwhelmed by the notion that they must take into account history, economics, politics, as well as the psychological knowledge they started with. However, any endeavor that seeks to work with persons must acknowledge the contexts in which they are embedded. Human beings lead social lives rooted in a historical, political, and economic system, and effective therapeutic work must take this complexity into account. It is difficult to work successfully with a client who is a refugee without knowing the specific details of that refugee experience, the specific political and social context of the chaos from which the client seeks sanctuary, as well as particular aspects of his or her culture of origin. The acquisition of specific knowledge is an ongoing task for practitioners. In many cases, what we start with are the tools to access and research quickly and efficiently to be able to respond to clients, rather than already coming equipped with the knowledge. This is primarily because of the variety and diversity of clients who we may see, and the unique combinations of issues they may present with. Any capsule of content knowledge must always be a starting point, to prevent it from becoming a way to generalize and stereotype. As the therapeutic relationship develops, we research more and fine-tune our knowledge to be applicable and relevant to the particular unique client we have.

REFLECTION QUESTIONS 12.4

- Which historically oppressed groups would you say you know the most about in terms of both their historical experience and their current experience and culture in general?
- How accurate is what you know, and how do you know?
- How have you learned what you've learned, and how could you find out more?

TABLE **12.2**
AMCD Multicultural Counseling Competencies

I. Counselor Awareness of Own Cultural Values and Biases		
Attitudes and Beliefs	Knowledge	Skills
1. Culturally skilled counselors believe that cultural self-awareness and sensitivity to one's own cultural heritage is essential.	1. Culturally skilled counselors have specific knowledge about their own racial and cultural heritage, and how it personally and professionally affects their definitions and biases of normality and abnormality and the process of counseling.	1. Culturally skilled counselors seek out educational, consultative, and training experiences to improve their understanding and effectiveness in working with culturally different populations. Being able to recognize the limits of their competencies, they (a) seek consultation, (b) seek further training or education, (c) refer out to more qualified individuals or resources, or (d) engage in a combination of these.
2. Culturally skilled counselors are aware of how their own cultural background and experiences have influenced attitudes, values, and biases about psychological processes.	2. Culturally skilled counselors possess knowledge and understanding about how oppression, racism, discrimination, and stereotyping affect them personally and in their work. This allows individuals to acknowledge their own racist attitudes, beliefs, and feelings. Although this standard applies to all groups, for White counselors it may mean that they understand how they may have directly or indirectly benefited from individual, institutional, and cultural racism as outlined in White identity development models.	2. Culturally skilled counselors are constantly seeking to understand themselves as racial and cultural beings and are actively seeking a nonracist identity.
3. Culturally skilled counselors are able to recognize the limits of their multicultural competency and expertise.	3. Culturally skilled counselors possess knowledge about their social impact upon others. They are knowledgeable about communication style differences; how their style may clash with or foster the counseling process with persons of color or others different from themselves based on the A, B, and C dimensions; and how to anticipate the impact it may have on others.	

(continued)

TABLE **12.2** (Continued)

II. Counselor Awareness of Own Cultural Values and Biases		
Attitudes and Beliefs	**Knowledge**	**Skills**
4. Culturally skilled counselors recognize their sources of discomfort with differences that exist between themselves and clients in terms of race, ethnicity, and culture.		

II. Counselor Awareness of Client's Worldview

1. Culturally skilled counselors are aware of their negative and positive emotional reactions toward other racial and ethnic groups that may prove detrimental to the counseling relationship. They are willing to contrast their own beliefs and attitudes with those of their culturally different clients in a nonjudgmental fashion.	1. Culturally skilled counselors possess specific knowledge and information about the particular group with which they are working. They are aware of the life experiences, cultural heritage, and historical background of their culturally different clients. This particular competency is strongly linked to the "minority identity development models" available in the literature.	1. Culturally skilled counselors should familiarize themselves with relevant research and the latest findings regarding mental health and mental disorders that affect various ethnic and racial groups. They should actively seek out educational experiences that enrich their knowledge, understanding, and cross-cultural skills for more effective counseling behavior.
2. Culturally skilled counselors are aware of the stereotypes and preconceived notions that they may hold toward other racial and ethnic minority groups.	2. Culturally skilled counselors understand how race, culture, ethnicity, and so forth may affect personality formation, vocational choices, the manifestation of psychological disorders, help-seeking behavior, and the appropriateness or inappropriateness of counseling approaches.	2. Culturally skilled counselors become actively involved with minority individuals outside the counseling setting (e.g., in community events, social and political functions, celebrations, friendships, neighborhood groups, and so forth) so that their perspective of minorities is more than an academic or helping exercise.
	3. Culturally skilled counselors understand and have knowledge about sociopolitical influences that impinge upon the life of racial and ethnic minorities. Immigration issues, poverty, racism, stereotyping, and powerlessness may impact self-esteem and self-concept in the counseling process.	

(continued)

TABLE **12.2**
AMCD Multicultural Counseling Competencies (Continued)

III. Culturally Appropriate Intervention Strategies		
Beliefs and Attitudes	Knowledge	Skills
1. Culturally skilled counselors respect clients' religious and/or spiritual beliefs and values, including attributions and taboos, because they affect worldview, psychosocial functioning, and expressions of distress.	1. Culturally skilled counselors have a clear and explicit knowledge and understanding of the generic characteristics of counseling and therapy (culture-bound, class-bound, and monolingual), and how they may clash with the cultural values of various cultural groups.	1. Culturally skilled counselors are able to engage in a variety of verbal and nonverbal helping responses. They are able to send and receive both verbal and nonverbal messages accurately and appropriately. They are not tied down to only one method or approach to helping, but recognize that helping styles and approaches may be culture bound. When they sense that their helping style is limited and potentially inappropriate, they can anticipate and modify it.
2. Culturally skilled counselors respect indigenous helping practices and respect help-giving networks among communities of color.	2. Culturally skilled counselors are aware of institutional barriers that prevent minorities from using mental health services.	2. Culturally skilled counselors are able to exercise institutional intervention skills on behalf of their clients. They can help clients determine whether a "problem" stems from racism or bias in others (the concept of healthy paranoia) so that clients do not inappropriately personalize problems.
3. Culturally skilled counselors value bilingualism and do not view another language as an impediment to counseling (monolingualism may be the culprit).	3. Culturally skilled counselors have knowledge of the potential bias in assessment instruments, and they use procedures and interpret findings keeping in mind the cultural and linguistic characteristics of the clients.	3. Culturally skilled counselors are not averse to seeking consultation with traditional healers or religious and spiritual leaders and practitioners in the treatment of culturally different clients when appropriate.
	4. Culturally skilled counselors have knowledge of family structures, hierarchies, values, and beliefs from various cultural perspectives. They are knowledgeable about the community where a particular cultural group may reside and the resources in the community.	4. Culturally skilled counselors take responsibility for interacting in the language requested by the client and, if not feasible, make appropriate referrals. A serious problem arises when the linguistic skills of the counselor do not match the language of the client.

(continued)

TABLE **12.2** (Continued)

III. Culturally Appropriate Intervention Strategies		
Beliefs and Attitudes	Knowledge	Skills
		When this is the case, counselors should (a) seek a translator with cultural knowledge and appropriate professional background, or (b) refer to a knowledgeable and competent bilingual counselor.
	5. Culturally skilled counselors should be aware of relevant discriminatory practices at the social and community levels that may be affecting the psychological welfare of the population being served.	5. Culturally skilled counselors have training and expertise in the use of traditional assessment and testing instruments. They not only understand the technical aspects of the instruments but also are aware of the cultural limitations. This allows them to use test instruments for the welfare of culturally different clients.
		6. Culturally skilled counselors should attend to as well as work to eliminate biases, prejudices, and discriminatory contexts in conducting evaluations and providing interventions, and should develop sensitivity to issues of oppression, sexism, heterosexism, elitism, and racism.
		7. Culturally skilled counselors take responsibility for educating their clients to the processes of psychological intervention, such as goals, expectations, legal rights, and the counselor's orientation.

Source: Adapted from Arredondo, P., Toporek, M. S., Brown, S., Jones, J., Locke, D. C., Sanchez, J. and Stadler, H. (1996). Operationalization of the Multicultural Counseling Competencies. (Alexandria, VA: AMCD).

CASE STUDY **12.1**

The Case of Maria Henderson

Ms. Henderson is a 27-year-old African American single mother seeking therapy. When asked what brought her in, she replied, "The school psychologist who works with my 9-year-old son said I should look into therapy because it would be a good way to help me deal with my stress." Ms. H went on to explain, "I'm a single parent and it's hard. My son is failing school, he's constantly being suspended for fighting, and I don't know what to do. Recently, I started working a second job, so when I come home, I'm exhausted. I have no time for myself. I just feel like my life is falling apart. Over the last 2 years, I have gained 40 pounds, I can't seem to make a relationship work, and I'm starting to have all kinds of health problems that I've never had before, like high blood pressure." In further conversations, Ms. H relates that she is the oldest of four, with two younger brothers and a sister who is still in high school. She and her siblings were raised by her grandmother and aunts when her mother died in a domestic violence conflict when she was 13. She has not known her biological father, who she shares with one brother, though other siblings have different fathers. The father of her son is currently incarcerated, and although she has some contact with him, she does not see him in any parental role with her son.

Case Discussion
Questions for Reflection
1. How would you characterize Ms. Henderson's presenting problem?
2. What are some aspects of knowledge that would be helpful to know before going in to see the client?
3. What are some knowledge areas that would be helpful to research after the intake assessment?

Areas of Knowledge
If you were to acknowledge and attend to the client's ethnic, cultural, and racial heritage, it would be important to investigate and acknowledge her kinship support systems, particularly of female relatives given her own upbringing. Ms. Henderson might be burdened by a belief that she needs to be strong while also having great fears about her son's future as a young Black man. You would want to explore her racial identity and discrimination experiences. A possible source of support might be achieved through accessing faith-based support systems. Finally, it might be important to recommend medical screening for weight gain and possible type II diabetes.

Skills

In developing aspects of skills, practitioners must be able to develop and use interventions that are culturally appropriate and sensitive. Skills in this domain include establishing a respectful relationship, through appropriate addressing and naming, and sensitivity to boundaries around touch and cultural rules about gender-appropriate behavior. Conducting appropriate assessments, making diagnoses that are accurate and take into account contextual factors in the presentation and explanation of symptoms, and then implementing responsive therapies are the other components in this area. Hays (2009) developed a set of 10 guidelines to incorporate multiculturally sensitive ways to use empirically based practices with clients. These are listed in Example 12.1.

REFLECTION QUESTIONS 12.5

- What particular skills or interventions do you have that you feel are effective with clients from diverse backgrounds?
- What makes those skills or interventions effective, and with which clients?
- How did you acquire those skills, and how did you become aware that they were effective?

SOCIAL JUSTICE AND ADVOCACY

Although multicultural counseling historically focused on counseling across racial and cultural lines, such that the competencies developed therein concentrate on the ability to work effectively in racially and ethnically diverse arenas, the movement for **social justice counseling and advocacy** goes beyond that. Similar to multicultural competency, there are elements of raising awareness, such that Love (2000) discusses the need to develop an intentional consciousness of systems of oppression. But social justice tends to focus most strongly on action in responding to systemic inequalities that marginalize various groups of people (Vera & Speight, 2007). This response is also not neutral, in that practitioners are called to advocate for change in societal values, policies, and practices that serve to marginalize and disadvantage oppressed groups (Goodman et al., 2004).

Manis, Brown, and Paylo (2009) remind us that the heart of counseling contains the desire to relieve suffering. When we recognize that the harm is due to conditions that lie outside an individual in systemic modes of discrimination and oppression, we move into the realm of acting as advocates and to equalize and strive for access and justice for our clients. In response to the need to distinguish social justice and advocacy from multicultural counseling per se, Lewis, Arnold, House, and Toporek (2002) developed competencies that provide a framework for addressing issues of oppression on individual and systemic levels (see Figure 12.1).

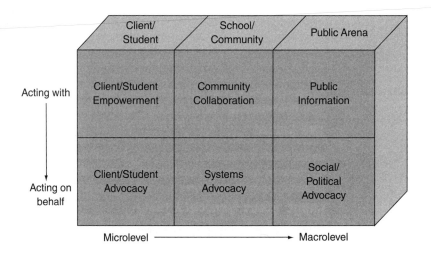

FIGURE **12.1** Advocacy Competencies Framework

Source: Adapted from Lewis, J., Arnold, M. S., House, R. & Toporek, R. L. (2002). *Advocacy Competencies: Task Force on Advocacy Competencies.* (Alexandria, VA: American Counseling Association).

REFLECTION QUESTIONS 12.6

- What does social justice mean to you?
- What has social justice meant to you in terms of your experiences in life and in counseling specifically?
- Can you think of instances when you stood up for someone in a way that empowered them?
- Can you think of instances in which you wished you stood up for someone and didn't? What kept you from acting? What did you learn from that experience?
- What changes have you been a part of making on an individual level? On a group level? On a systemic level?
- What changes could you be a part of on individual, group, or systemic levels, and how could you be part of that process?

Client and Student Advocacy Level

The two subsets here are empowerment and advocacy. In the first, the helping professional implements direct counseling strategies based on understanding the social, political, economic, and cultural contexts in which clients live, and facilitating self-advocacy on the part of the client. For instance, a helping professional might join an organization offering counseling services to returning veterans and their families. In the second, the counselor may directly address external barriers that impede the client's development that the client him or herself is unable to address due to lack of resources, access, or power. For example, a school counselor might intervene directly with a health education teacher who has failed a student for turning in a paper on indigenous healing methods.

School and Community Advocacy Level

In this domain, the first subset involves working directly with community organizations that are working for changes, such as developing a cultural sensitivity training program for volunteers at a food bank. The second subset involves going to a larger stage to maintain a direction for change that will impact on macrolevels of access and resources. An example of this may be to join in ongoing lobbying efforts to maintain funding and services for ex-offender employment and rehabilitation programs.

Public Arena Advocacy Level

In the first instance, disseminating information widely to raise social consciousness assists in deepening understanding. So, helping professionals might write an article for the local newspaper on Muslim mental health concerns, sensitizing public awareness of ongoing discrimination. The second subset involves working on large social issues that will then indirectly trickle into impacting the experience of marginalized groups. An example might involve efforts to bring about mental health parity in health insurance, so that mental health services are covered equally, ultimately enhancing access to services.

CASE STUDIES

This is a good place to start putting together the complexity of awareness, knowledge, and skills that you will need to use in counseling. In the following case studies, think deeply about possibilities, hypothesize freely, and then always remember to check out your assumptions.

CASE STUDY **12.2**

Betty Cadeau: A Native American Child

Eight-year-old Betty Cadeau lives with her parents, 13-year-old sister, 15-year-old brother, and elderly grandmother. The family lives in the city, some distance from the reservation. Although the family is above the poverty level, money is often a problem. Both parents have a high school education and work long hours at minimum wage jobs. Betty's grandparents moved off the reservation in an attempt to better their finances, and her parents traveled back and forth. She herself has visited relatives on the reservation, and she hears stories from her grandmother about traditional life. When her grandmother is sick, Betty often chooses to stay home with her. She speaks with her grandmother in their indigenous language.

Betty has been referred to you by her teacher, who reports that Betty is not doing well in school. The African American teacher says that Betty does not seem to listen to her, and she can never tell if Betty is paying attention; also, Betty hardly participates in class and is frequently absent. Her schoolwork is often incomplete, and her homework is not turned in. In class, she does not socialize much with the other students, who are mainly European American and African American.

In your first meeting with Betty, she is silent, does not meet your eyes, and looks down while you are talking with her. She appears both unresponsive and anxious. Her speech is halting and punctuated with long silences.

Case Discussion
Thinking About This Case
Based on the information provided about the client, briefly describe the clinically relevant cultural,

historical, and sociopolitical background to the client's status in the United States currently. Consider using the ADDRESSING framework as a way of organizing the information you deem most significant according to the following:

- Age,
- Developmental and acquired disabilities
- Religion,
- Ethnicity,
- Socioeconomic status,
- Sexual orientation,
- Indigenous heritage,
- National origin, and
- Gender

1. What are some specific cultural issues a counselor might need to attend to with this client? Are there other aspects of identity that you will need to address, and how will you do it? What clues in the case study will you need to follow up on, and why?
2. How might you identify the client's racial and cultural identity development and its potential impact on the counselor–client relationship? What evidence did you use to arrive at your conclusions? How would you establish rapport?
3. Explore how your own identities of race and ethnicity, culture, gender, age, sexual orientation, class, religion, disability, and so on might impact your work with this client. Consider implications for building rapport as well as obstacles.

CASE STUDY **12.3**

Susie Dinh: A Vietnamese American Teenager

Sixteen-year-old Susie is a second-generation Vietnamese American girl in high school. She lives at home with her parents. Her parents came over to the United States, but Susie was born here much later. She knows she had an older brother who died before she was born. The family owns and operates a Laundromat and dry-cleaning business, and Susie spends most of her after-school hours working there. She is doing well in school, and also takes piano lessons twice a week. Susie has come in to see you, the school counselor, reluctantly on the urging of some of her friends.

Susie says she is sad. She spends time with her friends in school, because of having no time out of school. Most of her friends are also Asian, but only girls. She cannot date like her peers do, because her father will not allow it. However, she reports that she wouldn't want to date boys anyway, though she feels embarrassed to say that. She enjoys the piano lessons, but her piano teacher, a young Russian American woman, is the real reason she keeps going. According to Susie, she is the one person who seems to really understand her. She reports feeling like crying most of the time, but is unable to really think of a reason. "After all," she says, "it's not like some tragedy has happened. Actually, nothing has changed except me." She reports that her parents are concerned and urge her to work harder, but they would never understand about counseling. She considers them very traditional, and though she does not want to fight them, she often feels that they do not understand what life is like for her as an American.

Case Discussion
Thinking About This Case
Based on the information provided about the client, briefly describe the clinically relevant cultural,

historical, and sociopolitical background to the client's status in the United States currently. Consider using the ADDRESSING framework as a way of organizing the information you deem most significant according to the following:

- Age,
- Developmental and acquired disabilities
- Religion,
- Ethnicity,
- Socioeconomic status,
- Sexual orientation,
- Indigenous heritage,
- National origin, and
- Gender

1. What are some specific cultural issues a counselor might need to attend to with this client? Are there other aspects of identity that you will need to address, and how will you do it? What clues in the case study will you need to follow up on, and why?
2. How might you identify the client's racial and cultural identity development and its potential impact on the counselor–client relationship? What evidence did you use to arrive at your conclusions? How would you establish rapport?
3. Explore how your own identities of race and ethnicity, culture, gender, age, sexual orientation, class, religion, disability, and so on might impact your work with this client. Consider implications for building rapport as well as obstacles.

OPENING THE DIALOGUE ON MULTICULTURAL COUNSELING COMPETENCY

With all of the topics discussed in this chapter, you are now challenged to think through how you would utilize this information in sessions with any number of clients from a variety of cultural backgrounds and worldviews. Questions for reflection offered to you throughout this chapter also serve as excellent process questions for opening the dialogue with clients on issues of

CASE STUDY **12.4**

Rafael Garcia: A Puerto Rican Elder

Señor Garcia, age 75, came into the community clinic where you are a counselor to explore some of his medical complaints, and he was referred to you because the doctor believed they might be psychosomatic. He complains of shortness of breath, difficulty sleeping, and pain in his heart. He walks with a cane, and has severe arthritis. He has never seen a counselor before and is not sure what you can do. He is primarily fluent in Spanish, but is able to understand and speak English with a heavy Spanish accent for which he frequently apologizes.

Papa Rafael, as he is known in the community, lives with his son, daughter-in-law, and two grandchildren. His wife, Luisa, died several years ago, and he still sighs and speaks of her with sadness. Both of them had come from the island and often visited their families back there. His son was born here, but is also very connected to his relatives on the island.

Recently, his son, Oscar, lost his job at the local construction company. His daughter-in-law, Carla, has been talking about finding a job to clean offices at night to keep the family afloat, and Papa Rafael has given his opinion that it would not be good for the family because it is a man's role to support his family. After all, Luisa stayed at home and raised the children while he worked as a factory worker. Papa Rafael is also concerned about his grandchildren, both Luis who is 15 and seems to be hanging out with a bad crowd on the streets, and Elena, who is 12 and hardly speaks any Spanish. His goddaughter, Angela, who is turning 15 in the next year, also preoccupies him. He is afraid they are losing their culture and complains about their lack of respect. Overall, he sighs, he has no place in their world, and no one listens to him anymore.

Case Discussion
Thinking About This Case
Based on the information provided about the client, briefly describe the clinically relevant cultural, historical, and sociopolitical background to the client's status in the United States currently. Consider using the ADDRESSING framework as a way of organizing the information you deem most significant according to the following:

- Age,
- Developmental and acquired disabilities
- Religion,
- Ethnicity,
- Socioeconomic status,
- Sexual orientation,
- Indigenous heritage,
- National origin, and
- Gender

1. What are some specific cultural issues a counselor might need to attend to with this client? Are there other aspects of identity that you will need to address, and how will you do it? What clues in the case study will you need to follow up on, and why?

2. How might you identify the client's racial and cultural identity development and its potential impact on the counselor–client relationship? What evidence did you use to arrive at your conclusions? How would you establish rapport?

3. Explore how your own identities of race and ethnicity, culture, gender, age, sexual orientation, class, religion, disability, and so on might impact your work with this client. Consider implications for building rapport as well as obstacles.

multicultural counseling competence. Some of these questions are listed here to assist you in terms of opening the dialogue with your clients:

- Considering our identities around race, culture, class, gender, sexual orientation, disability status, age, and spiritual affiliation, what would make it easier for us to work together? Based on these, what might create some challenges, and how can we deal with these in a way that is most helpful to you?

CASE STUDY **12.5**

David Washington: An African American Man

Mr. Washington is in his mid-40s and has come in for career counseling. He is dissatisfied with his current position as an accounts manager in the local bank, especially because he sees no hope of promotion. It is, he says, a glass ceiling, and he's gone about as high as they will let him, after 7 years.

He is currently also upset because of a long-term relationship that recently ended, and acknowledges feeling some grief about the way things turned out. He also says that he doesn't have anyone with whom to talk about this. He says his mother often complains that he will never be married and provide her with grandchildren, but then again, he says, she just doesn't get it, and she never will. His sisters' children will have to make her happy. He lives in a predominantly African American middle-class community, and several relatives live close by.

Currently, his niece and nephew are living with him, and he is taking care of them for his sister, who is sick. He says his own aunt is too frail to cope with teenagers, but she helps out in terms of meals. Meanwhile, he juggles his work schedule to be available for the teenagers. He wants to show them a father figure, especially his nephew because it's an important role model to have. After all, he says, he was lucky to have a father who was there and thinks he wouldn't have turned out half as successful without that. It was a tough upbringing, he admits, but that's life for Black folks.

Case Discussion
Thinking About This Case
Based on the information provided about the client, briefly describe the clinically relevant cultural,

historical, and sociopolitical background to the client's status in the United States currently. Consider using the ADDRESSING framework as a way of organizing the information you deem most significant according to the following:

- Age,
- Developmental and acquired disabilities
- Religion,
- Ethnicity,
- Socioeconomic status,
- Sexual orientation,
- Indigenous heritage,
- National origin, and
- Gender

1. What are some specific cultural issues a counselor might need to attend to with this client? Are there other aspects of identity that you will need to address, and how will you do it? What clues in the case study will you need to follow up on, and why?
2. How might you identify the client's racial and cultural identity development and its potential impact on the counselor–client relationship? What evidence did you use to arrive at your conclusions? How would you establish rapport?
3. Explore how your own identities of race and ethnicity, culture, gender, age, sexual orientation, class, religion, disability, and so on might impact your work with this client. Consider implications for building rapport as well as obstacles.

- What could I do in our work together that would show respect and responsiveness to your culture and needs as a client?
- What could we do in our work together that would be most empowering to you?
- Are you familiar with the term *micro-aggressions*? Have you dealt with any micro-aggressions, and would it be helpful to talk about some of those experiences?
- What do you think would be most important for me to know about your culture and who you are as a person based on that?

- Can you think of instances when you stood up for someone in a way that empowered them? How could I do that with you now?
- Can you think of instances in which you wish you'd stood up for someone and didn't? What kept you from acting? What did you learn from that experience?
- What changes have you been a part of making on an individual level? On a group level? On a systemic level?
- What changes could you be a part of on individual, group, or systemic levels, and how could I help you be part of that process?

CONCLUSION AND IMPLICATIONS

We began this process of this book by using the metaphor of a journey to imagine you, the reader, getting on board this "multicultural express." We explored the implications of the baggage you bring with you that might be both something you need along the way, and something that could prove to be obstacles rather than assets. We also explored the fact that you might be beginning this journey with a mixture of emotions in terms of excitement about new experiences and possible apprehension about difficulties that arise when dealing with the unknown and leaving behind whatever is most familiar, whatever you may call home literally or symbolically.

We asked you to be aware of your experience along the way and encouraged you to neither suppress your feelings nor label them as right or wrong. We also encouraged you to consider what you were bringing on this journey, and to take a good conscious look around at your fellow passengers. This meant opening yourself to the diversity of experience, opinion, values, and attitudes that exist around you and within you, and working to create an environment of honesty, authenticity, and congruence both in your learning process and in the healing process with clients from diverse backgrounds.

We've come to the end of this part of the journey together, which may, in some ways, be only the beginning of the journey that lies ahead for you as a person

and as a professional, multiculturally competent counselor who works to improve and empower the lives of all clients. In this chapter, we provided an overview of the need for cultural competence, moving beyond awareness to enter the domains of knowledge and skills. We offered some models of practice that add effectiveness, and introduced you to concepts of social justice and advocacy as part of the tools and demands made of a culturally competent practitioner.

As we mentioned from the start, this journey embodies the lifelong nature of a process of developing and refining multicultural competence. Therefore, you are being invited and challenged to view this text and other experiences you have had as stops along the way of gathering awareness and content knowledge you have found on various aspects of identity such as culture, race, gender, sexual orientation, class, religion, disability, and age, and translate this into positive, intentional action. We ask you to continue this critical journey and continue turning to those who both challenge and support you along the way, with the hope that you will offer the same to them in a process of ongoing growth. Thank you for making the journey and for the work you have done, are doing, and will continue to do for the benefit of all those in need. Again, this journey has an important destination: your ever-present effectiveness as a professional counselor in a diverse world.

GLOSSARY

ADDRESSING framework: A framework of cultural assessment that enables therapists to better recognize and understand cultural influences as a multidimensional combination of Age, Developmental and acquired Disabilities, Religion, Ethnicity, Socioeconomic status, Sexual orientation, Indigenous heritage, National origin, and Gender.

Multicultural competence: The ability to work effectively and sensitively within various cultural contexts.

Multicultural counseling competencies: A set of practices that enables people to work effectively and sensitively, honoring and respecting cultural worldviews and behaviors in the context of persons receiving services.

Social justice counseling: Therapeutic practice that focuses most strongly on action in responding to systemic inequalities that marginalize various groups of people.

REFERENCES

Arredondo, P., Toporek, M. S., Brown, S., Jones, J., Locke, D. C., & Sanchez, J., et al. (1996). *Operationalization of the multicultural counseling competencies*. Alexandria, VA: AMCD.

Balkin, R. S., Schlosser, L. Z., & Levitt, D. H. (2009). Religious identity and cultural diversity: Exploring the relationships between religious identity, sexism, homophobia, and multicultural competence. *Journal of Counseling and Development*, 87(4), 420–428.

Evans, R. (1996). *The human side of school change: Reform, resistance, and the real-life problems of innovation*. San Francisco: Jossey-Bass.

Gainor, K. A. (2005). Social justice: The moral imperative of vocational psychology, *The Counseling Psychologist*, 33(2), 180–188.

Goodman, L. A., Liang, B., Helms, J. E., Latta, R. E., Sparks, E., & Weintraub, S. R. (2004). Training counseling psychologists as social justice agents: Feminist and multicultural principles in action. *The Counseling Psychologist*, 32, 793–837.

Hays, P. A. (2008). *Addressing cultural complexities in practice: Assessment, diagnosis, and therapy* (2nd ed.). Washington, DC: American Psychological Association.

Hays, P. A. (2009). Integrating evidence-based practice, cognitive-behavior therapy, and multicultural therapy: Ten steps for culturally competent practice. *Professional Psychology, Research and Practice*, 40 (4), 354–360.

Hogan-Garcia, M. (2007). *The four skills of cultural diversity competence: A process for understanding and practice* (3rd ed.). Belmont, CA: Thompson Brooks/Cole.

Johnson, S. (1998). *Who moved my cheese? An amazing way to deal with change in your work and in your life*. New York: Putnam.

Lewis, J., Arnold, M. S., House, R., & Toporek, R. L. (2002). *Advocacy competencies: Task force on advocacy competencies*. Alexandria, VA: American Counseling Association. Retrieved from http://www.counseling.org/Files/FDashx?guid=680f251e b3d0-4f77-8aa3-4e360f32f05e

Lorde, A. (1984). The master's tools will never dismantle the master's house. In A. Lorde *Sister outsider* (pp. 110–113). Trumansburg, NY: Crossing Press.

Love, B. J. (2000). Developing a liberatory consciousness. In M. Adams (Ed.), *Readings for diversity and social justice* (pp. 470–474). New York: Routledge.

Manis, A. A., Brown, S. L., & Paylo, M. J. (2009). The helping professional as advocate. In C. M. Ellis & J. Carlson (Eds.), *Cross-cultural awareness and social justice in counseling* (pp. 23–44). New York: Routledge.

Paz, O. (1978). The labyrinth of solitude: The other Mexico, return to the labyrinth of solitude, Mexico and the United States, the philanthropic ogre. New York: Grove Press.

Pedersen, P. B. (1991). Multiculturalism as a generic approach to counseling. *Journal of Counseling and Development*, 70, 6–12.

Pedersen, P. B. (2003). Multicultural training in schools as an expansion of the counselor's role. In P. B. Pedersen & J. C. Carey (Eds.), *Multicultural counseling in schools* (pp. 190–210). Boston: Pearson.

President's New Freedom Commission for Mental Health. (2003) *Achieving the promise: Transforming mental health care in America: Final report* (DHHS Pub. No. SMA-03-3832). Rockville, MD: U.S. Department of Health and Human Services.

Smith, T. B., Richards, P. S., & Granley, H. M. (2004). Practicing Multiculturalism. In T. B. Smith (Ed.), *Practicing multiculturalism: Affirming diversity in counseling and psychology* (pp. 3–16). Boston: Pearson Education.

Vera, E. M., & Speight, S. L. (2007). Advocacy, outreach, and prevention: Integrating social action roles in professional training. In E. Aldarondo (Ed.), *Advancing social justice through clinical practice* (pp. 373–390). Mahwah, NJ: Lawrence Erlbaum.

GLOSSARY

Ableism: A pervasive system of discrimination and exclusion that oppresses people who have mental, emotional, and physical disabilities based on beliefs about health, beauty, and productivity, leading to an environment that is often hostile to those whose physical, mental, cognitive, and sensory abilities are considered nonnormative.

Ableism: Individual, interpersonal, and institutional discrimination toward and subordination of people based on their physical or mental abilities. Those people designated as able-bodied have status and privilege compared to those designated as disabled.

Acculturation: The process by which a person responds to the influence of the dominant culture or a second culture.

Acculturation: The process of adaptation from one's country of origin to a new country of residence. Defined by Marín (1992) as the process of attitudinal and behavioral learning and change after coming in contact with a different culture.

Addressing framework: A framework of cultural assessment that enables therapists to better recognize and understand cultural influences as a multidimensional combination of Age, Developmental and acquired Disabilities, Religion, Ethnicity, Socioeconomic status, Sexual orientation, Indigenous heritage, National origin, and Gender.

African American: All persons having origins in any of the Black racial groups of Africa.

Age: The whole duration of a person since beginning.

Ageism: Individual, interpersonal, and institutional discrimination toward and subordination of people based on their age, such that the very old and very young have little power or status.

Ageism: Negative perceptions and/or behaviors toward an individual exclusively based on age; this can be unintentional, operating at the unconscious level of awareness.

Alexithymia: The inability to describe emotions in words.

Anima: Carl Jung's archetype for the feminine side of the self.

Animus: Carl Jung's archetype for the male side of the self.

Anti-Semitism: A system of prejudice and discrimination against Jewish people.

Asexual: One who does not have, for a variety of reasons, sexual responses to either sex.

Asian American: All persons having origins in any of the original peoples of the Far East, Southeast Asia, or the Indian subcontinent including, for example, Cambodia, China, India, Japan, Korea, Malaysia, Pakistan, the Philippine

Islands, Thailand, and Vietnam. Also, sometimes considered within this category is Native Hawaiian or Other Pacific Islander—All persons having origins in any of the original peoples of Hawaii, Guam, Samoa, or other Pacific Islands.

Asian American identity development: A model proposed by Kim (2001) that describes Asian American identity development in five stages: (a) ethnic awareness, (b) White identification, (c) awakening to social political consciousness, (d) redirection to an Asian consciousness, and (e) incorporation.

Assimilation: A shift toward the dominant culture together with a rejection of one's culture of origin, with a goal of complete absorption and acceptance by the dominant culture.

Attitudinal barriers: Stereotyped beliefs or prejudices regarding people with disabilities that result in categorizing, blaming, limiting, or discriminating environments.

Bicultural competence: An individual's ability to effectively utilize "dual modes of social behavior that are appropriately employed in different situations" (LaFromboise & Rowe, 1983, p. 592).

Biculturalism: A flexible balancing of some dominant culture attitudes and practices with retention of culture-of-origin practices and identity.

Bi-gender: Some gender variants in which people reject the choices of male–female and man–woman and feel that their gender encompasses "both" genders. Within some American Indians cultures, expressing both genders is referred to as *two-spirited*. Within contemporary urban life, bi-gendered people often refer to themselves as *gender queers, gender benders, third sex*, and *gender* perverts as terms of pride.

Biracial identity development: A process of accepting and integrating more than one culture and racial identity into one's sense of self.

Bisexual: One who has sexual responses to either sex.

Black identity formation: A process of Black identity development conceptualized by Cross (1971, 1995; Cross & Vandiver, 2001) as consisting of four stages: (a) preencounter, (b) encounter, (c) immersion and emersion, and (d) internalization.

Brujeria: Witchcraft practiced in Spanish-speaking countries, and in some Latino communities in the United States.

Celibacy: Describes the lifestyle of someone who chooses not to act upon sexual responses.

Child of deaf adult: A Child Of Deaf Adult is a person who was raised by a Deaf parent or guardian. Many CODAs identify with Deaf and hearing cultures.

Chronological age: Describes age related to the passage of time.

Classism: Individual, interpersonal, and institutional discrimination toward and subordination of people based on their socioeconomic status. Those peoples designated as ruling class, upper class, or rich have status and privilege compared to those designated as poor or working class.

Classism: Prejudicial attitudes and behaviors toward other people who are members of a particular class.

Collectivism: An orientation emphasizing group cohesiveness and group goals rather than individual goals. The group is considered more important than the individual.

Coming out: The process of revealing, to self and others, one's sexual orientation.

Core belief: A fundamental faith-based belief.

Cross-dresser: Going beyond the older and more pathological term *transvestite*, this describes someone who prefers to wear clothing of the other sex for a variety of reasons, including eroticism and recreation. Crossdressing is not necessarily linked to being attracted to members of one's own gender.

Cult: Often used to refer to a group that has (a) a common set of beliefs different from the mainstream, (b) a specific leader who directs and guides the group, (c) strong coherence among its members, and (d) members who separate themselves from the mainstream society. The term cult has negative connotations.

Cultural identity: Affiliation with the culture of origin (e.g., cultural values, beliefs, practices, and language).

Cultural identity: The embodiment of the cultural norms, beliefs, values, and worldview and one's sense of affiliation and belonging to a group identity.

Cultural worldview: A system of beliefs, perceptions, attitudes, and values held in common by the individual in a culture.

Culture: A total way of life held in common by a group of people who share similarities in speech, behavior, ideology, livelihood, technology, values, and social customs.

Culture: Culture is the personification of a worldview through learned and transmitted beliefs, values, and practices, including religious and spiritual traditions and psychological processes. It is a way of living shaped by historical, economic, ecological, and political forces on a group. All individuals are cultural beings and have a cultural, ethnic, and racial heritage.

Culture: Values, beliefs, customs, traditions, language, and other behaviors that are passed on from one generation to another within a particular group.

Culture-bound syndrome: A combination of psychiatric and somatic symptoms that are considered to be a recognizable disorder only within a specific society or culture.

Curanderismo: The use of natural remedies, such as herbs to cure an illness. It is practiced in Latino communities across the United States, and in Spanish-speaking countries such as Mexico.

Curandero/a: A folk healer who practices *cuanderismo*.

Disability: Describes, with respect to an individual, a physical or mental impairment that substantially limits one or more of the major life activities, a record of such impairment, or being regarded as having such an impairment.

Distal aging: Effects that have taken place over the life span, such as the gradual loss of hearing.

Emic: A view of culture as specific and distinguishing between humans.

Enculturation: The process by which a person is socialized into his or her primary culture, receiving primary cultural knowledge, awareness, and values.

Esoteric expression: The inner sense of consciousness, sometimes referred to as a *spiritual state of enlightenment*.

Espiritista: A spiritual healer who has the ability to call spirits for assistance in curing an illness or personal problem.

Essentialism: A theoretical perspective focusing on differences between men and women based on genetic, biological, and physiological differences.

Ethnic identity development model: A model developed by Phinney (1992) for adolescents in which an individual moves from complete acceptance of cultural values, beliefs, and behaviors of the dominant culture to an identity based on one's ethnicity (beliefs, customs, traditions and values of one's culture of origin). Achieving an ethnic identity is characterized by positive feelings of self and others. The stages in Phinney's model are (a) unexamined ethnic identity, (b) ethnic identity search, and (c) ethnic identity achievement.

Ethnicity: A common sociocultural heritage that includes similarities of religion, history, and common ancestry.

Ethnicity: A group of people who share a particular social and cultural heritage, which includes language, customs and traditions, clothing, and history.

Ethnicity: Similar to the concepts of race and culture, the term ethnicity does not have a commonly agreed upon definition, but includes sociocultural heritage based on commonalities represented in such dimensions as collective history, common ancestral origin, religion, nationality, and language.

Ethnocentrism: The belief that one's worldview is normative and universal.

Ethnorelativism: The ability to acknowledge and value cultural differences.

Etic: A view of culture as a commonality shared by all humans.

European American (sometimes referred to as White, Not of Hispanic Origin): All persons having origins in any of the original peoples of Europe, North Africa, or the Middle East.

Exoteric expression: The external or public that is expressed through organized religion and religious beliefs.

Female-to-male transsexuals (FtM or FTM): Female-born people who live as men. This includes a broad range of experience from those who identify as "male" or "men" and those who identify as transsexual, *transmen, female men,* or FTM as their gender identity. FtMs are often contrasted with *biomen,* or biologically born men.

Gay: Male sexual responses predominantly to one's own sex.

Gender: An expression of self as female or male, including socially constructed roles, behaviors, and characteristics that define men and women in a given society. The definition may include the human body's anatomy and physiology.

Gender identity: The perception of self about one's gender that may or may not be related to the person's biological characteristics. It may incorporate personal manifestations of masculinity and femininity and sexual orientation.

Gendered difference: An aspect of Gilbert and Scher's (1999) model of gender, which is defined as how we see men and women as having different roles (e.g., women as nurturers and men as providers).

Gendered discourse: An aspect of a model proposed by Gilbert and Scher (1999), which refers to the ways in which gender expectations influence what we talk about, the language we use, and our assumptions about men and women.

Gendered process: An aspect of Gilbert and Scher's (1999) model, in which there are specific ways in which men and women interact with others.

Gendered structure: An aspect of Gilbert and Scher's (1999) model that focuses on the differences between men and women in opportunities, access to resources, and policies.

Handicap: A disadvantage for a person with a disability that occurs when they encounter cultural, physical, or social barriers that prevent their access to the various systems of society that are available to other citizens. Thus, handicap is the loss or limitation of opportunities to take part in the life of the community on an equal level with others.

Heterosexism: Individual, interpersonal, and institutional discrimination toward and subordination of people based on their sexual orientation. Those people designated as heterosexual are considered normative, and have status and privilege compared to those designated as gay, lesbian, bisexual, or transgender.

Heterosexism: The belief that heterosexuality is the only legitimate form of sexuality, together with institutional policies and practices that privilege heterosexuality and discriminate openly or subtly against gays, lesbians, and bisexuals. Heterosexism leads to homophobia.

Heterosexual: Sexual responses predominantly to the other sex.

Hispanic: A U.S. government term created to classify a group of people who come from Spanish-speaking countries.

Homophobia: An irrational fear and hatred of anyone perceived to be, or associated with, gays or lesbians.

Homophobia: Fear of and hatred toward people identified as gay, lesbian, bisexual, or transgender, expressed in prejudice and discriminatory acts, including emotional and physical violence.

Homosexual: A term used to label individuals who are attracted to someone of the same gender. This term was popularized in the 19th century and is currently used less and less due to its derogatory nature and negative stereotypes.

Identity development for People of Color: A model of racial identity development for Asian Americans and Pacific Islanders, Latinos, and Native Americans proposed by Helms (1990, 1995) in which individuals from these various groups undergo a process of achieving a sense of self that is internalized, integrated, and satisfying. The process involves a series of statuses: (a) conformity, (b) dissonance, (c) immersion and emersion, and (d) internalization.

Immigrant: A person who leaves one country to settle permanently in another.

Individual worldview: A unique way in which an individual sees, interprets, and ascribes meaning to the world. It is based on a cultural context and unique life experiences.

Individualism: An orientation emphasizing individuality, independence, and self-reliance. Individual rather than collective group goals are desired.

Internalized classism: The acceptance of classism by individuals in a given social class. It can be manifested by feeling inferior to those in higher social classes, or superior to those lower on the class spectrum. Individuals internalize prejudicial attitudes and behaviors toward people in a given social class.

Jewish American: The majority of Jewish Americans are Ashkenazi, having a common origin of Central and Eastern Europe, and fit the physiognomy of Whiteness in terms of skin pigmentation and morphology; they also have a common language of Yiddish (combining mostly Hebrew and German elements).

Kwanzaa: A 7-day celebration that honors African culture and history based on seven fundamental principles known as *nguzo saba.* During this time, people gather to celebrate ancestors, community, and family.

La Raza: Means "race" in English; however, the term encompasses culture, heritage and political consciousness.

Latino/Hispanic American: All persons of Mexican, Puerto Rican, Cuban, Central or South American, or other Spanish culture or origin, regardless of race. The term, "Spanish origin," can be used in addition to "Hispanic or Latino."

Latino ethnic identity development: A process of identity development for Latinos characterized by Ferdman and Gallegos (2001) as consisting of orientations rather than stages. They are (a) Latino-integrated, (b) Latino-identified, (c) subgroup-identified, (d) Latino as "other," and (e) undifferentiated.

Lesbian: Female sexual responses predominantly to one's own sex.

Locus of control: The degree to which the individual has the ability to master his or her environment.

Locus of responsibility: The degree to which the individual can take ownership for his or her actions and life circumstances.

Machismo: Male chauvinism.

Mal puesto: An illness or abnormality caused by a hex in Latino culture.

Male-to-female transsexuals (MtF or MTF): Male-born people who live as women. This includes a broad range of experience including those who identify as "female" or "women" and those who identify as transsexual women. Some words used to refer to transsexual women are *Tgirls* and *new women* as compared to *GG's,* or genetic women.

Marginalization: A rejection of both the culture of origin and the dominant culture; such individuals have difficulty with social functioning and acceptance, and may lack a sense of cultural identity and self-efficacy.

Masculinity ideology: The endorsement of beliefs, attitudes, and behaviors about masculinity and the male gender that socially constructed and grounded in the differences between males and females. It may be viewed as the extent to which males endorse traditional male roles in society.

Mestizaje: The mixing of races (e.g., Spaniards from Spain and indigenous peoples, Blacks and Spaniards from Spain, Europeans and indigenous peoples from Spanish-speaking countries).

Microaggressions: Persistent verbal, behavioral, and environmental assaults, insults and invalidations that can occur in such subtle ways that they are hard to identify. Micro-aggressions can be unintentional or intentional and convey hostility and intolerance.

Mindfulness: A state of being present in the here and now and owning oneself as grounded in the body.

Multicultural and diversity: The terms *multiculturalism* and *diversity* have been used interchangeably to recognize the broad scope of dimensions of race, ethnicity, culture, language, sexual orientation, gender, age, disability, class status, and religious and spiritual orientation as critical aspects of an individual's personal identity.

Multicultural competence: The ability to work effectively and sensitively within various cultural contexts.

Multicultural counseling competence: The ability of a counselor to recognize, acknowledge, and respond sensitively and appropriately to clients in their cultural contexts.

Multicultural counseling competencies: A set of practices that enables people to work effectively and sensitively, honoring and respecting cultural worldviews and behaviors in the context of persons receiving services.

Multidimensional model of racial identity (MMRI): A model of racial identity proposed by Sellers et al. (1998) that focuses on the self-concept and personal meaning of being Black. It is not a development model of ethnic identity, but rather focuses on how racial identity influences behavior in different situations.

Multiple heritage identity development model: A model developed by Henriksen and Paladino (2009) that focuses on multiple identities including race, identity, sexual orientation, national origin, religion, spirituality, language, and indigenous heritage.

Multiracial identity development: Development of a sense of self that incorporates more than one racial and cultural heritage. This term has often been used interchangeably with biracial identity; however, it has included other identities and dimensions such as gender, social class, physical characteristics, and spiritual beliefs as outlined in the factor model of multiracial identity.

Native American: (sometimes referred to as American Indian or Alaska Native): All persons having origins in any of the original peoples of North and South America (including Central America), and who maintain tribal affiliation or community recognition attachment.

Nguzo saba: The seven principles of African culture, which are *umaja* (unity), *kujichagulia* (selfdetermination), *ujima* (collective work and responsibility), *ujamaa* (cooperative economics), *nia* (purpose), *kuumba* (creativity), and *imani* (faith).

Oppression: The domination of subordinate groups in society through prejudice, discrimination, and access to political, economic, social, and cultural power. Oppression is exemplified by specific manifestations of racism, sexism, classism, ableism, ageism, heterosexism, anti-Semitism, and religious discrimination.

Orishas: An African spirit or deity that has specific roles and purposes, such as Shango, the male warrior representing power, and Oshun, the female representing fertility, beauty, and love (Wikipedia, n.d.-b).

People of color: A term used, primarily in the United States, to describe persons who are not of European heritage. In other words, people who belong to ethnic groups identified as African American, Hispanic and Latino/a, Asian, and Native American peoples. The term is meant to be inclusive, emphasizing a commonality of experience, particularly with racism.

Personal dimensions of identity (PDI): A model of identity developed by Arredondo and Glauner (1992) consisting of a variety of dimensions that interact and influence how a person thinks, behaves, and views the world.

Personal identity: The way an individual defines himself or herself in the context of his or her culture of origin and present culture, which is influenced by personal experiences. Personal identity can encompass a wide variety of dimensions such as age, gender, race, ethnicity, social class, sexual orientation, and personal agency.

Primary aging: Changes in one's body due to age (e.g., bones becoming more brittle).

Privilege: Advantages, favors, or immunities specially accrued through membership in a dominant group that are withheld from members of subordinate groups.

Probabilistic aging: Features that are common with aging but not universal, such as arthritis.

Proximal aging: Effects that have happened recently, such as the recent development of back pain.

Race: A construct that classifies persons by shared genetic history and/or physical characteristics such as skin color.

Race: Originally based on biological characteristics based on skin pigmentation, physical features, hair and body type. Race was used to classify people into groups based on these characteristics. A contemporary view defines race as a "social construction," which encompasses the sociopolitical and historical contexts of racial classification.

Race: The categories to which individuals are assigned based on physical characteristics, such as skin color or hair type, and the generalizations and stereotypes made as a result. Although race may have some basis in shared genetic history and heritage, there is much empirical evidence that there are as many within-group variations as there are across so-called racial groups, leaving it a powerful social construct rather than a biological one.

Racial identity development: Development of an identity based on race and responses to experiences of oppression. Often characterized by movement in stages in which individuals achieve a sense of racial identity that is more internalized, integrated, and satisfying.

Racism: Individual, interpersonal, and institutional discrimination toward and subordination of peoples based on their racial classification. Those people designated as White have status and privilege compared to those designated as People of Color.

Refugee: One who comes to a new country unable or unwilling to return to his or her home country due to war, famine, political instability, or persecution due to race, religion, political opinion, or membership in a particular social group.

Religion: A set of beliefs and devotion to some organized faith. It is also the social vehicle and organizational framework to express and practice specific faith-based beliefs.

Religious discrimination: Individual, interpersonal, and institutional discrimination toward and subordination of people based on their religious affiliation. In the United States, those people designated as Christian have status and privilege compared to those who are affiliated with Judaism, Islam, Hinduism, Buddhism, Zoroastrianism, Wicca, and other indigenous or nature-based spiritual belief systems.

Santeria: A belief system that comes from the Yoruba religion, which is a combination of African, indigenous, and Roman Catholic traditions and practices. It is practiced mostly in the Caribbean. Practices include animal sacrifices, communicating with ancestors, and spirits (Orishas) such as Obatalá, Oggún, and Changó.

Secondary aging: Processes that are influenced by aging but not the direct processes of aging (e.g., a weakened bone breaks from stress).

Separation: A mode that describes those who retain their cultural values and identity while rejecting those of the dominant culture.

Sexism: Individual, interpersonal, and institutional discrimination toward and subordination of people based on their gender classification. Those peoples designated as male have status and privilege compared to those designated as women.

Sexuality: The way in which individuals express themselves as sexual beings, including practices, behaviors, and relationships.

Shadow: Carl Jung's archetype for the part of the self that is impulsive, instinctual, and viewed as the dangerous or dark side of the human experience.

Sign language: A sign language is a language which, instead of acoustically conveyed sound patterns, uses visually transmitted sign patterns to convey meaning—simultaneously combining hand shapes, orientation and movement of the hands, arms or body, and facial expressions to fluidly express a speaker's.

Social class: An individual's position in an economic hierarchy based on income, education, and occupation. Social class is membership in a particular group (e.g., middle class, working class, or upper class). Social class structures vary across societies and countries.

Social class worldview: The beliefs, attitudes, and behaviors of an individual in a particular social class.

Social class worldview model (SCW): A framework developed by Liu (2001) and Liu et al. (2004b) that consists of the individual's relationship to property, social class behaviors, lifestyle, referent groups, and awareness of social class. The model consists of the following:

- *Social class referent groups*: Key people in an individual's life who help to shape the person's worldview such as friends, family members, and aspirational peers.
- *Relationship to material objects*: Material possessions that represent a certain social class
- *Social class lifestyle*: Specific actions and behaviors tied to economic resources
- *Perceived class and status position*: A subjective sense of one's location within a particular socioeconomic hierarchy.

Social constructionism: A postmodern ideology perspective emphasizing that individuals are influenced by the social environment. It focuses on contextual, historical, and historical perspectives.

Social justice counseling: Therapeutic practice that focuses most strongly on action in responding to systemic inequalities that marginalize various groups of people.

Socioeconomic status: Based on quantifiable measures of income, occupation, and education that stratify people in our society. SES does not include belonging to a particular group such as the "middle-class" or "upper-class" group.

Sojourner: A temporary resident who holds on to one's culture of origin and may make only surface adaptations to the host culture.

Spirituality: A desire to understand human existence, the universe, and a sense of connectedness or wholeness beyond the physical; not tied to any one religion.

Straight: A term used to describe someone who is attracted to the opposite sex.

Theory of Nigrescence: A framework developed by Cross (1971, 1995) in which African Americans and Blacks undergo a process of identity formation. The theory also proposes that Black identity is continuously challenged by the dominant society and different social contexts.

Transgender: One who identifies with both male and female roles or as a member of an alternative gender. Often identified as a sexual orientation issue, transgenderism is more a gender identity issue.

Transsexual: A more medical term than *transgender*, the term *transsexual* describes someone who has a long-standing desire to live as the sex other than his or her biological sex. Sex reassignment is a complex process that includes therapy, electrolysis, hormonal therapy, and living in the new gender role for a prescribed period of time based on the Harry Benjamin standards.

Universal aging: Features that all will experience with aging, such as wrinkled skin.

Vodou: The worship of deities and ancestors that includes rituals and magic. Sometimes referred to as *voodoo*.

White privilege: Advantages that are assigned based on being designated as White.

White racial attitudes toward People of Color: A framework developed by Helms (1995) in which Whites undergo a process of attitudinal change toward people of color (e.g., African Americans, Asian Americans, Latinos, and Native Americans). It consists of stages: (a) contact, (b) disintegration, (c) reintegration, (d) pseudo-independence, (e) immersion and emersion, and (f) autonomy.

White supremacy: An entire system designed to maintain White economic, legal, political, and social privilege.

Worldview: How an individual sees himself or herself, others, and his or her environment. Lonner and Ibrahim (2002) define it as the way in which an individual perceives his or her world from philosophical, ethical, social, and moral contexts.

NAME INDEX

SUBJECT INDEX

Page numbers referring to tables are rendered in **bold**.
Page numbers referring to figures are rendered in *italics*.